Understanding Adult Family Relationships

CW00384810

Attachment theory has become a key focus of both research and practice in understanding and treating psychological and social risk for marital and relationship problems, parenting and clinical disorders. In particular, adult attachment style is a major explanatory factor for understanding problems in human relationships.

This practical book introduces and explains an easily accessible assessment tool for adult attachment style: the Attachment Style Interview (ASI). Based on extensive research over ten years, it discusses appropriate interventions and case assessments that can be made to help families in need. Simpler than the Adult Attachment Interview, which requires expert administration, the ASI is an invaluable and evidence-based resource. Presenting clear and concise descriptions of the measure and summaries of the attachment models developed, this text provides discussions of its relevance for different practice contexts, and uses a range of worked case studies to illustrate its principles and applications. It details attachment issues in different relationship domains to cover areas of risk and resilience relevant for practice such as:

- adult depression and anxiety and stress models;
- partner difficulties including domestic violence;
- childhood neglect and abuse as a source of attachment problems;
- parenting and intergenerational transmission of risk;
- interventions, service application and use in family therapy.

Understanding Adult Attachment in Family Relationships provides an important reference for all practitioners working with children, adolescents and families, especially those undertaking further study.

Antonia Bifulco is Professor of Lifespan Psychology and Social Science, Director of Lifespan Research Group, Centre for Abuse and Trauma Studies at Kingston University, London, UK.

Geraldine Thomas is a specialist therapeutic service provider and consultant working in partnership with Early Help Services for Children, Young People and Families and Looked After Children in Kensington and Chelsea, London, UK.

Understanding Adult Attachment in Family Relationships

Research, assessment and intervention

Antonia Bifulco and Geraldine Thomas

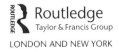
Routledge
Taylor & Francis Group

LONDON AND NEW YORK

First published 2013
by Routledge
2 Park Square, Milton Park, Abingdon, Oxon, OX14 4RN

Simultaneously published in the USA and Canada
by Routledge
711 Third Avenue, New York, NY 10017

Routledge is an imprint of the Taylor & Francis Group, an Informa business

British Library Cataloguing in Publication Data
A catalogue record for this book is available from the British Library

Library of Congress Cataloging-in-Publication Data
Bifulco, Antonia, 1955–
Understanding adult attachment in family relationships : research,
assessment, and intervention / Antonia Bifulco and Geraldine Thomas.
p. cm.
Includes bibliographical references.
I. Thomas, Geraldine, 1951– II. Title.
[DNLM: 1. Object Attachment. 2. Adult–psychology. 3. Anxiety–therapy.
4. Family Relations. 5. Family Therapy. WM 460.5.O2]
616.89'156–dc23
2012013178

ISBN13: 978-0-415-59432-5 (hbk)
ISBN13: 978-0-415-59433-2 (pbk)
ISBN13: 978-0-203-09455-6 (ebk)

Typeset in Baskerville by
FiSH Books Ltd, Enfield

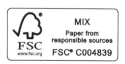

Printed and bound in Great Britain by the MPG Books Group

Contents

Preface

The purpose of this book is to provide an accessible but informed account of attachment in families, for use by both practitioners and researchers, with a particular focus on support-based adult attachment style. Whilst there are many acclaimed publications on the issue of attachment, this book will emphasise a social approach to balance the psychodynamic, cognitive, neuroscientific and other contributions already available. It approaches attachment style from the point of view of the adult or young adult, and takes a lifespan perspective, tracking experiences from childhood to maturity. It looks backwards from adulthood to childhood in order to capture early life experiences crucial for attachment-based models. It also looks forwards to examine change in attachment and to the parenting of the next generation, to look at transmission inter-generationally. Partner relationships and the role of fathers are taken to be of critical importance, although the reporters here are mainly women, with accounts of adult males in the family provided by female partners and daughters and sons. The retrospective reconstructions of childhood and adolescence are used because of the measurement and ethical challenges obtaining complex information from children. However to approach the issue of younger children's development, case material from practice examples describing the experience of children living with parents with problem attachment styles is provided.

The research findings presented are based on two five-year Medical Research Council-funded UK programmes conducted during the 1990s, which researched vulnerability to depression in community women, and tracked their lifetime attachment experience and vulnerability to clinical depression. The second programme re-interviewed a proportion of the mothers to look at attachment change, and to also interview their 'emerging adult' offspring. This enabled investigation of intergenerational transmission of risks around attachment, but also to reassess experiences from a younger age group closer to childhood, and to include males as well as females. Given lengthy biographical interviews were undertaken in both generations, extensive case material was generated in addition to reliable quantitative data. This allowed for parallel description of numeric findings illustrated with case material to further understand the linkages found. This book attempts to give equal weight to both.

The Attachment Style Interview (ASI) is used throughout. This support-based interview of attachment style is very different in content but not in overall classification from the more widely used Adult Attachment Interview (AAI). There were various reasons for utilising this measure, designed by the first author and the Lifespan Research team. First its content involves ongoing relationships to assess relating-ability and support in parallel to the attitudes held around Secure, Anxious, Avoidant or Disorganised attachment styles invoking issues of autonomy, trust, fear and anger in relating. Assessing ongoing relationships and attitudes is useful for a social and contextual-based approach, and its focus on the here-and-now means in it can be used to predict future risk, and change as social experiences change. The ASI is used in models as an independent outcome of childhood adverse experience. It is a transparent and relatively easy measure to use both in research and in health and social care practice. In the latter it is used to assess clients, parents or prospective adoptive/foster parents to look at the stability of close family relationships and the context in which a child is raised. It is similarly useful in adolescent and adult clinical practice, family therapy and marital therapy.

The book aims to enhance understanding of attachment from a psychosocial perspective through discussion of the research literature, and the presentation of findings from the MRC programme of research in London. It also extends this to discuss interventions, focusing on those most representative of particular approaches, those best evaluated or those more commonly used. It also focuses on child and family services, particularly those relevant for child safeguarding and child protection. In each instance it attempts to link these back to the models proposed around psychosocial causes of attachment difficulties at different lifestages. The penultimate chapter looks at the use of the ASI in a Filial Therapy context in order to illustrate some of the issues that arise when working with parents with Insecure styles and children who are showing emotional or behavioural difficulties. This seeks to explore the dynamics involved and to show the inter-relation of various risk factors. It does not, however, provide instructions for implementing Filial or any other therapy. Neither does it in itself provide training in the ASI, although providing an effective primer for the four-day courses held nationally for practitioners and researchers.

By taking a social approach, we emphasise the very large impact of the adverse social environment, whether involving neglect or abuse in childhood, adult domestic violence, stressful life events, lower social class position, single parent status or other markers of deprivation and stress emanating from the external world. This is to underline the damage to healthy development often caused by factors external to the individual over which they may have little control. This is not to overlook the fact that adult attachment itself emanates from within the individual as a psychological construct including cognitive, emotional and behavioural aspects centred around the 'internal working models' described by John Bowlby, but rather to look wider at the individual in context. We also discuss the impacts of gender and culture. Both are limited in our own samples, but amplified by other studies using the ASI or other attachment measures. The ASI is now being used internationally, particularly across Europe and Asia, and where possible we have included findings from these studies to extend the reach of the ASI, and our London attachment findings. Also, where appropriate we have outlined the biological underpinnings of attachment, although our expertise is greater on the psychosocial side and we can present no new data on the complex and fascinating interplay between the mind and body. We have included enough, we hope, for a constant reminder that the genetic, hormonal and brain-related elements to an individual's behaviour may provide critical input to risk or resilience to psychological disorder and in future is likely to become a routine aspect to disorder profiling. We look forward to greater use of the ASI in those investigating biological risk factors to add yet a further dimension to the contextual life-history approach.

Antonia Bifulco
Geraldine Thomas
March 2012

Acknowledgements

Research is always teamwork and we owe a large debt to our research colleagues involved with the London studies over a ten-year span, between 1990 and 2000, and our work with health and social care services over a further 10-year span since 2000. The MRC programme was originally headed by Professor George Brown, and we acknowledge his role in initiating the individual-in-context approach to social psychiatry and developing the distinctive measurement utilised. In this he was aided by Tirril Harris who contributed a lifespan and psychodynamic approach, with a concern for implications for clinical practice. The first author (AB) programme managed these studies throughout and took over their direction when Professor Brown retired. We are also grateful to the numerous research assistants who laboriously collected thousands of hours of interview data and meticulously re-listened to and scored the material with diligent attention to consensus reliability. They were responsible for lively discussions aimed at understanding the case material and extending measurement and the developing models. We are particularly in debt to Dr Patricia Moran who was responsible for developing screening self-report instruments, and leading the intergenerational work on the sons investigated. We are also grateful for the continued support of Catherine Jacobs and Amanda Bunn who worked not only on this programme, but also on the development of the ASI training packages now used to aid social workers in their difficult task of assessing parental risk.

We also owe thanks to our various collaborators over the years who have used both the ASI and the Childhood Experience of Care and Abuse (CECA) measure of childhood in their various studies and provided stimulating discussion about their findings and experiences. An important boost to the ASI was provided by Professor Channi Kumar from the Institute of Psychiatry, Kings College, London (KCL), who included it in his European Transcultural – Postnatal Depression (TCS-PND) project in 2000. We also owe a debt to Dr Odette Bernazzani from Montreal, Quebec, Canada who worked with us in London for three years on this and related projects and TCS-PND partners Dr Vania Valoriani, Dr Barbara Figueirido, and Dr Nichole Guedeney who continue to use it in different research and practice contexts.

We also acknowledge the important contribution of our Italian collaborators to the analysis and use of the ASI in the Italian context. This was initiated by Professor Vincenzo Caretti who has been generously supportive of our endeavours and provided Italian translations of our work. We are also grateful to Professor Adriano Schimmenti who has provided skilful and insightful understanding of both ASI and CECA in Italian samples and clinical work, we also owe him a debt for his excellent statistical skills. Our Japanese colleagues Professor Keiko Yoshida, Dr Junko Kihara and Professor Momoko Hayashi have also provided wonderful cross-cultural insight using the ASI in Japan and provided training opportunities there. In Malaysia Dr Nor Bayah Abdul KIadir has extended the cross-cultural dimension by using the ASI in Moslem Malaysian mothers.

We would never have ventured into training practitioners but for the insight of Karen Irving, then Chief Executive Officer of Parents for Children, who foresaw the importance of 'translating' research into practice and providing standardised and reliable interview measures for social workers assessing prospective and adoptive parents. It was through Karen that we were introduced to St Christopher's Fellowship (SCF) who run fostering and residential care services, and they have been loyal sponsors of the adolescent ASI in their care homes and also sponsored the development of the child ASI. Under the leadership of Jonathan Farrow, we owe particular thanks to Ron Giddens, Gordon Parker and Maxine McBriar for operationalising its use.

We would also like to thank our many collaborators and sponsors in the social care practice field including Mark Jowett and Katie Kerr. Professor Arnon Bentovim and Liza Bingley Miller provided a wonderful catalyst for extending the ASI training into social care practice by including it in their portfolio of child- and family-assessment tools, and continue to roll out training of the ASI nationally. Their dedicated trainers regularly illuminate social workers on attachment models and social approaches to its measurement. This includes Dorothy Porter, Elaine Rose, Carol Joliffe, Sue Skrobanski and a number of others who are highly committed to the ASI. From Royal Holloway, University of London we want to thank Professor Jane Tunstill and Professor John Turner, who helped us survive as a research group and to Martin Kelly, Lydia Daniels and Philip Johnson for simplifying licensing and entrepreneurship principles to further extend the ASI, as well as to Professors Paula Nicolson and Duska Rosenberg for personal support. At our new home in Kingston University we want to thank Professor Peter Scott, Professor Martin McQuillan and Professor John Davis for providing us with a new home with alacrity, graciousness and trust for the work of the group. We also thank Professor Julia Davidson, for helping to make the Centre for Abuse and Trauma Studies possible and providing the Criminology element that extends our understanding of psychosocial models of abuse so elegantly. Finally our thanks go to Professor Jon Allen of the Menninger Clinic in Houston, Texas, USA for giving us very valuable feedback on an earlier draft of this manuscript. Any errors or opaqueness which remain are all our own!

We of course owe an immeasurable debt to all the individuals who contributed their views of attachment through narrative accounts, and to the children who did so through dynamic play, and thus provided us with the rich tapestry of directly experienced personal attachment in family relationships.

Finally on a personal note and to illustrate the prime importance of attachment, we would like to thank our husbands and children: Vincent and Lucy Bifulco, and George, Georgiana and Morgan Thomas for providing support and security in this endeavour.

Dedication

This book is dedicated to John Bowlby for his vision in promoting the study and practice around attachment, which has proved so beneficial to children and families.

A research note

The research samples and data analysis outlined in this book have been simplified for purposes of readability. In most instances articles published in scientific journals are cited as sources for greater detail on the samples and statistical analysis. Further details are also produced in the appendices of the samples utilised and of prevalence rates of risk and disorder variables. The following points are noted here to explain the findings presented.

Background to the studies: The ASI was introduced into a programme of research which had been undertaken over three decades under the direction of Professor George Brown and Tirril Harris and by Antonia Bifulco on their retirement (grant G702833 and G9827201). They were responsible in the 1970s for establishing the key role of vulnerability factors and severe life events in the onset of episodes of disorder in women living in the community. The vulnerability identified in the early studies involved lack of confiding in partner or close other, lack of employment, having three or more children at home or loss of mother under age 11. Any one of these factors increased the likelihood of a major depression occurring when a severe life event strikes. Over time these vulnerability factors were refined – the partner variable developed into negative interaction, as did the parenting factor, and this added to lack of a close confidant, and low self-esteem as providing the best vulnerability markers in prospective studies for onset of depression. The childhood factor moved from loss of mother to the quality of care in childhood, with neglect and abuse proving to be a major early life risk factor for later vulnerability and disorder. Given the role of conflict and lack of support in close relationships, and the importance of childhood experience, an attachment approach was later adopted and in turn adult attachment style examined. The original aim was to establish the mechanisms by which conflict and poor support increase risk of disorder, and relate to low self-esteem, and how all emanate from adverse childhood experiences.

The London samples: These are described in detail in the appendix and in the text are referred to as the 'midlife' sample of women, the 'follow-up' of these women, the 'mother-offspring dyads' or the 'offspring' samples. These largely represent high-risk individuals and families in the London community. There was no prior selection for presence of psychological disorder and the high rates reported are a reflection of the psychosocial factors present. The midlife samples are exclusively women, although the offspring younger series were both male and female. Therefore much of the analysis can only be said to reflect female experience although reference is made where possible to other ASI studies where males are included. We believe the models developed hold for both males and females.

Measurement: The standardised semi-structured interviews used cover a range of experiences and vulnerabilities across the life course. These measures are described in the text, but references are provided for the reader to search out more detail. They all have acceptable levels of inter-rater reliability, and validity. Most have been used on prior representative community studies.

Statistical analyses: Those described in the book are relatively simple and highly summarised to aid reading the text. The book is not a statistical exposition of the findings. Further details can be found in publications listed, or by contacting the first author. The main statistics presented are correlations (usually Pearson's 'r' or Kappa) to show the association between dimensional variables or occasionally dichotomised ones. The chi square statistic is used to test the differences between variables, or groups, particularly in relation to disorder outcomes. Four-point scales are often dichotomised for simplicity and because of the dichotomised clinical disorder outcomes, or to build into indices. Usually the top two ratings 'marked' or 'moderate' are contrasted with 'some' or 'little/none'. For most of the analysis an index of Insecure attachment style is used, those Insecure styles at 'marked' or 'moderate' levels are included, those with 'mild' levels of insecurity are combined with Secure. The reason for this is the lower risk levels of those with mild levels. Binary logistic regressions have been used in the analysis, usually with disorder outcomes, to determine the most parsimonious model when examining several independent variables. These are not presented although the most parsimonious models are described. A few examples of path analysis (and one partial Structural Equation Model) are provided for the childhood and parenting models and more details of these can be found in published papers. Only significant pathway coefficients are shown here. Mostly significance levels in the analysis up to 5% level are utilised, but occasionally those up to 10% are shown to avoid type 2 errors on relatively small numbers. The latter are described as 'showing a trend' in relating. Various controls are made in the analysis for social class, ethnicity, gender and these are briefly referred to in the text but figures are not usually presented. In addition, for the midlife sample, the inclusion of sisters for half the sample has been entered elsewhere as a control in all analyses, and their presence does not affect the findings and models presented. For ease of reading, findings and figures are presented in bulleted sentences, mostly in percentages, and with 'p' values given. This is to avoid 'clunky' text heavily laden with figures. Tables have been avoided since this would entail much more statistical detail, and therefore findings are presented graphically where possible. We have provided various summaries of findings, since there are many throughout the book as an aid to absorbing the rich material.

New and summarised findings: The findings presented are a mix of previously published findings which have never been collated before, together with new findings and original case material which has not been published elsewhere. Each chapter contains some new analyses from the London samples described; for example, the analysis of life events and coping; domestic violence; and different types of childhood experience, resilience factors and attachment change are all newly presented here.

The final models: Various models are shown in Chapter 1 to illustrate different aspects of attachment theory. It was not feasible to develop a single model which would highlight the many findings presented. However, a model indicating the confluence of bio-psychosocial factors in the different attachment styles is shown in the concluding chapter for each style, as well as an overall lifespan model and an intergenerational one. These models are schematic and conceptual, not statistical, and aim to summarise the various elements described in the analysis to work towards a more integrated view and one that practitioners can easily absorb to aid in their work.

Case material and ethics: All case examples presented are taken from actual research interviews or clinical or social work practice. In all instances these have been anonymised and any distinguishing details masked. For ease of identification all the cases are described by a first name beginning with the same letter as the style (for example Fearful Felicity) and their key characteristics are summarised in the appendix. Clinical or social work cases have been taken from a variety of sources with permission of the social workers or clinicians involved. Ethical permission for the research studies was granted by the relevant Local Health Authority prior to the programme of research start. All those participating signed informed consent, and for the offspring interviews, maternal consent was also provided. All agreed to anonymised use of their interview material for research purposes.

Labelling attachment styles: For simplicity, when referring to research studies utilising a variety of different labels for adult attachment style the simplified labels of Secure, Anxious, Avoidant and Disorganised have been used, with greater specification added when necessary.

Ten key findings

The research findings are described in detail in Chapters 2–7 covering a range of factors associated with adult attachment style including different role domains (partner, support figure, parenting), functioning (self-esteem, coping, resilience, clinical disorder) as well as adversities (childhood neglect/abuse, adult adversity, recent severe life events).

Ten main findings are outlined here to orientate the reader, and these summarised in more detail in the conclusion and throughout the book.

1. **Measurement:** Measuring adult attachment style with the ASI involves categorising the quality of partner and close support (family or friends) as a basis for determining level of insecurity. This provides a behav-

ioural as well as attitudinal basis for attachment categorisations with attention to context. Two Anxious styles (Enmeshed or Fearful) and two Avoidant styles (Angry-dismissive or Withdrawn) as well as those Dual/disorganised and those Secure are identified.

2. **Clinical Disorder:** Insecure attachment styles (Dual/disorganised, Enmeshed, Fearful and Angry-dismissive) at 'marked' or 'moderate' levels of insecurity relate to major depression and anxiety disorders and to lifetime recurrent depression. In the Offspring sample Angry-dismissive style additionally related to Deliberate Self-Harm (DSH) behaviour and Dual/disorganised style to substance abuse. Withdrawn or Secure style is unrelated to disorder in either sample.

3. **Self-esteem:** Insecure attachment style is related to Negative Evaluation of Self (NES). In particular, Enmeshed and Fearful styles have high rates in both generations. Adult women with Angry-dismissive style also have high rates of NES. Withdrawn or Secure style is unrelated to low self-esteem.

4. **Stress and coping:** Those with Insecure attachment style are more prone to severe life events, particularly those involving interpersonal, and financial events, and exhibit poorer coping skills with such events, involving helplessness, denial and anger. They also have higher rates of lifetime adult adversity. Those with Anxious styles (Enmeshed or Fearful) showed more avoidant strategies (cognitive avoidance or denial) as well as helplessness. Those with Angry-dismissive styles exhibit blame and anger, in addition to emotional distress. Those with Dual/disorganised styles used an array of negative coping responses. Those with Withdrawn or Secure styles have low levels of negative coping behaviour.

5. **Partner relationships:** Insecure attachment style was related to problem partner relationships as well as to single parent status. Those with Fearful styles were less likely to be in a partnership, and more often single parents, with those Enmeshed and Angry-dismissive most often with a partner. Those Dual/disorganised were more likely to have been separated from their partner. Problem partnerships related differentially: those with Enmeshed or Withdrawn styles were most likely to lack partner support through conflict or indifference respectively. Those with Angry-dismissive styles also had a high rate of partner conflict. Those with Enmeshed style were more likely to have been in a violent partner relationship whilst those Dual/disorganised were more likely to have had partners with antisocial behaviour, disorder or criminality. Those with Angry-dismissive styles also had high rates of antisocial partners and those with Fearful styles had partners with disorder or criminality. Improvement in partner relationship, or change to a new supportive partner was a factor in positive attachment change.

6. **Family and friends support:** Having Very Close Others (VCOs) who are confidants contributed to ratings of 'ability to make and maintain relationships' and hence to security. These included adult family members

or friends. Those with a Withdrawn style were the least likely to have a close confidant and Enmeshed the most likely of the Insecure styles to have a close confidant. Acquiring a new close confidant was a factor in positive attachment change.

7. **Childhood adversity:** Severe neglect or abuse was a major early life factor associated with all adult Insecure attachment styles, apart from Withdrawn style. Insecure attachment style was shown to mediate between early neglect/abuse and adult depression/anxiety. Whilst the overlap of different neglect or abuse experiences made differentiation difficult, evidence was found of lack of care experiences relating to Anxious styles (Enmeshed or Fearful) and Dual/disorganised styles, with abuse relating to Angry-dismissive style. In the young sample, there was a significant relationship between maternal antipathy, neglect or physical abuse and emotional disorder. There was also some association of fathers' antipathy, neglect or physical abuse and Angry-dismissive and Dual/disorganised style in relation to substance abuse.

8. **Problem parenting:** Mothers with Insecure styles had higher levels of estimated incompetent parenting and this in turn was associated with offspring independent accounts of maternal neglect or abuse. There was, however, no direct link between mother's attachment style and offspring neglect or abuse other than through incompetent parenting. Fathers/substitute fathers also play a critical role, and problem part-ners (those criminal, disordered or violent) increased the likelihood of the mother showing incompetent parenting, with marital adversity also contributing to the child's neglect/abuse context. Attachment elements highlighted were hostile and helpless or anxious parenting styles. Enmeshed and Angry-dismissive styles had the highest rates of incompetent parenting.

9. **Resilience and Attachment change:** Secure, mildly Insecure and Withdrawn style were all related to lower rates of emotional disorder, even when childhood adversity was present, indicative of resilience. Positive childhood and teenage experience contributed to Secure outcomes. Around a quarter of adult women changed attachment style significantly over a three-year follow-up period, half in a positive direc-tion. An increase in partner or close other support was associated with positive change to more security.

10. **Attachment and services:** The use of the ASI in child and family serv-ices has shown its utility in assessing adoption carer suitability, in conceptualising family and parent–child problem interactions in attachment terms and in identifying attachment difficulties in young people in residential care. Case examples highlight patterning of different attachment styles and behaviours drawing out the implica-tions for family disruption and conflict and pointing to ways in which these might be helped or repaired in different interventions.

1 Introduction to attachment

1.0 Introduction

The importance of close relationships for psychological health and well-being is widely accepted. Attachment theory provides a critical developmental framework for understanding how individuals form close relationships, first as children and later as adults. Driven by the need for a protective bond with the main carer, usually the mother, the child's internalised experience of this early relationship develops as a cognitive–emotional template that continues to inform expectations of future relationships. The effects thus become observable across the lifespan. One of attachment's primary functions is around the management of stress. Thus individuals' regulation of emotions at times of stress, particularly around life events involving loss, abandonment, rejection or conflict, by seeking out help from close others, gives us an insight into psychological attachment mechanisms at play. The good quality of attachments first enacted during childhood is continued through the acquisition of trust, ability to seek help from others and development of appropriate levels of autonomy into adulthood. How these actions vary in individuals with different attachment styles is critical to understanding risk and resilience profiles. When attachment styles in adulthood are distorted, psychological disorder becomes more likely, through the combined psychosocial elements of greater interpersonal stress, poorer coping skills, lower self-esteem and less social support. Such styles and behaviours are typically underpinned by biological vulnerabilities derived from early life adversity. Their impact is not only on individuals but also on their families, which in turn leads to transmission of risk to offspring.

Whilst much has been written on attachment from the point of view of the developing child in relation to its parents and carers, there has been less systematic focus on adult attachment style utilising a lifespan and intergenerational approach which integrates historical relationship difficulties going back to childhood and ongoing adult experiences to understand risks for adult clinical disorder. There is relatively little integrated study from a social perspective of adult relationships which examines childhood as an independent contributor and looks closely at the context of ongoing close relationships in relation to Anxious, Avoidant and Disorganised as well as to Secure styles. This is the purpose of this book.

1.1 Background to attachment theory

The belief that developing close attachment in childhood to parents or carers is essential to human wellbeing is now a well-established principle which underlines much of the research, clinical and social care practice involving child and family and mental health services (Rutter and O'Connor 1999). It was not always so. In past times attachment was rarely made a priority in policy or practice involving children and adults, with a greater priority given to issues of physical safety, or utility of services. For example, in the Second World War children were evacuated from London and major cities to the country without their mothers with no particular psychological risk being anticipated from the separation and potential disruption of this bond (Rusby 2005). Priority was given instead to physical safety (the children deemed to be safe from bombing) and the utility of having mothers freed up to work in munitions factories and other services to aid the war effort. Whilst the children's experiences proved to be varied (in some cases damaging and in some cases an improvement on prior care), the distress associated with losing the mother and with substitute care was not taken into the calculation of future mental health or wellbeing as it would be today.

Other examples from previous decades include young children being kept in hospital with only limited contact with their mothers or close relatives. Parents were seen as an impediment to efficient running of the hospital wards, and little official importance was given to the distress caused by the separation until this was observed to hamper recovery (Robertson and Robertson 1971). Until relatively recently children looked after by the state were accommodated in large institutions with little opportunity to develop attachments and attachment capacity in personal relationship with carers, leading to the disorders of attachment and relating, evident at the most extreme in Romanian orphanage adoptees (Rutter and ERA team 1998; Rutter, Beckett *et al.* 2007). Also, children's stressful experience of fragmented care by strangers in unfamiliar settings during prolonged stays in residential nurseries in the earliest months of life, was only retrospectively acknowledged as provoking anxiety. Only in later years after attachment was recognised as of importance were arrangements made for greater parent–child contact and frequent visits, much deriving from the film evidence of children showing distress on separation, undertaken by the pioneering work by the Robertsons (Robertson and Robertson 1971). These scenarios of children's responses following reunions with their mothers, were the real-life versions of the experience Mary Ainsworth sought to recreate in her laboratory technique the Strange Situation Test

(SST) to measure the variations of response in terms of Secure or Insecure styles in the infants (Ainsworth, Blehar *et al.* 1978).

John Bowlby formulated the importance of attachment in child development, in adult functioning and in relation to psychiatric disorder. His development of attachment theory, further enhanced by collaboration with Mary Ainsworth, expanded and refined a scientific framework which encompassed biological, ethological, sociological, psychological and psychiatric principles (Bowlby 1969; Bowlby 1973; Bowlby 1980).

Basic precepts of attachment theory state:

- Attachment is a basic human need, required for optimal human development.
- Close relationships with parents or caregivers, promotes actual and felt security in the infant which forms the trust template for later relating-ability.
- The close parent provides a 'secure-base' (or 'safe haven') in which the child is loved and cared for, encouraged to develop skills and to explore its environment. In turn the child develops other attachments to close family and friends to whom, when experiencing threats to its safety and wellbeing, the child can signal for help and communicate need to gain practical and emotional support.
- The child learns appropriate levels of autonomy – when to cope alone and when to ask for help, as well as a measure of trust that others around will help when needed.
- The child also develops optimal capacity for self-reliance to aid exploration which lead to new learning and the development of coping skills. Such support can allay emotions of fear and anger in relation to the set-backs and trials which occur in everyone's life.
- The psychological development which accompanies such experience is a positive 'internal working model', a cognitive, or mental template, or road plan, which mirrors experience to encapsulate a view of the social world as responsive, supportive and benign. This psychological roadmap sets the scene for approaching new relationships in later life with an expectation of positive and companionable interaction, and selecting appropriate others to become close to. It is typically accompanied by a parallel positive internal working model of the self – viewing the self as lovable and worthy and having positive self-esteem.
- Such positive internal working models then promote better care and a capacity for attunement and 'reflective function' or mentalising behaviour (Fonagy, Gergely *et al.* 2002) in parenting roles which lead to greater security in the next generation.

It now seems self-evident that close attachment in childhood is imperative for the child to survive and thrive. Secure attachment to parents or caregivers has been shown to ensure both physical and emotional safety for the child and to provide a Secure context for healthy development. The same principle of security in close relationships as a key to healthy functioning and development applies throughout the life course. Having close attachments helps individuals negotiate key points of development and change across the lifespan – for example the ability to negotiate age-appropriate autonomy in toddlerhood; the capacity for developing positive peer relationships in middle childhood or adolescent move towards independence and leaving home; adult embarking on sexual and partner relationships; taking on parental roles; finding enduring friendships; negotiating work roles and then retiring from these. All these change-points can be negotiated more easily with the help of supportive, enduring, harmonious and mutually rewarding relationships with close others. Each optimal developmental phase is promoted by healthy attachment behaviour.

The negotiation of stress is an important feature of attachment. One of the key factors in successfully dealing with stressful events is through support. Such events can involve the losses and dangers, entrapments and humiliations, trauma and bereavements that occur during the life course. Having close, reliable, attentive support can mitigate many of the effects of these stressors on our functioning, mental health and coping. Attachment is therefore a fundamental need for human resilience throughout the life course and in relation to myriad stressors. Without attachments the quality of life is greatly depleted, day-to-day functioning is reduced and psychological difficulties and damaging social interactions more likely.

However, the concept of attachment and its role in a wide range of life situations is in danger of becoming so broad that its utility is devalued by an over-usage and over-valuation of its role. The question 'what does attachment not relate to?' becomes a refrain from researchers as more and more aspects are included in its remit. An important issue remains: how can it be easily measured at different life stages, preserving continuity but amenable to different levels of development? Whilst its absorption into professions such as social work is heartening in relation to promoting children's development and loving family relationships, here too, attachment has become a loosely applied by-word for an inferred bond between parent and child. So when an adult or child is referred to a service because of problems in attachment, the referrer is assumed to have made an accurate judgement of the individual's attachment behaviour. But this is often in the context of a loose model of attachment behaviour and without the benefit of reliable and valid instruments through which such evaluation can be substantiated. So while it is encouraging that the relevance of attachment theory to practical areas of support and intervention is acknowledged, and recognition of different patterns of attachment behaviour have become absorbed into mainstream thinking, the absence of empirical back-up to claims of attachment problems is concerning. In this way, as prophesised by some of its early researchers, attachment has indeed become a victim of its own success

(Waters, Corcoran *et al.* 2005). The popularity of attachment concepts has been such that personal judgement of what constitutes attachment has been permitted to become acceptable as the preferred method for assessing quality of attachment in many services. The purpose of this book is to look in close detail at a particular type of standardised assessment interview for adults and its use in a range of studies which have looked at attachment style in relation to risks for psychological disorder in families to inform both research and practice applications. This will seek to inform a model of attachment which will examine its early life sources and its relationship to later clinical disorder.

Summary of key attachment concepts

Attachment: The protective bond the child develops first to the mother or main carer and then to other family members involving proximity seeking, responses to the child's emotional state, dyadic soothing and understanding and acceptance of the child's emotional experience.

Attachment figure: Someone who provides safety, responsiveness to distress, support, understanding, protection and care. In childhood the primary and secondary carers are usually the parent figures. In adulthood other close figures who provide support such as partners and close family or friends.

Attachment behaviours: In infancy this includes crying, smiling, clinging, searching, proximity seeking and other adaptive responses to the experience of distress related arousal and/or separation from primary attachment figure. In adults this involves seeking out the attachment figure for support, comfort and acceptance.

Attachment behavioural system and style: Secure styles involve an organised strategy optimising approach or avoidance of others to find a balance of autonomy and safety/support. Insecure styles maximise either the approach or avoidance to others for purposes of emotion-regulation, mistrust of care or harm-avoidance developed in childhood in relation to caregiver behaviour and other experience. Disorganisation, or absence of organised strategy, can occur due to overwhelming fear or powerlessness. The behavioural system leads to a distinct pattern of interaction with the caregiver or close other in childhood as well as in later adult life.

Safe-haven: The physical and emotional security provided by the mother or main carer to the infant to promote healthy development. In adulthood this is provided by adult close relationships.

Secure base: Feelings of safety transmitted through close proximity to the caregiving parent from which the child has the confidence to explore.

Internal working model: A cognitive template (or roadmap) which develops in childhood about others and of the self based on early experiences of care or neglect/abuse which determine future expectations of relationships. These continue into adulthood but are open to change and adaptation.

When children do not have attentive caring in early life, damage is done to their development and to their capacity to relate to others which endures into adult life although this is capable of re-alignment. Expectations that others are hostile, unpredictable or cold, or untrustworthy, arise from real experiences of neglect, emotional, physical or sexual abuse from carers and others. In these situations the internal working models developed similarly reflect that the social world is cold and hostile, and that others will not be available for help or support. This is frequently accompanied by the belief that the self is unworthy and unlovable. Such expectations inhibit the ability to develop close attachments and builds up negative expectations for future social encounters.

Problems in attaching in adulthood lead to a range of social problems. For example, attachment theory can help us to understand the behaviour of a woman in a violent partnership who continually returns to the abusive relationship despite danger to herself, because of her overly high need for attachment proximity, however misplaced. Alternatively, there is the older age person living alone who will not ask for help from services having learned over a lifetime to be self-sufficient and not accept charity, and has to endure isolation. Or the single mother who has been let down in her partner relationship and so becomes fearful of starting another relationship in case she is rejected or abused again. Or the abused individual who uses anger to combat adversity and rejections. In these instances distortions in attachment behaviour can lead to remaining in damaging relationships, or avoiding potentially positive relationships. In each case these individuals would also find it difficult to seek professional help effectively, to communicate need effectively or welcome support. Understanding the nature of attachment and the styles individuals develop helps us to see where such behaviour comes from, and aids practitioners in their assessment and care plans for such individuals.

Attachment theory and the research which has arisen from it, allows us greater understanding of the circumstances and psychological response of individuals whose attachment style and behaviour does not fall within the usual adaptive range. It helps us to understand the tolerance or perpetration of hostility and violence in relationships; the extreme avoidance of others through heightened self-sufficiency or fear of contact; the increased dependency of individuals on relationships which provide them with little support or reward. It also helps us understand how such adult relationships impact on parenting and the experience of children who are born into families where Insecure attachments are instilled.

The scope of attachment theory and its applications are therefore very broad and central to services which provide for health and social care (Howe, Brandon *et al.* 1999). The aim of this book is to outline details of attachment theory as it applies to adults, provide research findings which help explain non-adaptive and non-supported social relationships and their origins in adverse childhood experience, describe assessment tools for attachment style with emphasis by explaining one interview assessment in particular detail (the ASI) and illustrating the styles and related experience through case material. In the course of expounding attachment style in adults, issues of gender, culture and mental health will be addressed. In addition the implications for interventions and best practice in relation to some of the social problems arising from attachment difficulties will be addressed. Figure 1.1 shows the experiences and behaviour related to adult attachment which influence the organisation of this book. Each of these will be briefly summarised below.

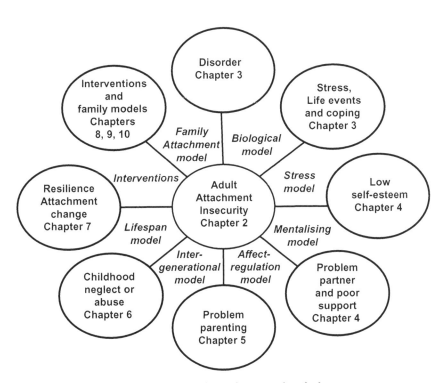

Figure 1.1 Illustrative scheme of social attachment-related phenomena

1.2 Outlining adult attachment styles

John Bowlby outlined those attachment styles which were dysfunctional (or Insecure) in his trilogy on Attachment and Loss, encompassing, for example, Compulsive Caregiving as an Anxious style and Compulsive Self-Reliance as an Avoidant style, but current typologies used owe more to the categorisations developed by collaborations with Mary Ainsworth (Ainsworth, Blehar *et al.* 1978). In observing the effects of maternal separation on children in field work undertaken in Africa where she studied mother-child interactions, Ainsworth developed the SST, as a research tool to investigate infants' responses to brief maternal separations, as a basis for classifying their attachment patterns. The children reacted differently, but in definable patterns and from these she derived a three-fold classification of different attachment styles in children: Anxious-resistant, Anxious-avoidant and Secure. These represented a protesting, clinging style; a cool dismissive style and a healthy style with temporary distress followed by effective comforting, respectively. A fourth style of Disorganised was later added (Main and Solomon 1986) with a mixed and disorientated response to the mother's absence. These styles were adopted for classification of adult styles, both by Mary Main and colleagues in working on parent–child interactions (George, Kaplan *et al.* 1984; Main and Cassidy 1988), and later by Cindy Hazan and Phil Shaver when seeking to understand attachment in partner relationships These style classifications have since spawned a large and fertile area of research (Hazan and Shaver 1987).

The concept of attachment style in adults relates to:

- How individuals' preconceptions, based on earlier life experience and influenced by the internal working model, dictate how individuals act, think and feel in relationships (Waters, Crowell *et al.* 2002).
- Those Secure feel comfortable with both autonomy and closeness, have reciprocal relationships, value attachment and feel able to confide and seek help when needed.
- Those Insecure Anxious-ambivalent (variously called Enmeshed or Preoccupied) have a great fear of separation and abandonment, and so cling onto relationships with very high levels of attachment need, requiring high need for company and closeness, have low levels of self-reliance and can express anger when their needs are not met (Feeney 2007).
- Those Insecure-avoidant (or Dismissive) express very high levels of self-reliance, have psychological barriers to getting close, can be mistrustful, have low need for company and can be angrily dismissive or denigrating of others (Bartholomew 1990).
- Those with Insecure-disorganised styles are variously labelled as Unresolved around issues of prior loss or trauma or unclassifiable (Main and Solomon 1986), or have dual categorisations (Crittenden

1997). These individuals have attitudes and behaviours more difficult to classify, showing often contradictory behaviours or fulfilling both Anxious and Avoidant characteristics (Lyons-Ruth and Jacobvitz 1999).

There are a number of categorising schemes for attachment style, relating to different measures of attachment style, and whether interview- or questionnaire-based. Not all include the Disorganised/dual style (for example the questionnaire assessments) and the schemes variously subdivide Anxious styles (e.g. whether or not including Fearful) and Avoidant (e.g. differentiating Angry-dismissive from Withdrawn). These will be described in more detail when the measures of attachment style are outlined in Chapter 2. However, for ease of identification when discussing the research literature, reference will be made to Anxious, Avoidant, Disorganised and Secure styles as general categories rather than specific labels for different styles in different measures.

Adult attachment categories

Secure (or Autonomous): Comfortable with closeness; trusting; moderate levels of autonomy; ability to relate to close others; ability to seek support; resilient under stress.

Anxious (or Enmeshed, Preoccupied): High need for closeness, and the company of others; low autonomy; fear of separation; dependency and ambivalence in relationships sometimes expressed as anger, other times as possessiveness or jealousness.

Avoidant (or Dismissive): Low need for company of others, overly high autonomy; discomfort at closeness; angry mistrust of other's intentions; blaming of others.

Disorganised (or Unresolved, Can't Classify, Dual–Insecure styles): No integrated strategy for dealing with attachment difficulties; unintegrated anxious and avoidant attitudes and behaviour; dissociated anger.

1.3 Attachment style and psychological disorder

Insecure attachment styles are highly associated with psychological disorder, with Secure style consistently found in most studies to be associated with the absence of disorder (Mickelson, Kessler *et al.* 1997). Insecure styles are related to depression both in terms of depressive symptomatology as assessed by checklist (Gerlsma and Luteijn 2000) and with clinical levels of disorder (Hammen, Burge *et al.* 1995; Mickelson, Kessler *et al.* 1997;

Bifulco, Moran *et al.* 2002a; Bifulco, Kwon *et al.* 2006). However, there is little consistency in linking specific attachment styles with particular disorders. Whilst it is expected and supported that Anxious styles relate to depression (Gerlsma and Luteijn 2000; Murphy and Bates 2000), some studies have identified Avoidant styles (McCarthy 1999). Others have shown no differentiation between any Insecure style and depression (Mickelson, Kessler *et al.* 1997). This may be a result of different types of measures used or other factors such as chronicity or co-morbidity (duality) of disorder. There are findings which indicate that those with Avoidant/Dismissive styles are more prone to substance abuse, conduct and antisocial problems (Murphy and Bates 2000). Insecure styles relate to new onsets of depression and anxiety disorder prospectively, thus acting as vulnerability factors for disorder (Bifulco, Moran *et al.* 2002b), and Insecure styles are also associated with personality disorders, for example with Anxious styles relating to Borderline or Hystrionic styles and Avoidant with Antisocial or schizoid styles (Fonagy, Leigh *et al.* 1996).

1.4 Attachment style and the self

Individual's with Insecure attachment styles are more likely to have a negative view of themselves which can also serve to inhibit the formation of successful relationships and good parenting (Bartholomew and Horowitz 1991). A model has been proposed by Bartholomew and Horowitz that a negative or positive view of self and other is differentiated in the different styles. For example whilst Secure have a positive view of others and of the self, Anxious/Enmeshed styles have a positive view of others but negative of the self, Dismissive have a negative view of others but positive of the self and Fearful have a negative view of both self and other. It is clear that belief in the self as worthy of love is bound up with the expectations of others as loving (Bartholomew 1994).

Related to internal working models of self and other is the notion of mentalising, which is a key determinant of self-organisation, which together with affect-regulation and attention control mechanisms is acquired during early relationships, and involves 'holding mind in mind' (Allen and Fonagy 2006). It is related to empathy, emotional intelligence, psychological mindedness and insight. It is defined as '*the mental process by which an individual implicitly and explicitly interprets the actions of himself and others as meaningful on the basis of intentional mental states such as personal desires, needs, feelings, beliefs and reasons*' (Bateman and Fonagy 2004, p.21). Mentalising accurately in attachment relationships is needed for better management of relationships for example in resolving conflicts, and those Secure are judged to have better mentalising skills (Fonagy 2006). Secure attachment provides a level of positive emotional arousal that increases interest in mentalising, with the attachment figure continually mentalising the other and actively stimulating mentalising. Attachment is thus a generally non-competitive relationship where learning about minds can be safely practised (Fonagy 2006).

For Insecure styles, those Avoidant who deactivate negative emotion and emotional memory centres might manifest an unthinking or inconsiderate approach to relationships. For those Anxious, these aspects are hyperactivated with easy access to emotional memory and negative affect and preoccupation with relationships. However, for those with Disorganised styles the situation is more complex. Given the child scans the mental states of the carer who threatens to undermine him or her, this can create an alien presence within the self-representation which leads to re-externalising parts of the self onto the attachment figures rather than internalising and containing affect. Thus childhood adversity causes the breakdown of attachment-related mentalisation (Allen and Fonagy 2006).

Whilst the research findings reported later in this book do not involve measures of mentalisation, it is important to bear in mind this underlying component which may inhibit the development of good relationships with problems in affect regulation and sense of self.

1.5 Attachment style and stress

At the heart of attachment theory, is a model of stress and coping. The purpose of attachment in evolutionary terms is for the parent to protect the child from external threat and harm. The parent thus provides a 'safe haven' for such protection and the child learns the parent is a 'secure base'. In addition a good parent will teach the child to cope with adversity and will model emotional-regulation to minimise distress. As attachment behaviour becomes activated by stress, the child, and later the adult, seeks support from close others to regulate their distress levels. Various stressors are also viewed as threats to attachment security. These include threatened or actual losses of close others, rejections, abandonments, conflicts and other interpersonal events. These are also termed 'attachment injuries' which are harmful to relationships, as well as interpersonal trauma which in childhood can be the basis of Insecure attachment styles developing (Johnson and Whiffen 2003).

Adult models of stress and clinical disorder identify both longer-term vulnerability factors which can emanate from childhood adversity, and recent provoking agents in the form of severe life events, which interact to create onset of disorders such as depression. In such models Insecure attachment style is identified as a vulnerability factor which can become activated by interpersonal severe life events to lead to emotional disorders such as depression (Bifulco, Brown *et al.* 1988; Bifulco, Moran *et al.* 2002a). In social approaches to adult attachment style a focus on the relationship with partner and other close adults and the capacity for seeking support, in relation to stressors which require such support, and further stressors which may emanate from the very relationships deemed to be close, requires examination in exploring attachment styles in adult life (see Figure 1.2).

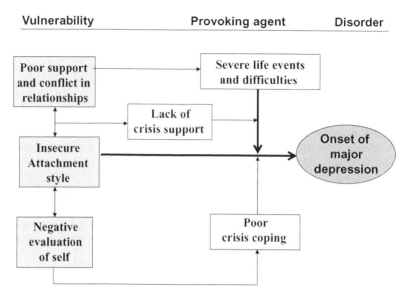

Figure 1.2 Model of stress and attachment style

1.6 Attachment style, partner relationships and support

Insecure attachment styles are associated with difficulties in partner relationships, particularly difficulties that are repeated over time and in
different relationships (Feeney 1996; Davila and Bradbury 2001). These
can include conflict in relationships with a high level of negative interaction but accompanying feelings of attachment (Kobak and Hazan 1991).
The styles can also include distance with little sharing and feelings of closeness. Secure styles in contrast are associated with high confiding in
relationships, good mutual support and feelings of attachment and good
interaction. Even choice of partner relationship and age at first cohabita-
tion is associated with attachment style, with those with Insecure styles
having more inappropriate choice of partner and earlier first age of cohab-
itation (Lapsley 2000).

Insecure attachment style is also associated with having fewer confiding
relationships (Mikulincer and Nachshon 1991). Those with Avoidant style
tend to have fewer social contacts in general, those with Anxious style have
more superficial and briefer relationships with less meaningful interaction.
For some who are insecure, reliance is put on family relationships only for
support, for others family are avoided and only non-kin relationships developed (Runtz 2007). For individuals who have experienced abusive
parenting in childhood, sometimes those same abusive parents are counted
as close confidants with resulting ambivalent interactions. Where those with

Insecure styles also have mental health problems sometimes the close others selected are those with similar problems making for less-effective support. Other behaviours are associated with the type of style – clinging and need for company in those Anxious and withdrawal or hostility for those Avoidant (Muller 2000). For Secure individuals support figures will be selected for their support capacity, relationships will be close (but not overly relied on) and be high in confiding, with typically two or three confidants with whom high levels of disclosure and consistent closeness is achieved.

A key effect of good support is that of emotional regulation which is linked to proximity seeking and occurs when close others are available:

- In Secure individuals, seeking out the attachment figure relieves any distress resulting from encountering life events which involve threat or negative change and thus becomes a positive factor in affect-regulation.
- For those with Insecure styles, such proximity cannot be achieved and distress and anxiety following from threatening events is not automatically relieved. This leads to two scenarios: one deactivating and one hyper-activating.
- Deactivating (Avoidant Style) is where the attachment figure is avoided and the individual learns to use deactivating strategies, distancing themselves from the stressor and its impact and so 'shuts down' the affect by blocking feelings and perceptions of threat.
- Hyper-activating (Anxious Style) is when proximity seeking is viable but there is a hyper-activation of threat and affect such that the proximity seeking whilst very active, is unable to regulate the affect.

A model has been developed of the process of events activating proximity seeking and resulting in regulation of emotion differentiated by adult attachment style (Shaver and Mikulincer 2002; Mikulincer, Shaver *et al.* 2003) and is highly instructive for support-based approaches to attachment style in adults. For this model, three components are critical:

- The monitoring and appraisal of threatening life events responsible for the activation of attachment leading to potential proximity seeking behaviour.
- The availability of attachment figures to whom the individual can go for support to aid with affect regulation or soothing
- The monitoring and appraisal of the viability of proximity seeking.

In other words, does the individual trust the close other to provide support and soothing? Different individual responses, related to attachment style involve hyperactivating versus deactivating strategies. The pathways through which proximity seeking are sought or avoided, where support figures are available or not and the impacts on regulation of affect are delineated (see Figure 1.3).

This model outlines the classic Anxious and Avoidant attachment approaches versus Secure, but does not allow for some of the other possibilities such as anxious avoidance or anger in the behaviour and emotion regulation. Also, as with other social approaches to adult attachment it does not identify effects of Disorganised attachment style on affect dysregulation. Figure 1.3 is based on the model proposed by Mikulincer and Shaver (2008).

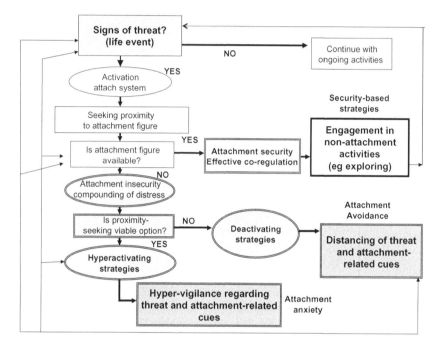

Figure 1.3 Model of affect regulation and attachment style

1.7 Attachment style and parenting

Insecure parental attachment style is highly associated with poorer parenting behaviour (Steele, Steele *et al.* 1996). This can occur as early as in the postnatal period – in fact mothers identified as having Insecure styles even in pregnancy are found to have poorer interaction with children after birth (Fonagy, Steele *et al.* 1991). The different attachment styles have variously been shown to relate to more intrusive interactions with infants and children (Anxious, Enmeshed) or distant (Avoidant) with both indicating insensitivity (Murray, Stanley *et al.* 1996; Simpson, Rholes *et al.* 2003; McMahon, Barnett *et al.* 2006). Abusive parenting has been related to Insecure attachment style (Crittenden 1988), and, by contrast, effective fostering and adoption by carer's Secure style shown to mitigate the effects of prior damaged attachment (Dozier 2003).

Attachment theory has now influenced the development of family therapy, and models have been developed which bring together attachment styles in the caregiving couple and the nature of the caregiver alliance, as well as the problems in child care around disruption, parental helplessness or anger and rejection. Thus the primary caregiver may have reduced availability, reduced empathy and attunement or may be prone to making coercive demands on the child as a function of their attachment style. If the secondary attachment figure is also Insecure then not only will the caregiver alliance be damaged but also the caregiving will be impaired, either with disengagement, or through coercive control. Impacts on the child will include perceived threats to availability and abandonment, failure to protect or rejection. This in turn leads to child symptoms and problem behaviours.

Kobak and Mandelbaum argue that attachment approaches in family therapy emphasise that caring for the child occurs in the context of the parent's relationship with each other and other adults and that the parents own adult attachment relationships need to be examined in their capacity to provide a secure base for the raising of children (Kobak and Mandelbaum 2003). The three elements in the relational system: the parent–child, the caregiving alliance and the adults' relationship can enhance or impede caring for children. Security and cooperation in one system can enhance functioning in the others. Alternatively, distress in one subsystem can influence the others and may divert attention from the source of the difficulty. For example, feelings of anxiety, anger and distress that accompany an insecure adult relationship may be misdirected towards the child or may absorb the caregivers' attention in ways that reduce the child's security. Failures to contain the stress generated from the adult–carer relationships increases the likelihood of added burden to children. Such 'boundary violations' often result in failed problem-solving that further increases the caregiver's sense of frustration and helplessness (Kobak and Mandelbaum 2003). Figure 1.4 shows the family model developed.

1.8 Attachment style and childhood experience

Attachment theory is a theory of human development and identifies childhood experience as the mainspring of developing Secure or Insecure attachment styles (Shaver and Rubenstein 1980). For a Secure style parents need to provide continuous, consistent, close care and protection (Asendorpf 2000). Insecure styles relate to inconsistent, hostile, emotionally unavailable parenting, separation from parents or experiences of neglect or

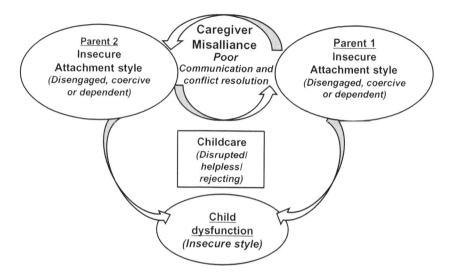

Figure 1.4 Family attachment model

abuse (Belsky 2002). Attempts have been made to relate the styles to differ-ent experiences; for example, Anxious styles to inconsistent parenting involving both warmth and rejection, hostility and role reversal and Avoidant styles to punitive, cold, distant parenting and separation. This is difficult to test, in part because the experiences themselves are highly corre-lated, and in part because adult attachment styles can go through change and be influenced by other more recent experiences (Runtz 2007). Yet research findings are consistent in showing that any Insecure adult attach-ment style is highly associated with adverse childhood experience.

Key elements in adult attachment style are those around trust and autonomy. Erikson's lifespan developmental theory encompasses both of these within stages (Erikson 1950). Whilst this theory is not mainstreamed in developmental theory, its focus both on lifespan development and on trust as a key element in development is relevant to attachment. Its concep-tualisation of psychosocial 'crises' which can impair lifespan development and reference to both strengths and weaknesses in development still has merits. Erikson viewed the course of development to be determined by the interaction of the body (genetic biological programming), mind (psycho-logical) and cultural (ethos) influences. In his stages of development, the establishment of trust is ascribed to the first 18 months of life, with mistrust developing when care is not forthcoming. If a child successfully develops trust, he or she will feel safe and secure in the world. Inconsistent, emotion-ally unavailable or rejecting care contributes to feelings of mistrust. Failure to develop trust results in fear and a belief that the world is inconsistent and unpredictable. Issues of autonomy arise in infancy where the infant learns a sense of personal control in developing physical skills and a sense of independence which, when successful, leads to feeling secure and confident and, when not, to a sense of inadequacy and self-doubt.

In understanding the development of different attachment styles, the patterning of early maltreatment to the different styles is required. In broad terms that involves fear of abandonment or rejection in the Anxious styles, mistrustful detachment in the Avoidant styles and a chaotic dysregulated response in Disorganised styles. A mediation model hypothesises causal links between childhood maltreatment and disorder in individuals mediated by attachment style. Whilst in general terms this is easy to test, for example any maltreatment and any Insecure attachment style as mediator to a specific disorder, differentiating particular childhood experiences as mediated by particular attachment styles, possibly for different clinical disorders is a much more difficult task.

1.9 A social and lifespan approach

Finally, the social dimension also needs highlighting. Issues here concern the role of social adversity and socio-economic factors, particularly when these are relationship based. Thus in childhood poor parenting is known to relate to social disadvantage, the impact of stress worsening parenting competence. Following from disadvantage in childhood the opportunities for having close and supportive relationships may be diminished by reduced opportunities. For example the availability of positive partnerships may be reduced among those teenagers leaving residential care (Quinton, Pickles *et al.* 1993). Thus attachment is not only about the individual's capacity for forming good relationships, but also the availability of suitable support in terms of situational factors. Sometimes support is unavailable for extraneous reasons – the single mother who moves into a new area, leaving family behind with no immediate access to support – the immigrant or asylum-seeking individuals socially excluded – the teenage runaway. The number of interacting factors between the social environment and the individual capacity for relating is complex, particularly when taking a life-course perspective, but developing a framework will help to illuminate the expression of the attachment system in different settings.

The model shown below is derived from the Brown and Harris work (Harris 2003), is both a lifespan and social model which incorporates psychological elements (see Figure 1.5). It also subsumes the adult stress model shown earlier (right-hand side of the model) with the influence of socio-economic status and adult adversity interacting with lack of social support and low self-esteem, leading to clinical depression. Extending this model to incorporate adult attachment style could readily show that following from childhood neglect/abuse, Insecure attachment style is a psychological driver of poor social support and low self-esteem. Using such a model helps to bring the social adversity and psychological vulnerability together in a coherent fashion in an extended stress model.

Socio-structural strand

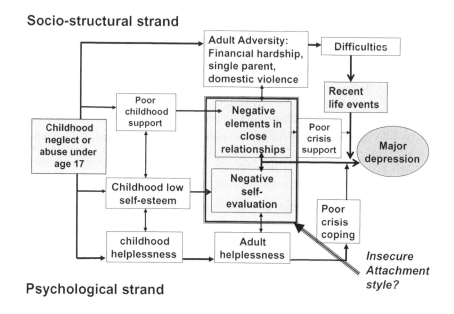

Figure 1.5 Lifespan psychosocial model

1.10 Attachment and biological processes

The past two decades have contributed sophisticated understanding about how life events and attachment-related stress change brain organisation, leading to complex attachment-related behaviours and altered psychological processes and behaviours to the point of dysfunction (Perry, Pollard *et al.* 1995). At the core of these changes lie the effects that early stressors, including attachment-related stress, have on multiple brain circuits and the way in which the individual is, or is not, able to make use of stress-attenuating interpersonal support to help socially regulate the response to perceived threat. Advances in mapping the biological underpinnings of psychological disorder, have encompassed neuroscience, brain development, and the endocrine system with stress hormones, such as cortisol, and the genetic bases of behaviour involving the production of oxytocin and dopamine. Those have provided evidence of neural impacts related to attachment phenomena including stress responses, proximity seeking, reward and attachment, social recognition and maternal sensitivity.

Most of the advances have come from both the investigation of the physiological impact of childhood neglect and abuse, and from human response to stress in general, both in childhood and its lasting impact in adults. These include developments in neuroscience, where deficits in early brain development as a result of maltreatment (Insel 1997) result in reduced volume of the hippocampus and the smaller volume of corpus callosum leading to reduced white matter and grey matter in the adult brain (McCrory, de Brito *et al.* 2010). Similarly, early adversity can lead to individual differences in oxytocin and vasopressin neuropeptide production for stress buffering. In parallel developments in endocrinology, particularly the Hypothalamus–Pituitary–Adrenal axis (HPA) show how chronic use of stress hormones in early life related to adversity can affect adult response to stress and failure of mechanisms to regulate stress hormones (Quirin, Preuessner *et al.* 2008). The aim of the HPA axis is to produce an optimal amount of cortisol: too much or too little can cause problems. Over- or under-production is termed 'toxic stress' and can lead to psychopathology and vulnerability. Infants with Insecure or Disorganised attachment have raised cortisol levels (Lyons-Ruth and Jacobvitz 2008). Evidence for this is provided by Oskis and colleagues using the ASI in school adolescents showing an association between Anxious styles (Enmeshed or Fearful) and cortisol dysregulation (Oskis, Loveday *et al.* 2011). Accessing the relational and pleasure-mediating neural system activates the hypothalamus and sets in train a chain reaction of pituitary and adrenal HPA-axis activity. As the hypothalamus goes into overdrive to deal with the stress response, the amygdala mediates fear responses and the prefrontal cortex is mobilised to activate memory templates (of expectations) that have encoded earlier experiences of managing stress in threatening contexts. These templates appraise the attachment figure's capacity to provide the soothing required to attain a feeling of safety and security. The mechanism by which HPA soothing can be achieved is regulation by 'another' so that stress becomes manageable.

Oxytocin, a neurotransmitter, plays a role in attachment due to its known connection to social recognition, trust, love and caregiving behaviours, and is usually present in large quantities after childbirth. Tests show that being given a sniff of oxytocin before the 'Reading the mind in the eyes' test of recognising emotion from photographs increases accuracy and speed of response (Domes, Heinrichs *et al.* 2007). Oxytocin levels increase in response to massage, stroking and pleasant sounds and smells and enhanced calm in a crisis. Low oxytocin levels have been linked to emotional abuse (Heim, Young *et al.* 2009). Similarly, dopamine is a neurotransmitter that regulates reward and attentional strategies. Parenting brings into play a series of neural circuits in the child in reward-seeking and stress-regulation.

Underpinning observable attachment behaviours are complicated neural response patterns associated with proximity seeking and the experience of reward in successful attachment formation as contrasted to those associated with the disregulatory processes of unassuaged stress induced by failed attachments. Involved are networks of biochemical processes which respond to the experience of reward by releasing dopamine, the hormone responsible for the feel-good factor associated with a sense of competence, energy and power to achieve goals. Distress through failed proximity seeking restricts the flow of this hormone and results in a surge in adrenaline and noradrenaline which prepare the body for fight (need) or flight(dismissal of need).

So far, physiological measurement has not shown a capacity for identifying causal brain-behaviour relationships in human attachment processes (Norris, Coan *et al.* 2007). Most of the studies investigating neural pathways in modulating attachment behaviour are focused on non-human animal populations so that findings that implicate neuropeptides, specifically oxytocin in males and vasopressin in females, in providing stress-buffering effects are still to be accepted as also modulating human attachment behaviour (Insel 1997). Even so, neural correlates to Bowlby's concept of proximity seeking as an evolutionary response to threat are likely to play an important part in dealing with stressful experiences and thus activate different human attachment behaviours. Key are the connections in the brain that link decrease in distress with the experience of survival and feelings of pleasure, or those that link increase in risk with increased threat and feelings of distress (Perry, Pollard *et al.* 1995). Such associations of pleasure and the experience of security with attention and approval, or the experience of insecurity with loss of attention, rejection and abandonment, are retrieved from the amygdala, the brain's 'storage room' for pleasure or fear-related experiences and attachment transactions.

Relevant biological responses are:

- Feelings of reward and pleasure (increase in dopamine release).
- Feelings of disincentive and distress (decrease in dopamine release).
- Both further contribute to encoding understanding of relational experiences as reliable – or not – to provide social- and biological-soothing.
- If dominated by dopamine decrease, the stress response system will be over-loaded and the axes of Avoidance and Anxiety related to security will remain primed or sensitised to danger so that even small stressors provoke large responses.
- Loss of ability to regulate the HPA-axis activity may lead to reduced capacity to regulate social interactions and abstract cognitions.
- Gradually changes at the neurochemical level accumulate and eventually start to get in the way of cortical or cognitve functioning. The effects on individual behaviour can be profound leading to psychopathology.

Parental regulation of physiological need in infancy as a necessary function for survival assumes an equally salient function when, in adulthood, heightened emotions in relation to stressful life events require interpersonal support to help regulate feeling responses to threat. Proximity seeking in response to stressful events thus implies a process in which the individual is guided behaviourally to find a way of having emotions (i.e. hyper-arousal in relation to danger) that arise in response to threat regulated within a relational context (Carter and de Vries 1999; Mikulincer and Shaver 2008). Regulated stress leads to controlled release of the stress hormone cortisol from the hypothalamus whereas unmanaged stress involves uncontrolled release of the chemical messages in turn triggering high HPA activity.

The attachment behavioural system thus responds by endeavouring to achieve a physiologically soothing and security-restoring social experience with respect to stressful life events through close proximity with those available for providing such a stress-buffering response. From the perspective of behavioural neuroscience, supportive social behaviours contribute to reduced stress-related activity in the autonomic nervous system (ANS) and the HPA axis (Coan 2008). Specifically, HPA-axis activity which heightens emotional distress is attenuated through the presence of trusted close others, resulting in oxytocin and vasopressin release.

Depending on how memory templates have encoded the availability of the 'close other' to provide this vital decrease in HPA-axis activity, behaviour is guided by high anxiety associated with overwhelming fear of losing the regulating relationship or, conversely, by low proximity seeking in moments of stress as the added threat of punishment or rejection leads to feeling dismissive of the need of others. Low anxiety and low avoidance denote a capacity to seek proximity and security from others as well as to self-soothe and maintain a sense of emotional homeostasis.

From a neurobiological perspective each of the behaviours that contribute to the 'attachment behavioural system', specifically the approach or withdraw strategies linked to Anxious or Avoidant attachment behaviours are visible manifestations of complex neural activity activated by the emotional stimulus of stressful life events. Sensing threat, the emotionally responsive amygdala is activated to retrieve short- and long-term memories of the availability and capacity of close others to provide HPA soothing.

Even if the precise mechanism by which these activities achieve social soothing are not fully understood, a major contribution to the way in which the threat response – and interactions with attachment figures – are managed comes from the hypothalamus where metabolic processes are regulated through cortisol release via the HPA axis and behavioural systems activity is coordinated. Therefore the understanding of biological correlates of a variety of attachment behaviours, including those emerging from early life maltreatment has been transformed in recent years such that a fully developed bio-psychosocial model of attachment is likely to soon be achieved.

1.11 Attachment style and resilience

The study of resilience is now an important theme in psychological research for understanding normal development in conditions of adversity, and is required by practitioners who need to assess both strengths and weaknesses of clients in their care planning and decision-making. It is generally acknowledged that Secure attachment style provides many benefits for the individual in terms of mental health, rewarding relationships and good parenting skills. Research evidence demonstrates that Secure style protects against adversity, leading to better outcomes in the face of stress and therefore constitutes a resilience factor (Fonagy, Steele *et al.* 1994). However, conditions under which Secure adult attachment style can emerge from adverse childhood is not fully understood. The concept of 'earned security' has been developed in the context of adult attachment approaches which emphasise working through vulnerabilities emanating from childhood adversity in adult life (Hesse 2008). This does not, however, explain the phenomenon of childhood Security arising because of early positive experiences co-existing with those negative. But many individuals survive childhood adversity in terms of their mental health status, with little vulnerability and this needs to be investigated in relation to Secure outcomes (Bifulco and Moran 1998). Using adult attachment measures with a focus on current relationships and attitudes to closeness, and a separate retrospective assessment of childhood adverse experience makes this an easier analysis to undertake. In addition, positive changes in attachment style in adulthood need investigating in relation to experience. Recent research has shown approximately 30% of adults report change in their attachment style over time (Hazan, Hutt *et al.* 1991) and such change is shown to be related to life events or new relationship experiences (Kirkpatrick and Davis 1994). Identification of the personal and interpersonal factors that predict meaningful change in attachment styles over time remains a challenge (Cozzarelli 2003) within contextual approaches which can incorporate social cognitive or individual-difference perspectives (Davila, Karney *et al.* 1999).

1.12 Attachment interventions and psychotherapy

In the last 10 years or so, there has been a burgeoning of therapeutic treatments that seek to deal with attachment-related difficulties of adults, children, parent–child and family settings (Slade 2008). Most approaches argue that attachment theory enriches a therapist's understanding of their patient but does not dictate a particular form of treatment. Indeed the breadth of attachment theory and attachment-related aspects of functioning means that a range of attachment-related elements are selected for the focus of therapy.

Attachment style has been shown to predict the patient's willingness to engage in therapy, with Secure the most willing to commit (Dozier 1990; Dozier, Lomax *et al.* 2001). By contrast, those Avoidant are shown as denying their need for help and those with Anxious styles have such a high level of neediness that it makes it difficult to engage with the therapist effectively. In terms of therapeutic alliance, Bradley and colleagues describe a typology of transference dimensions (angry/entitled; anxious/preoccupied; avoidant/counterdependent and secure/engaged) which map onto attachment-style categories (Bradley, Heim *et al.* 2005). Whether psychotherapy leads to change in attachment categorisation shows mixed findings. Fonagy and colleagues report on 82 in-patients insecure at start of treatment with 40% becoming securely attached as an outcome (Fonagy, Steele *et al.* 1995). Travis and colleagues found a reduction in Anxious (Fearful) styles, but with most patients moving from one type of Insecure attachment style to another (Diamond, Clarkin *et al.* 1999; Travis, Bliwise *et al.* 2001). A 12-month randomised controlled trial (RCT) investigation of transference-focused psychotherapy showed a significant increase in those classified as Secure with improvements in narrative coherence and self-reflective function (Levy, Meehan *et al.* 2006).

Fonagy and colleagues found that Avoidant (Dismissing) patients did better than Anxious (Preoccupied) or Unresolved (Fonagy, Leigh *et al.* 1996), a finding echoed by McBride and colleagues with depressed patients showing those with Avoidant style improving more than those with Anxious styles (McBride, Atkinson *et al.* 2006). It is speculated that the therapy exposes Avoidant (Dismissing) patients to their emotional experience in a new way, whereas those Anxious (Preoccupied) who habitually dwell on their feelings have already well-formed often 'self-serving' views harder to shift (Daniel 2006). However, there is little agreement concerning which type of patient does better in which treatment, with arguments made for Avoidant patients doing better both with psychoanalytically orientated psychotherapy (Fonagy, Leigh *et al.* 1996) and cognitive behaviour therapy (CBT) (McBride, Atkinson *et al.* 2006) and Anxious (Preoccupied) patients with binge-eating doing better with CBT and non-psychodynamic approaches (Borman-Spurrell 1996) (Slade 2008). The underlying assumption is that a therapy non-complementary to the patients attachment style would perform better – thus the more deactivating therapy such as CBT may be better for Anxious (Preoccupied) patients and psychodynamic for those Avoidant (Daniel 2006). Therefore, whilst attachment theory is becoming influential for practice, there is still some degree of uncertainty about how it should be applied. Utilising attachment classification in patients has not proved an approach favoured by most clinicians, with the categories seen as limiting. For example, Slade argues that patients for whom attachment is a primary issue are best understood in terms of fear in general, with the therapist providing the secure base, rather than in terms of attachment subtypes.

Many interventions used in attachment frameworks focus on related elements such as insensitive parenting (Bakermans-Kranenburg, van Ijzendoorn *et al.* 2003) or mentalisation in relation to personality disorder (Allen and Fonagy 2006) or changing biological vulnerabilities to stress in foster care contexts (Dozier, Lindheim *et al.* 2005). There are also a number of community-based interventions using attachment frameworks (e.g. Marvin, Cooper *et al.* 2002). Many of these show good levels of success in improving outcomes for children and parents although with less emphasis on adult attachment style.

Summary

This chapter has outlined some of the different approaches to attachment style in adults, topics which relate to the organisation of the remaining chapters.

- The four usual attachment categories in adults (Secure, Anxious, Avoidant and Disorganised) were outlined as well as the relationship of attachment style to stress models, to psychological processes such as self-esteem, and support aspects including close partner relationships and others in stress management and emotion-regulation.
- Childhood adversity is a prime cause of difficulties in attachment behaviour in adult life with attachment style posited as a key mediator for disorder. Whilst patterns of poor and unpredictable care are posited for Anxious attachment styles, hostile and cold parenting for Avoidant and abusive parenting for Disorganised styles, these require further confirmation by research.
- Attachment insecurity is a key factor in parenting capacity and maternal sensitivity. This in turn is related to the carers' relationship, their emotion-regulation and how this affects family systems.
- Lifespan social models looking at effects of adversity over the life course add a new dimension to the study of adult attachment style, providing opportunities to study how Insecure attachment style is maintained, or maybe overturned.
- Biological underpinnings of attachment behaviour involve neuroscience, endocrinology and genetics. Many problems in biological development are related to childhood maltreatment and the developing infant brain and physiology are distorted by experiences of severe stress. Thus under-development of brain structures, under- or over-production of cortisol, genetic factors relating to the production of oxytocin and dopamine are all implicated. These have implications for stress-alleviation, affect regulation, caregiving, proximity seeking and other attachment-related behaviours.

- Resilience and attachment style need further investigation, but Secure style is identified as resilient either as 'earned' through adult effort, or emerging from positive elements in negative childhoods. Change in adult attachment style also occurs for around 30% of individuals. Factors influencing positive change need to be identified to inform interventions.
- Attachment interventions show positive impact on attachment insecurity. There is some limited evidence that those with Anxious style do better with structured CBT style approaches, and those Avoidant with psychotherapeutic approaches. However, other aspects of functioning related to attachment insecurity, such as insensitive parenting and poor mentalising are also shown to benefit from tailored interventions and treatments.

1.13 Discussion

This chapter has outlined attachment theory, particularly from the point of view of adult attachment style, and summarised key aspects of attachment style which are used to organise the rest of the book. Various models were shown of attachment-related phenomenon, and biological, social and psychological elements are outlined. Attachment theory has always been an integrative theory, and the aim and challenge of the book is to explore and integrate a lifespan psychosocial approach with an emphasis on adult relationships and support.

However, childhood experience of adversity, including neglect and abuse will be a core aspect explaining the origins of adult attachment style. Depending on early life experiences, and previously laid down templates or working models around relationship expectations, attachment activation can lead to effective proximity seeking and supportive response for those with adaptive or Secure attachment styles. Less adaptive styles are Anxious styles with hyper-activation of the system and hyper-vigilance leading to excessive proximity seeking, but with little soothing response achieved. Alternatively, Avoidant styles with low expectation of support availability utilise 'shut down' attachment responses, with self-soothing behaviour and distancing from stressors.

In the models presented here in the overview of attachment theory most involve adversity or 'signs of threat' or life events to trigger attachment behaviour. Thus any model of attachment activation needs to take into account life stress both in early life and in adulthood. The biological model involves appraisals of threat together with activation of prior memory of both event-response and expected support, ultimately leading to the bodily responses of flight or proximity seeking. Psychological models outline differential proximity seeking or avoiding responses for affect-regulation from support figures. Social support is a source of 'soothing' as a means of regulating stress through proximity seeking in most models, but the stress model would also see it as an additional resource for positive coping input. The lifespan model extends the interplay of stress, support-seeking, self-esteem and coping from childhood to adulthood. Whilst these models all give different perspectives on the underpinning of adult attachment styles, all have themes in common. The aim of this book is to try and synthesise these further.

Secure, Anxious, Avoidant and Disorganised styles in early and later adulthood will be a core feature of the data presented and discussion in the book. Whilst not measured directly, affect-regulation and mentalising, will be referred to as explanatory mechanisms. Similarly while no data will be presented on biological correlates of insecure attachment behaviour or response to stress, these are introduced at different points as a reminder of the more extensive model. The next chapter will look at how attachment style in adulthood is defined and measured, with particular reference to the ASI.

2 Assessing attachment styles in adults

2.0 Introduction

Progress in adult attachment-based research has grown with the development of measures to reliably reflect the different categories of Secure, Insecure and Disorganised attachment proposed by attachment theory. Some of these measures have additionally moved across for use in services and interventions to aid family assessments. The onus of measurement, both in self-report questionnaires and interviews, has been to identify relationships between Insecure attachment categories and clinical status, self-esteem, support, and parenting as well as the intergenerational risks between parents and their children. The aim has been to verify the predictions made from attachment theory to add to our understanding of human behaviour. This chapter will first briefly outline some of the most prominent measures in the field, but then describe the ASI which will be the focus of the rest of the book, and provide case material to illustrate its attachment categories.

Adult attachment measures have emerged from two distinct research traditions: first, developmental/psychodynamic psychology with a focus on parenting and predicting intergenerational patterns of attachment quality, and, second, social psychology with an interest in personal adjustment, partner/support relationships and mental health risks (Fraley and Shaver 2000). Whilst the measures differ substantially on whether the focus is childhood reporting or ongoing support, whether interview or self-report, in dimensional or categorical systems, all have overlap of basic classification including Secure and varieties of Anxious and Avoidant attachment style, with the interviews also including apects of Disorganised style.

The methods divide into self-report questionnaires and narrative-style expert-rated interviews. Self-report questionnaires belong mostly to the social psychology tradition and assess adult perceptions of relationships (particularly romantic ones) or attitudes about others in general. The interviews include those aimed at tapping states of mind (including unconscious processes) that focus on current representations of childhood relationships with parents (George and West 1999) and the ASI which examines relationships with partner and other support figures and attitudes to closeness and autonomy.

2.1 Self-report attachment measures

The first measure historically is the Adult Attachment Questionnaire (Hazan and Shaver 1987) which has been widely used and adapted (Stein, Jacobs *et al.* 1998). This is a simple one-page format which uses brief vignettes to represent the summaries of Ainsworth's Secure, Anxious and Avoidant styles. The respondent rates each style as more or less like him or her, and then chooses the style which reflects his/her own style best overall. The Relationship Questionnaire has built on this, but with the addition of a Fearful vignette (Bartholomew and Horowitz 1991) and the very recent Clinical Version a Mistrustful vignette (Holmes and Lyons-Ruth 2006). The first two versions have been used extensively in survey studies of relationships, parenting and psychopathology. Their advantage lies in their simplicity, brevity and transparency.

Other questionnaires are dimensional, utilising Likert scales (giving a choice of items, for example from 'not at all like me' to 'very like me') of items reflecting issues around closeness or autonomy and scored around two factors denoting Approach/Avoidance, or in the case of the Vulnerable Attachment Style Questionnaire (VASQ) of Security/Insecurity and Approach/Avoidance. The Relationship Style Questionnaire (RSQ) (Bartholomew and Horowitz 1991) and the Vulnerable Attachment Style Questionnaire (VASQ) (Bifulco, Mahon *et al.* 2003) are used for any adolescent or adult, regardless of partner status and in relation to styles in general, whilst the Experiences in Close Relationships (ECR) (Brennan, Clark *et al.* 1998) was originally designed for partner relationships specifically. Other attachment questionnaires based on the partner relationship include the Adult Attachment Scale (Simpson 1990), and its revised version (Collins and Read 1990).

The advantages of all these self-report measures are those common to all questionnaires – their brevity, and having no requirement for training in administration. The disadvantages include reliance on self-report which assumes the respondents can report accurately on their attachment attitudes, a problem with insecurely attached adults. Inconsistent categorisation of style is a problem, but this holds for all adult attachment measures. Another problem is that Disorganised styles are not formally reflected.

Summary of Attachment style questionnaires

Categorical vignette style

Adult Attachment Questionnaire (AAQ) (Hazan and Shaver 1987). – Three vignettes representing Secure, Preoccupied and Dismissive. The overall style most like respondent is selected. Originally referred to partner relationship only. It has 70% stability test–retest.

Relationships Questionnaire (RQ) (Bartholomew and Horowitz 1991). As above but with additional style of Fearful. Each of the four vignettes is rated on 7-point scales as 'most like' the respondent, and overall 'most like' style selected.

RQ-Clinical Version (RQ-CV) (Holmes and Lyons-Ruth 2006). As above but additional vignette of severely mistrustful added for use in clinical samples.

Dimensional scales

Relationship Style Questionnaire (RSQ) (Bartholomew and Horowitz 1991). Thirty item, 5-point Likert scale regarding feelings about close relationships. Items denoting approach-avoidance in relationships. Scoring is dimensionals. Test–retest range 0.49–0.71.

Experiences in Close Relationships (ECR) (Brennan, Clark *et al.* 1998). Thirty-six item Likert scale of items derived from meta analysis of other scales and rated according to relationship with partner. Two scoring dimensions denoting Anxious and Avoidant attachment. Reliability in terms of internal consistency is good (alpha 0.91, 0.94).

Adult Attachment Scale (Simpson 1990). Thirteen statements on 7-point Likert scale regarding feelings towards romantic partners. (Revised version seventeen items). Alphas range from 0.42–0.79. Test–retest not available.

Vulnerable Attachment Style Questionnaire (VASQ) (Bifulco, Mahon *et al.* 2003). Twenty-two item 5-point Likert scale of items derived from ASI interview, two factors denoting insecurity and approach-avoidance in relationships. Reliability alpha=0.82 and 0.67, test–retest 0.73 and 0.65. Sensitivity 70% and specificity 67% against the ASI Interview. Correlation with RQ r=0.53 and 0.43 for each factor.

2.2 The Adult Attachment Interview and related tools

The AAI (George, Kaplan *et al.* 1984; George and West 1999) is probably the best known of the research interviews. It is a face-to-face semi-structured, recorded interview which questions about childhood experience, transcribed for evidence of coherence, idealisation and denigration in reporting. From this, four basic styles are derived each with subcategories: Secure, Preoccupied (Anxious[1]), Dismissive (Avoidant) and Unresolved or 'Can't Classify' (Disorganised) (Main and Solomon 1986). This psychodynamic interview was devised with the aim of unmasking defences associated with the individual's overall state of mind in relation to their reports of childhood experiences of parental care. It seeks to identify security in adulthood in terms of the respondent's ability to speak clearly about their early life experiences of attachment, their ability to acknowledge the influence of attachment-related experiences and support the choice of adjectives to describe parental relationships with matching memories of specific events (Hesse 2008). It shows good inter-rater reliability (75%–100%) although only after extensive training and has good test–retest over 12 months (77% stability). Its validity in parent studies has largely been tested in relation to concordance with the infants' categorisation in child attachment measures such as the SST (Ainsworth, Blehar *et al.* 1978).

The AAI has provided an important catalyst for the expansion of attachment-based research. Its use of an investigator-based approach (distinct from self-report) allows for subtle categorisations of individuals' reporting, to reveal responses linked directly to their internal working models of attachment, through their representations of parental behaviour in childhood. However, its complex scoring system and high level of approved-rater qualification make it amenable only to key experts and virtually inaccessible for use by most mental health and social work practitioners. Also, its reliance on tapping into unconscious processes makes it difficult to provide transparent feedback to clients. Its use in research has, however, contributed important insights into many aspects of attachment behaviour in adults. In addition, the Self-Reflective Function measure for mentalising capacity is an important offshoot from this interview (Fonagy and Target 1997).

Another variation of the AAI is the Adult Attachment Interview Revised (Crittenden 1988) which uses a different categorisation of attachment style and is argued to be somewhat easier to score. This version utilises further interview questions concerning mildly threatening experiences in childhood to access procedural, imagined, semantic and episodic working memory around the issues of protection and danger. A social-ecological approach is incorporated that stresses the contribution and effect of culture on the organisation and function of the individual's attachment in relation to danger. The approach has leaned much more towards measuring attachment in high-risk and child-protection contexts.

Other interviews include the Current Relationship Interview (Crowell 1996) which is designed to investigate the nature of attachment relationships in adult partnerships. Its scoring also relies on patterns of adult discourse used for describing mentally represented attachment in romantic relationships. The focus of the assessment is on the individual's state of mind regarding romantic relationships. Three major classifications of Secure, Preoccupied and Dismissing are identified on the basis of verbalised statements and descriptions of the represented relationship with partner, own behaviour and extent to which attachments are valued with the Dismissing and Preoccupied categories both denoting insecurity. Whilst this approach belongs to the more psychodynamic rather than social tradition, it remains a potential bridge between the two.

2.2.1 Comparison of measures

Comparisons between different attachment measures show significant but modest correlations between questionnaires, or between questionnaires and interviews (Bartholomew and Shaver 1998; Stein, Jacobs *et al.* 1998; Bifulco, Mahon *et al.* 2003; Guedeney, Fermian *et al.* 2009). One of the problems about comparison is that most use somewhat different categories of attachment style, or use categorical rather than dimensional scores to yield attachment insecurity scores. It is likely that measures reflect Secure style fairly consistently, the problem arises in differentiating categories of Insecure style. This means that research has at times reflected the Secure versus Insecure dichotomy with positive results, but this loses the main underpinning of attachment theory around the different attachment strategies arising from problematic childhood experience linked to different vulnerability profiles and different disorder outcomes. To date there is no published study comparing the AAI and ASI as described below.

2.3 The Attachment Style Interview

This interview takes a social approach to measuring attachment style, by incorporating accounts of ongoing relationships with partners, family and friends and those named as 'Very Close' and asking about attitudes towards autonomy, closeness/distance, fear or anger in relationships. The questions about ongoing relationships and attitudes are scored in sections, each summarised to build to an overall profile which gives both the degree of insecurity (marked, moderate or mild) and the type of style Enmeshed or Fearful (Anxious) or Angry–dismissive or Withdrawn (Avoidant), in addition to Secure. Dual/disorganised style is denoted by the presence of two or more simultaneous Insecure styles. The inter-rater reliability of the measure is good with 0.80 for the overall scale and an average 0.75 for subscales, and this has been replicated in studies in continental Europe and Japan. Validity is also good as tested in terms of prediction of onset of major depression prospectively and as mediator for childhood neglect/abuse and disorder described in later sections.

Originally based on measures of partner relationship and close other support to identify risk and resilience for adult depression, the ASI extended these to encompass the attitudes which correspond to different styles identified in attachment theory. It is a semi-structured 60–90 minute interview which uses open probing questions to elicit full context and content of experience, after which the interviewer-estimated ratings are made according to benchmarked thresholds. Scoring is made on the basis of listening back to the interview recording, and selecting key comments for justifying ratings. Scoring typically uses 4-point scales to determine characteristics in three relationships reported as close (including confiding, emotional support, positive and negative interaction and felt attachment). Overall summary scales rate the quality of each of these relationships on 7 points from 'very close' confiding support, through 'good–average', to 'insufficient' and 'inadequate' support. These are also differentiated by whether the relationship is discordant or not. Key areas related to functioning are assessed, including 'Ability to make and maintain relationships' (which summarises the support capacity) as well as core attachment attitudes denoting Avoidance (mistrust, constraints on closeness, high self-reliance, low desire for company and anger) or Anxious (fear of rejection, low self-reliance, high desire for company and fear of separation). From these scales profiles can be reliably produced to reflect the different types of Secure, Insecure or Dual/disorganised styles.

2.3.1 Case example: Secure attachment style

Before describing the ASI in detail, a case study of a woman from the London studies rated Secure will illustrate the information collected. This is the most common attachment style in most measurement systems, is the most adaptive and resilient and is associated with better relationships, self-esteem, coping with stress, childhood experience and mental health in the various measurement approaches.

2.3.1.1 Secure Susan

Susan is a 26-year-old woman living with her long-term partner James. Both she and her partner work. She named three VCOs in whom she confides, and she has regular and positive contact with her family of origin. Susan is the eldest of four children and one of her sisters died as a young adult. She did have some difficulties in childhood (her mother was very critical, her father had a drink problem and was absent for part of her childhood) but this does not appear to have influenced her current relating style. She currently has positive interactions with her mother and siblings (closeness was rated 'moderate' and antipathy 'little/none'), and harbours no resentment about childhood.

Susan described confiding in her partner James: *'I can confide in him about anything. For the first few years we were together he just couldn't understand the problems I had with my family. He didn't really understand the deep emotions that are involved, because he never had experienced it himself. Now he does, and I can now talk to him very easily about anything, and he really does know how I feel. He knows everything about me and I've told him things I wouldn't tell anybody else. He's helped me through all the crises – the money problems, my health difficulties and when my sister died. He has been very supportive over me looking for another job.* James gives good emotional support: *'He's a good listener and always sympathetic'.* Their time together is positive: *'We do have interests in common and spend a lot of time together. We have lots of joint friends as well. We are involved with each other. We do argue occasionally – the flat is small and very claustrophobic, so we can get under each other's feet. But it tends to be forgotten quickly, and does not get heated. It becomes clear if there is a problem to deal with and then we tend to both be practical'.* She had strong felt attachment: *'He's reliable. I would feel lost without him. We're terribly, terribly close. If he wasn't there I would be quite lost. The relationship gets better all the time. He's had to live through the problems I've been having. We've both gone through things together and it's made us closer'.* Thus her partner relationship provides support and positive interaction and felt attachment was rated 'very high' on overall quality.

Susan selected two friends as VCOs: Jane from her university days, and Liz, who she works with. She felt close to both and could confide openly. About Jane she said: *'We've always been able to talk to each other about most things. There have been a number of times over the years where I've gone to her with practical problems for example my health issues, money problems, but also when my sister died. She was always there for me. She is always sympathetic. I think I would really miss her if we lost touch for any reason'.* (Rated 'very high' on quality of support). About her work friend Liz she says: *'We get on really well and since I see her most days, I do find I tell her things which are worrying me. I don't think I tell her as much as Jane, but if I had a worry I would tell her I think. I've talked to her a lot about my work problems and talked through my application for a new job. She was really helpful. She tends to know the right thing to say.'* (Rated 'good average, no discord' on quality of support).

On the basis of having three close confiding relationships, Susan was rated as having 'marked' ability to make and maintain relationships.

Susan was then asked about various attitudes to attachment. She described being trusting: *'I think most people can be trusted. I am not suspicious of people. Although some may be out for themselves, there is a lot of kindness in the world. I would say I can trust the people close to me.'* She does not find it very hard to get close to people and feels it is important to have someone close: *'having James is very important, and having my close friends also helps me a lot. I don't think having family close is particularly important. I think as you grow older you find your own people to love.'* She has no anxiety about getting close and no fears about being let down. *'I think everyone gets let down from time to time, but you can't live your life as though everyone will let you down. I have some very dependable people in my life, they would never let me down. If you find the right people, you can usually feel safe with them.'*

When asked about her self-reliance, she described being able to make decisions without others' help although *'sometimes it's a great help to be able to talk to somebody else.'* It is important to feel she has control over her life. *'I feel impatient and frustrated if things don't go the way I want them to'.* However, she can ask others for advice and values their help. When asked about her need for company, she explained that she enjoys meeting new people and can initiate new friendships, but doesn't want to be with friends all the time: *'It's nice to separate and then come back and compare notes at the end of the day.'* Susan was then asked if she felt anxious when those close to her were away for brief periods: *'Occasionally James goes away for the weekend for work reasons. That doesn't bother me. He will call when he gets there, but I don't feel I have to keep calling him. I am quite independent that way.'* Susan has no difficulties in saying goodbye to others: *'I am not one of those people who gets tearful at brief goodbyes. I know I can always get in touch with my friends when they go away. I don't usually expect any catastrophes!'* Finally, when asked about anger or conflict in her relationships, she expressed no resentments, even about her childhood: *'I think you just have to move on in life. I think I can now understand why my parents behaved as they did when I was young. But there's no point in holding a grudge. It just makes you more miserable.'* She does not have any arguments, fights or feuds with her partner, family or friends.

On the basis of this information Susan was considered to have a Secure attachment style. She has close relationships and can access support. She has a good level of autonomy in managing her life, and has a similar balance in her contact with close others. She had no fear of rejection, or of separation. Neither was she angry with the people around her. Therefore she had neither Avoidance nor Anxious elements in her view of other people or her behaviour in relationships. Her reporting style was clear and factual, with an understanding of her own psychological needs and those of others around her.

The information in this case study, shows what is covered in the ASI, and the type of responses expected if a person is exhibiting Secure attachment style. The next section will go through the ASI in detail explaining the questions asked and the scoring.

2.3.2 The Attachment Style Interview – Support

The demographic section includes basic background information about current relationships, assessments of closeness or antipathy with family of origin as well as a checklist of recent life events (Recent Life Events Questionnaire (RLEQ) (Brugha and Cragg 1990). The purpose of including the events is not only to place the ASI in line with a stress model (where the purpose of close attachments is to provide support at times of crises) but also a more pragmatic function of outlining recent severe events in order to aid confiding questions, and grounding these in actual recent examples. The section on partner and VCO follow with similar questions about confiding and support, quality of interaction and felt attachment. These are outlined below.

Summary of Attachment Style Interview Support scales

(All scales rated 1-Marked, 2-Moderate, 3-Some, 4-Little/None: 1 or 2 considered 'high')

Closeness to family of origin: Feelings of attachment, affection or pleasurable contact rated for mother, father (or substitute parents) and siblings.

Antipathy to family of origin: Feelings of anger, resentment, arguments or conflict rated for mother, father (or substitute parents) and siblings.

Support members: For (i) partner, (ii) first VCO, (iii) second VCO and (iv – if no partner, third VCO). VCOs can be family members or friends, excluding others under age 18.

Confiding: The extent to which the interviewee is able to talk to partner about personal feelings, crises and emotionally charged topics. Supporting evidence of examples of recent confiding required.

Active emotional support: The extent to which the partner has responded to confidences, strong personal feelings and/or crises in a sympathetic, helpful and understanding way. The rating is made on the basis of the frequency and strength of such supportive behaviour. Negative response will reduce the rating.

Positive interaction: The extent to which time spent together and enjoyment of joint activities is characterised by a positive tone. Intensity and pervasiveness of tone are taken into account.

Negative interaction/discord: The extent to which time spent together, including tension, rows, quarrelling or more-intense conflict is characterised by a negative tone. Intensity and pervasiveness of tone are taken into account.

Felt attachment: The extent to which the simple existence of the partner provides a particular kind of emotional reassurance for the interviewee in terms of a feeling of inner security and safety. Denotes an emotional dependency and bond with partner.

Overall quality of relationship (scale 1–7): summary of above scales (1 or 2 is high and 3 or 4 is low) to denote – **Good support:** very good (1) to good average, (2) with discord and (3) without. **Poor support:** insufficient support (4 with discord and 5 without discord) or inadequate support (6 with discord or 7 without). Two or more close support figures needed for Secure/mildly Insecure rating.

2.3.3 The Attachment Style Interview – Attachment Attitudes

The attachment attitudes are outlined below. High ratings are based on both the intensity of feeling (e.g. 'I absolutely hate my family') or generalisation ('there is absolutely nobody that I can trust'). Whilst most scales are uni-directional, self-reliance and desire for company, both have the middle point as most adaptive, with high and low denoting extremes of over autonomy or under autonomy. These scales also include a contradictory point for individuals who vacillate in describing themselves first in one way, then another.

Summary of Attachment Style Interview Attachment Attitudes

(Rated 1-Marked, 2-Moderate, 3-Some, 4-Little/None unless stated otherwise. 1 or 2 is summarised as 'high')

Mistrust: The extent to which lack of trust in people close, as well as in outsiders, and suspicion of others' motives and behaviour is present. Intensity of attitude and generalization to range of others determines the level. May include either angry or fearful components.

Constraints on closeness: The existence of attitudinal blockages inhibiting the development or maintenance of close confiding relationships and care eliciting. Barriers within the individual to achieving closeness and seeking help.

Fear of rejection: The extent to which constraints on closeness are based on fear of getting close, specifically on fears of rejection or being let down. Discomfort is rated at the lower levels, and generalisation to a wide range of others at the higher levels. Feelings of anxiety, rather than intolerance and irritation at closeness, with specific expectations of rejection determine this rating.

Self-reliance: The extent to which the interviewee feels able to cope well on his/her own, values his/her independence and whether dependent on others for practical and emotional help. Scaling here is different: a high rating (1) denotes over-self-reliance and low dependency. A low rating (3) denotes dependency and too little self-reliance. '2: Moderate/Average' is the midway, Secure rating. Occasionally 4-contradictory can be rated when the description veers between 1 and 3.

Desire for company: The extent to which the interviewee likes/needs to have a high degree of contact with close others; has high dependency on others; and likes/needs a high level of companionship. Scaling here is as for self-reliance: a high rating (1) denotes excessively frequent contact with others, whereas a low rating (3) indicates avoidance of social situations. '2: Moderate/Average' is the midway,

---

Secure rating. Occasionally 4-contradictory can be rated when description veers between 1 and 3.

Fear of separation: The extent to which there is distress at temporary separations from close others. The interviewee may fear being abandoned and losing people close to him/her. Fears of being alone, anxious searching behaviour when others are later than expected are taken into account and a high rating is given when concern for own safety/protection or that of the close other is expressed.

Anger: The extent to which the interviewee feels hostile, resentful, or jealous of others close to him/her, including parents and siblings, partners, children, VCO/confidants and other friends, is rated. This may also include resentment about the past. Negative interaction ratings and whether these emanate mainly from the respondent are taken into account. A high rating can be made even if the anger is present but not easily expressed to the persons concerned. If the anger is entirely provoked then it is rated lower than if it is an over-reaction to some minor slight.

2.3.4 Attachment Style Interview Overall attachment styles

The information collected from both the support and attachment attitude scales is combined into an overall attachment style categorisation. Rules for how to combine these scales are provided. However, as well as recognising the particular style from the patterning of attachment scales, the rating also requires a scoring of the intensity of the insecurity so that each Insecure style can be rated at 'marked', 'moderate' or 'mild' levels. The basis for this is the support summary and judgement about 'ability to make and maintain relationships'. Where there is only one, or no close confidant then 'moderate' or 'marked' insecurity of style will be rated respectively. Where there is 'moderately good' ability to relate but there is evidence of a profile on the different attachment scales, then a 'mildly' Insecure style is rated. Later analyses will show that those mildly Insecure belong in the Secure range, and have low rates of disorder and psychosocial risk, similar to those termed 'Clearly Secure'. The summary below provides a description of each attachment profile.

Summary of Attachment Style Interview attachment styles

Clearly Secure: (Lack of negative attitudes, good relationships)

This is the most stable and flexible style with a lack of negative attitudes denoting either Anxious or Avoidant attachment. There is comfort with closeness and appropriate levels of autonomy. There will always be 'good' ('marked or moderate') ability to make and maintain relationships and evidence of good support.

Anxious attachment styles

Enmeshed: (High fear of separation)

This is a dependent attachment style as exhibited by high desire for company, and low self-reliance and high fear of separation. These individuals tend to have fairly superficial relationships and despite a high number of social contacts may have few which are objectively close. Anger is sometimes present, denoting the ambivalence often associated with this style.

Fearful: (High fear of rejection)

This attachment style has fears of being rejected or let down which is generalised to others. This may relate to actual experiences of having been let down which have generalised to fear of future interactions. There is often a desire to get close to others, together with fear of doing so which can lead to loneliness. Fearful style will always have '1: Marked' or '2: Moderate' on fear of rejection, and is the only style that rates high on this scale. Anger is absent. Mistrust and constraints on closeness present.

Avoidant attachment styles

Angry-dismissive: (High mistrust and anger)

This style is characterised by high mistrust, high self-reliance and low desire for company. Its key characteristic is high anger. Individuals with this style usually need a high level of control over their lives, are extremely self-reliant and typically are in conflict with those around them. This is often reflected in individual negative interactions with close others and family as well as in feelings of anger and resentment about the past.

Withdrawn: (High self-reliance)

This is a detached style characterised by high self-reliance, high constraints on closeness and low desire for company. This is often expressed as desire for privacy and clear boundaries with regard to others. However, there is neither fear nor anger expressed. It can appear as very practical, rational and non-emotional style.

Anxious and Avoidant style

Dual/disorganised Insecure: This dual attachment classification is only considered for those rated 'markedly' or 'moderately' Insecure; it has no

Secure counterpart. It reflects those individuals who are unable to relate to others and for whom no single clear style can be determined from the subscales rated. Both 'primary' and 'subsidiary' attachment styles are rated with precedence given to the more pervasive style which affects wider relationships. An example of dual rating is when a high degree of both anger and fear in relationships fulfil both Angry-dismissive and either Fearful or Enmeshed types. Enmeshed and Fearful can also be included and unusually Enmeshed and Withdrawn. The autonomy scales (self-reliance and desire for company) may be rated as 'contradictory' to show the pull in both Anxious and Avoidant directions.

2.4 Case examples

Examples of each Insecure style will be given here, pointing out the key characteristics which contribute to the categorisations. These examples are all taken from the London study of adult women. Styles for men are rated in exactly the same way, and examples from males are provided in subsequent chapters. (See appendix for summary of all case examples used).

2.4.2 Ellie's Moderately Enmeshed style

Ellie is a 40-year-old single parent, of mixed heritage (English/West Indian) who lives alone with her children, and a previous partner's teenage child. She works as a typist and is holding down two jobs due to financial hardship but recently lost the second evening job. She was divorced from her second husband Graham two years ago, her youngest child age 13 is Graham's child and his daughter (aged 19) by another woman also lives with Ellie. Her older son is from her first husband. She was divorced from Graham because of his extreme unreliability, violence, criminal behaviour and extra-marital affairs; however, she is in contact with him and he is trying to regain close contact phoning her three times a day and sending her red roses. She views this as 'courting' behaviour and maintains there is a nice side to his personality. She has a new boyfriend, Lester, 10 years younger, who she described as close but is not cohabiting. In terms of family of origin, Ellie's mother died when she was aged 15, and she does not have contact with her father. She has an older sister, but is not close (closeness rated 'some', antipathy rated 'some'). She describes herself as very close to a number of friends and confides readily. Her events and difficulties include those financial which increased when she lost her second job, and her son lost his job. She also helps support Lester. Lester was recently charged with criminal damage, and Ellie accompanied him to court. She also has problems with her ex-husband Graham who is very unreliable about contact with the children and he has taken money from her for the children's holiday but then spent it on himself.

Ellie's support: Ellie does not confide in Lester. She likes his company because he is young and good looking, and she feels flattered by his interest in her. Whilst she says she can talk about '*everything and anything*' in fact she has not told him about her problems with Graham, and does not tell him the extent of her financial difficulties. Their interaction is good, although she finds he can be a bit demanding. She does not describe herself as being very close since they have only recently met. The relationship was rated as 'insufficient support, no discord'.

She named two VCOs who were close friends, Tricia from work and Angela to whom she mainly talks on the phone. She can talk to Tricia about her exhusband and says she can tell her most things. Whilst she was vague on detail, her confiding about her ex-husband and about her money difficulties was considered sufficient for a 'moderate' confiding rating. Tricia is described as very sympathetic and supportive. She will take Ellie's side and is a good listener. She feels close to Tricia and they do not have arguments or rows. This was rated as 'good–average' supportive relationship, with no discord.

There is less closeness and confiding in Angela: '*I haven't told her about this new relationship – I don't think she would be very pleased to hear about it. I would talk to her about problems but I would probably have spoken to somebody else and got a different view point before I ended up telling her. If I share a weighty problem with her she stops thinking about her own problems. I give it to her gladly because I know it brings her out of herself.*' However there was a problem in the relationship due to Angela's illness which Ellie thinks is imagined: '*I want to dissociate myself from her because I do not agree totally with why she is ill – I think she is a malingerer, but I still keep up with her because her other friends have all left her. But I would not miss her if she moved away, I would keep contact by telephone.*' This relationship was rated as 'insufficient' support, with no discord.

Thus Ellie effectively only has one close support figure (Tricia) and so was rated as having 'some' ability to make and maintain relationships which meant her attachment style was rated as 'moderately' Insecure.

Ellie's Enmeshed attachment attitudes: Ellie was not mistrustful but did describe starting new relationships as difficult. About her new boyfriend she says: '*I would like it to go well, I mean it's quite novel to me after two years on my own, but I think it's horrible getting to know somebody. I really hate it, it's diabolical. It's hard. But I think it's worth it because if you're a natural person then it's natural to be with somebody of the opposite sex. I do like to be in a relationship. I've come out of a bad relationship and I feel I'm totally in equilibrium now, and I can start something new and I can give an enormous amount. That is not because of what I've been through in the past, that is because I want to do that now, and if whoever I'm with doesn't respond to that, and share in that and give me back, then I don't think it would be a nice, equal sharing relationship.*' (Mistrust rated 'some').

Ellie had few constraints on getting close (rated 'little/none'): *'I'm not shy to talk to people about something that may be affecting me deeply. It may be the wrong person to talk to – but it invariably isn't because you get a view point. I was totally satisfied before I met a man, but that opens up a whole sphere, and of course I'm dissatisfied now because I've got to go through this awful process of getting to know him. It's important to have friends, because I'm very nosey, I'm very inquisitive, I love a good laugh and if you haven't got friends... you can't do that.'* Her self-reliance was rated 'low': *'I do find it hard to make decisions alone, I find I need to ask a lot of people before I can decide what to do. I don't really feel in control of my life.'* Her desire for company was rated 'high': She will not 'let go' of the relationship with her ex-husband and phones Angela daily: *'I believe in closeness with my friends, as well as the children. I'd say all my friends, all of them. I like them all.'* About Angela *'I can't turn my back on her, but I feel in a trap because I don't feel sympathy and then I'll just have to say to her, you've got to pull yourself together, you've got to try and do something.'* Her fear of separation was however moderately high: She is unable to break free of her relationship with her ex-husband – she does encourage him to keep in contact, and is unable to break off contact with her friend Angela. *'I hate it when people leave me – I can't bear being on my own.'* (Fear of separation rated 'moderate'). She was rated as only 'some' level of anger. She says: *'I'm very bolshy, very blunt. People think I'm quite severe until they get to know me. But I am not one to harbour resentments.'* In terms of her childhood relationships she feels that her parents did not do enough for her, and wishes her sister would help her out more. However, she also describes her childhood as 'happy' and does not have any arguments or rows with family.

Comment: Ellie shows typical features of Enmeshed style: she has a high need for closeness to others, a high fear of separation but little mistrust or constraint on closeness. She does not have high anger, but many with Enmeshed style will also have the anger often expressed as 'anxious-ambivalence'. She is rated at 'moderate' levels of the style because she does have one close support figure and because her attitudes are not at the highest extreme of Enmeshed style, for example, her fear of separation was 'moderately' rather than 'markedly' high. Her major depression and life-time adversity and coping is described in Chapter 3 as well and her partner relationships in Chapter 4. Ellie's reporting style was very full – she was talkative and lively in her descriptions. However, she was also contradictory at times and did not follow a logical course in all her answers.

2.4.3 Fiona's moderately Fearful style

Fiona is a 43-year-old married woman with four children. Her two oldest children have now left home leaving her son aged 16 and a daughter aged 7 at home. Fiona works full-time as a deputy in a day nursery where she has been employed two years. She is committed to working and she enjoys her job. Her husband Terry does shift work in the film business and often works nights. Fiona reports that because of this they do not often have time together. In terms of events and difficulties: Fiona's sister Jane who she is close to, was diagnosed as having thyroid cancer. In addition, Fiona has recently heard that she is going to lose her job as the nursery will close in a few months. She has not been offered any redundancy pay but she will be offered another job at the same salary. In terms of her family relationships: she remains close to her sister. Whilst in infrequent contact with her parents she is not close given adverse childhood experience (closeness: 'some', antipathy 'some').

Fiona's support: Fiona reports that she and her husband do not have much time to see each other and talk as her husband works nights. She does not confide much in him: *'Any decisions I want to make, that's up to me – it's what I want to do, not his concern, so I won't always discuss it. I don't talk to him about my work. I might say I've had a bad day, but that's all.'* Her husband was supportive of Fiona when she was on strike. *'He worked as much overtime as he could to in order to support us. When I don't tell him things until a long time later, he will say "why didn't you tell me, keeping that to yourself?"'* She did not tell him immediately about Jane's cancer. This is because she did not want to think about it and get emotional and *'there wasn't anything he could do.'* She described their interaction: *'I suppose we get on, we share things, talk to each other. We don't argue about money or anything like that.'* When asked what makes them irritable with each other, she said: *'Well, if he asks me to do something and I've already got enough to do then I do get annoyed.'* They do row at times: *'Sometimes. He's got a quick temper. I suppose it's because I don't always answer him. I'm in a bit of a world of my own. I'm not very responsive and I think that annoys him.'* They get irritable once or twice a week and have a blazing row from time to time *'my husband has got a temper'*. Fiona recognises she has been more irritable recently, feeling stressed. She complains: *'he works nights and we don't have that much time together'*. She can rely on him however, and he has never let her down. *'He is dependable about money, he gives me all of his wages including any overtime he's done.'* She mainly relies on him for: *'money, but I don't think I rely on him a lot really'*. What keeps you in the relationship? *'I think that we must think a lot of each other.'* What would you miss most? *'His company really.'* The overall relationship was rated as 'insufficient support, with discord'.

Fiona has one confidant, her friend Martha, who she confided in about her sister's cancer, which is a great worry to her, as well as about losing her job. Martha is supportive and a good listener and will offer advice. However, Fiona does not feel very close to Martha: *'she has been a good friend, but if she moved away, I suppose I would find someone else. It's not like family'*. (The relationship was rated as 'good–average support, no discord). Her other VCO, her sister Jane has recently been diagnosed with cancer. Fiona reports that she feels guilty that she was not there with her sister when the results came through. '*I feel guilty that she has the cancer not me, when I'm the older sister.*' She sees her sister and offers support but does not confide in her '*she has enough problems of her own. I wouldn't want to burden her.*' (The relationship rated 'insufficient support, no discord).

Given only one effective support figure, Fiona was rated 'some' on ability to make and maintain relationships and therefore moderately Insecure attachment style.

Fiona's Fearful attachment attitudes: She reported 'moderately' high mistrust: '*It's not trust... I just think I'm not a person to open up, it might be trust though. I don't know, deep down, I might have had experiences before where I've really trusted somebody and been let down. I think when you get older you hear people saying so-and-so and you think, "Oh God, I hope they aren't spreading my business around."*' She also had 'moderately' high constraints on closeness: '*I know I keep too much to myself, and find it difficult to share problems.*' She finds getting close difficult: '*I'm really shy and I think sometimes I talk too much through being nervous. Going into a new room... I really hate it.*' She had 'moderate fear of rejection', and when asked if she was afraid of being let down she said: '*I suppose underneath I am afraid of being let down. That if people knew the sort of person I was, they wouldn't like me. They would make fun of my worries, and laugh behind my back. It does stop me getting close.*'

She describes being let down by her parents in her childhood and recognises this has made her reluctant to get close. '*I think too much of the burden was on me. I had to be mother to the others.*' She does however like having other people around '*I'm not alone that much. I'm not really alone. I suppose for long periods alone I would hate it. But sometimes when I am alone it's heaven.*' She likes to cope on her own when she can '*I think I'm quite independent. But I can also ask my husband for help. He is reliable.*' She feels others rely on her: '*I'm like the eldest in my family, if anything happens they (siblings) come to me. I'm like their mother figure. I think I cope alright*'. (Self-reliance: moderate/average.) She did not have any fear of separation '*I have no problem with people being away – I know I will see them when they come back*', and low levels of anger (rated 'some'): '*I suppose I sometimes get into arguments, but I don't like to argue and avoid it when I can.*'

Comment: Fiona's attachment style was rated as Moderately Fearful with the key characteristic of fear of rejection, and this linked with mistrust and constraints on closeness. Since she does have some capacity for making relationships, and because her negative attitudes were not very extreme she was rated in the 'moderate' rather than 'marked' range. It can be seen that the anxious elements revolve around worrying that people have a negative view of her and will let her down, dislike her or reject her, but other features such as mistrust and constraints involve avoidant characteristics. However, she does not have the high levels of self-reliance, or low desire for company of the more avoidant styles. Her reporting style was straightforward, although reference to childhood difficulties and worry about her sister were minimised and stated quite briefly. Fiona will be described in more detail in Chapter 3 in relation to her stress, coping and disorder.

2.4.4 Alexa's markedly Angry dismissive style

Alexa is aged 32, of African-Caribbean background, having been born in Jamaica. She lives with her two young children aged two and six months in social housing. She is not working. She has had two previous cohabiting partners and her children are fathered by her current partner from Zimbabwe, who does not live with her. She knew from fairly early on in the relationship that her partner was living with another woman. When she found out he was about to marry someone else three years ago, she became pregnant just prior to the break-up. They came to an understanding that Alexa would have the child and, so that it wouldn't be an only child, she would have another by him at some future time. This had now happened and, although their relationship is an unconventional one and he gives her no financial support, they have maintained consistent contact and he sees the children every week. She went to Zimbabwe to meet his family recently, because she felt they should be involved in the children's lives, but does not keep in regular contact with them. Her relationship with her mother is very poor – she is still emotionally dependent, but also very hostile at her bad treatment in childhood. And they argue frequently (closeness: 'some', antipathy: 'marked').

In terms of her recent life events and difficulties, Alexa has financial problems and an ongoing difficulty of conflict with her mother. The relationship with her non-live-in partner also causes difficulties because of his other wife and family. Alexa was born into a large family of whom she is only in touch with one sister, Dana, but is not close. Her family life in childhood was very adverse and unhappy.

Alexa's support: She has no supportive relationships. Her relationship with her boyfriend is non-confiding. There is much conflict and little closeness. She says '*We had a good relationship to start with but I didn't want to live with him, or anybody else for that matter. He's very withdrawn, very self-centred, not selfish exactly, but self-reliant, self-contained, like I am. The relationship is very "off" rather than "on" at the moment. We had sex first time round three years ago and I got pregnant. At the beginning we had a brilliant relationship – really very good. I was always at his place, and he'd be here as well. We get on well. When we do argue, I shout – I'll be quick to shout, he'll just keep quiet.*' They argue once or twice a month. (Relationship rated 'inadequate support with discord').

She described having some friends, but could not name even one who was close, and none confiding. She was very taken up with the children and ruminated a lot about her mother and her past. With no close support figures, she was rated very low ('little/no') on ability to make and maintain relationships. This means her attachment style is 'markedly' Insecure.

Alexa's Angry-dismissive attachment attitudes: She was rated 'marked' on mistrust she said: '*I'll let people be close to me but I find it had to be close to them. I've not known really what it is to trust. I wouldn't say I had ever trusted anyone.*' She also had 'marked' constraints on closeness, consistent with the fact she had no close relationships at all. When talking about her partner she said: '*the truth is, it's the best I could manage as a relationship. The alternative would have to be a very strong man – more controlling towards me, but I'd resist it.*' She found it difficult to ask for help: '*I don't think I'd feel as apprehensive now about saying to a social worker "it's too much, I need a break . . . can I talk with you?"*' (But she has not done this).

She did not describe any fear of rejection, claiming she did not get close enough to get let down. She has 'high' self-reliance: '*I realised in adolescence and early years that I was on my own – doing things for myself. I was very self-sufficient I am self-contained. I'm happy to be a parent but I keep a distance. I hope my daughter grows out of me.*' She also had 'low' desire for company: '*I don't want to live with anybody unless there's a lot of space, I think it's claustrophobic. I feel I need space.*' Her partner is the same. '*We nudge each other and call it a relationship . . . we can do that because we're so self contained, we don't actually give very much of ourselves. I don't mind sharing my space . . . my mental privacy is very important – very. I'm a bit aloof and distant – but only on a very personal level. I am very friendly generally with people I meet.*' She was rated as 'marked' on anger. She described her anger towards her mother: '*I still can't forgive my mother for how she treated me. I get angry when we meet up, and we often row. I suppose the expression is that I haven't let go . . . I spent so many years when my needs weren't met and the implications have been very far reaching. The reality is that there is a point beyond which you can't return to your mother. As a child I didn't even know what it was to be needy. I still feel very angry about it. I'm reminded of it each time I see her.*' She also felt angry towards her partner's wife: '*she makes it difficult for him to come here, she's jealous of me and the children.*' She also had some anger towards her partner's family in Zimbabwe – '*They didn't really accept me. Didn't welcome me and the children when we went there.*'

Comment: Alexa has the combination of high mistrust and self-reliance which denotes Avoidant attachment style, but with high anger levels being denigrating and dismissive of others. She acknowledges her self-reliance, her inability to make good relationships and her anger levels. She even hopes that her child soon learns to stop needing her. She has selected a partner who cannot spend much time with her, but has another family, and seems detached. She resents this but also semi-acknowledges that the distance it creates in the relationship is all she can manage. She does, however, feel slighted by his wife and family. The characteristic feature is the high need for control and self-reliance, coupled with an angry denigration of others. Alexa's life events, coping and disorder is revisited in Chapter 3.

2.4.5 Whitney's moderately Withdrawn style

Whitney is a 45-year-old woman living with her husband Tony and their six-year-old son Simon. Whitney works as a nurse part-time, being available for her son after school. She trained as a nurse after leaving school and remained single and unattached until she married in her 30s, having her only son when she was aged 37. Her life events include her husband's drink problem as well as his physical health difficulties (he has been spitting up blood, but they do not yet have a diagnosis). She has tried to persuade him to get professional help but he refuses. The other difficulty is with their housing as their flat is too small and they cannot afford to move. Recently their water tank burst and caused water damage while they were away. Whitney is also having problems with her son who has speech difficulties and is falling behind with his school work. This also leads to displays of temper.

Whitney has regular contact with her mother, her father died a few years ago. She does not feel particularly close to her mother who she finds distant and unsupportive, (rated 'some' closeness) but they do not have any conflict with her ('little/no' antipathy). During childhood her parents were not close and her father was a disciplinarian and would hit her. Her mother was passive and did not protect her. She was close to her aunt in childhood, and retains more closeness to her ('moderate') and has no antipathy ('little/none'). She has one brother who she sees a few times a year but does not feel very close ('some') but to whom she has no hostility (antipathy rated 'little/none').

Whitney's support: When asked about confiding in her partner she says: *'No we don't talk very much. But he tends to talk a lot and he'll just go on and on and on. He doesn't listen very well. I tend to be the one who has to listen to him and I find that quite hard going sometimes. I have to pretend not to worry about our son so Tony doesn't know. I just don't tell him things that I think about because I know it will prey on his mind. I can't confide about my son, because he just gets too worried.'* In terms of closeness: *'I suppose my husband took over where my auntie left off. Well, yes I am, obviously, yes, very close . . . I am, yes and no, like every couple we have our differences.'* (Relationship quality rated 'insufficient support, no discord'.)

Whitney has had two close friends for years who she named as very close but they live away and only seen less than once a year. She therefore named another friend Sara who was not close, but who is seen every two weeks and in whom she can confide. She will talk about her problems with her son and her husband. Whilst she will not always describe the extent of her worry and concern, she can tell Sara the problem and ask for advice and help. Sara is helpful and suggests practical things Whitney can do and is sympathetic. The get on well together and never argue. However Whitney does not have high felt attachment: *'I think it is more of a practical arrangement. I don't think I would really miss her if she wasn't there. We've only known each other about two years. We met through nursing.'* (Relationship rated 'good-average, no discord').

Whitney also named her mother as very close, but is unable to confide in her: *'If you try to tell her about problems – what she does is say "alright dear, forget about it, it will work itself out tomorrow sort of thing", that is her whole philosophy of life. I find that completely frustrating. When Simon was young I used to ring her up and say "he is driving me nuts. He doesn't sleep, he doesn't eat, he cries all the time". And she would say, "oh never mind, don't worry dear, give him a kiss and say goodnight"'* (Relationship rated 'inadequate support, no discord'). Given Whitney had only one confiding relationship she was rated as 'some' on ability to relate and therefore 'moderately' Insecure style.

Whitney's Withdrawn attachment attitudes: She had 'moderately' high constraints on closeness. She describes how it is not easy for her to confide in people because it is not helpful: *'I think that a lot of people tend to gloss over your problems and you tend to simplify them when you tell them, and other people will just agree with anything you say, or else people have got the same problems and can't help.'* She also said: *'I would hate it if someone knocked on the door wanting to borrow money. That is why I don't make friends with the neighbours. Because they all do that. Once or twice I have loaned them money and never go it back. People are unreliable. Perhaps I expect too much of people.'* She is 'highly' self-reliant: *'I've had to be. I need to make my own decisions and have control over what happens to me. It's too important to ask other people what they think.'* She also had a low desire for company: *'I often think, I'd love some peace and quiet. It is important to have time for myself. I need peace and quiet to come home and be on my own, to recharge my batteries. I find that a lot, probably because I have been on my own so much in the past – I just need more space.'* However, she did not have high levels of mistrust (*'I don't really feel suspicious of people'*), fear of rejection (*'I can't really think of when people have let me down'*) or fear of separation (*'I quite like it when people go away'*). Also she had no anger in relationships.

Comment: Whitney's profile was consistent with Withdrawn style, rated at moderate level because she does have one confidant and because her attitudes were not at the most extreme of self-reliance. This style is the truly detached one, without the anger of Angry-dismissive or the fear of Fearful. She is very private, contained and does not readily open up to others. At interview she was unable to give expressive responses, but used short statements, often just saying 'sometimes' rather than anything more specific. She does, however, have awareness of her detached tendencies.

2.4.6 Deirdre's Dual Angry-dismissive and Enmeshed style

Deirdre is a 36-year-old Scottish woman married to her Cypriot husband with two children aged 13 and 11. She and her husband are unemployed. The main trauma in her recent past concerns the death of their 12-year-old son Paul three years ago, in an accident on a building site. She is still preoccupied with the loss. She also has difficulties with her teenage daughter aged 13 with whom she has negative interaction. Her clinical status and coping is described in Chapter 3. She comes from a large family. She has contact with all of them although only one sibling lives nearby. Her mother comes to visit her, but they usually end up arguing. She is still resentful of her early upbringing feeling her mother was lazy and neglectful of her ('some' closeness to mother; 'moderate' antipathy). She feels close to her father but does not see him as often ('moderate' closeness; 'little/no' antipathy). She suffered adversity in childhood mainly from her mother.

Deirdre's support: She and her husband have an unsupportive and conflictful relationship. They had grown apart after their son's death and she is now clear that she told him little in the way of confiding, although her initial statements were that she did confide. '*I can talk to him about my son. I can talk to him about anything really*'. However, when asked if she ever regretted telling him anything, she said: '*No, because I've never really told him anything. I don't think I really wanted him to help me then* (when her son died). *I would say he is sympathetic at the time of a problem. But if I were to mention money worries he says "don't worry, don't worry". Everything's always "don't worry" with him. He bottles it all up. He never ever confides in me, even about the way he feels about Paul's death. I don't know how he feels because he's never confided that in me. We don't really talk to each other abut anything meaningful.*'... '*He's not a bad husband, he does try, but he always does it wrong. Then again, it's my high standards. He irritates me, he irritates me something terrible since the accident. Now I think he just avoids me. You can stand there and bawl and shout at him and he wouldn't think of answering you back. He just goes "yes, yes" and that irritates me. He wouldn't retaliate. He is 10 years older than me, I think we argue about that too. We also argue because he doesn't like me going out. If I wanted to go out for a night with the girls he'd say "no, you're not going". He's very jealous. We row almost every fortnight. He always wants to know where I am and what I've been doing. That's why I feel so trapped. He doesn't shout back or threaten or get violent.*' She doesn't rely on him and she wouldn't miss anything if he went: '*I don't think there's anything. I really, honestly don't think there's anything I would miss.*' The relationship was rated as 'inadequate support, with discord'.

She described one VCO, her friend, Mary who lives locally and in whom she can confide about her children and marriage. '*I like to meet up with Mary and talk. She's a good listener and it makes it easier for me to tell her things. She's calm and not judgemental. We get on well together.*' This relationship is considered to be 'good-average support, no discord'. Her second VCO was her sister in Scotland who she sees every few months, and does not confide anything very personal in case she tells their mother. Their relationship is also rather volatile and they do fall out at times, but not in the last months. This relationship was rated as 'insufficient support, no discord'. Her overall ability to 'Make and Maintain Relationships' was rated as 'some' and therefore her attachment style as 'moderately' Insecure.

Dual Attachment attitudes: When asked about her attitudes, the picture that emerged was more complex than those described so far, showing both Avoidant and Anxious elements. Her Angry-dismissiveness was clear with moderately high levels of mistrust and constraints on closeness *'Yeah. I'm very suspicious. I'm suspicious of everyone. You can't rely on people – they are mainly out for themselves. I don't think it's right to be too close, really.* When asked 'What do you consider to be very close?' *'Telling them everything. I don't tell everything. Some of my business I don't tell even to Mary. I'm not really close to many people.'* When Paul died: *'I didn't confide much at the time. I never asked anyone for help. I have found myself sometimes telling people things I later regret.'* Her fear of rejection was low: *'No, I get close to people quite quick. I haven't been let down – I don't let people get close enough to let me down.'*

Deirdre made 'contradictory' statements on self-reliance: When asked if she saw herself as a loner, she said: *'It depends, really. I do rely on my husband being there, I don't think I could manage without him, but I like to make my own mind up about things. I don't rely on him if I have a problem to deal with. I would say I do rely on myself more than anyone. But I do feel I need people. I seem to flip from one to the other, needing help and wanting to cope alone.'* She was similarly rated as 'contradictory' about her desire for company: She has friends and family but says she doesn't enjoy socialising since her son's death. *'I don't really bother with other people. Yeah, I'd say I enjoy having people around me, but only when I want people around me. If I didn't see Mary for a couple of days I'd probably miss her. I'd take the kids and go there. I wouldn't miss my husband if he went away – no I never rely on him for anything. But I can get lonely if I spend time alone – I find I brood too much. Having people around stops me brooding.'*

Deirdre exhibited 'markedly' high fear of separation typical of Enmeshed style. Since her son's death she has felt panic and worry about the children, particularly if they come home late. *'I get very anxious about leaving the children . . . I don't like to do it. Even if they are only a little late I get nervous and start pacing up and down the house. I start to panic until they walk in the door and I know they are OK'.* She doesn't let them stay overnight at friends and needs to keep them close, even though they are now coming up to teenage and want more independence. Her anger is high: She has a difficult relationship with her daughter with high negative interaction. She also has a fraught relationship with her family of origin. When asked 'Do you often get into arguments?' *'Yes, my daughter and I are going through a rough patch. I suppose it has been ongoing for quite some time. We tend to argue a lot and she often tells me how much I upset her.'* Do you feel resentful about the past? *'My goodness yes, I blame my mother for all the things she put me through during my childhood. When we discuss it, it erupts into a fight. I just see no reason to forgive her.'* She argues with her husband, she still blames him for the loss of the son and the atmosphere *'simmers with resentment'*.

Comment: Deirdre's moderately Angry-dismissive style was considered the more pervasive style and her moderately Enmeshed characteristics were subsidiary since they are restricted to her children. Such dual rating is considered to be similar to the Disorganised style identified in childhood attachment styles and in this instance also the Unresolved loss of the AAI classification. These are linked to trauma, and the loss of Deirdre's child would constitute traumatic loss, and her coping is further discussed in Chapter 3. As will be seen in later chapters, unresolved recent loss is not, however, the only scenario for Dual/disorganised style.

In order to consider other possible similarities between the ASI and the AAI interview, the next section will examine reporting style at interview to see whether different characteristic styles relate to attachment styles in expected ways.

2.5 Attachment style and reporting at interview

Whilst the ASI ratings do not involve a discourse analysis of speech patterns, it was nevertheless possible to rate reporting style as a possible correlate. In the London sample of women four such ratings were made on the basis of the way the individual related information throughout the life history interviews. This included 'reluctance in reporting', 'stated inability to recall the past', 'emotional involvement in reporting' and as part of the attachment measure 'inconsistency between attachment behaviour and attitudes'. These would be expected to relate to Avoidant, Anxious and Disorganised styles respectively. Correlations between the scales and the degree of each attachment style (e.g. 'marked', 'moderate', 'mild' or 'none') showed:

- **Fearful style** was significantly associated with reluctance in reporting (0.18, $p<0.001$). Secure style was inversely related (-0.11, $p<0.04$)
- Both **Fearful style** (0.30, $p<0.0001$) and **Angry-dismissive** style (0.16, $p<0.01$) were significantly more likely to describe being unable to recall the past. Again, Secure style was inversely related (-0.23, $p<0.001$).
- **Enmeshed style** was related to emotional reporting (0.22, $p<0.0001$) as was Dual-disorganised (0.12, $p<0.02$). Withdrawn style was inversely related (-0.19, $p<0.001$).
- **Dual/disorganised** style was related to inconsistency in attachment behaviour and attitudes ($p<0.18$, $p<0.002$) and Secure style inversely related ($p<-0.16$, $p<0.005$).

These associations are consistent with predictions from the style profiles. There was no evidence, however, that stated inability to recall the past correlated with lower reports of neglect and abuse in childhood. As will be described in Chapter 5 those with such stated poor recall actually had highest rates of neglect and abuse measured.

Summary of adult attachment style measurement

- There are a number of questionnaires of adult attachment style. These are correlated with each other, although identifying different styles makes comparisons difficult.
- The best-known interview is the AAI which questions adults about their childhood experience with discourse analysis of the interview transcript for incoherence in narrative, idealisation, denigration and other characteristics allows for reliable categorisation of Preoccupied (Anxious), Dismissive (Avoidant) or Unresolved loss as Insecure styles. Secure style is characterised by coherent, factual and insightful descriptions of past experience. This interview has been responsible for a wealth of research studies internationally into adult attachment and has good psychometric properties. However, it is a complex measure requiring a high degree of training to acquire reliability and is costly and time consuming to administer and score. It also reflects nothing of current relationship context.
- The ASI is presented as a reliable and valid measure of adult attachment style which is based on the quality of ongoing relationships including partner, family or friends in terms of whether they are close and supportive. Those Secure in their styles require at least two close and confiding relationships. Attachment styles are determined by scored responses on a range of questions about mistrust and constraints of closeness as well as autonomy scales (self-reliance and desire for company) and anxious scales (fear of rejection, fear of separation) as well as anger. The combination of highly rated negative scales provide the overall classification. Disorganised style comprises a dual rating for those unable to make relationships.
- When reporting style of those with different attachment styles were examined, Fearful were the most reluctant reporters, and these together with Angry-dismissive had poorer stated recall of the past. Those Enmeshed and Dual/disorganised had the most emotional reporting with Withdrawn having the least. Only Dual/disorganised had contradictory elements in reporting on attachment behaviour and attitudes. Secure style was least reluctant to report, and had no inability to recall or inconsistency of reporting. This is consistent with Avoidant and Anxious elements.

2.6 Discussion

The challenge of attachment research and practice is to find reliable and valid assessment tools which differentiate attachment styles, and can test attachment theory predictions. These include the way information is processed, the way in which non-verbal social cues trigger feelings of safety or threat, the way perceptions of others are guided by trust or mistrust to maintain a sense of safety and protection, and the daily negotiation of social relations. Importantly it also influences the way in which stress is managed, feelings are regulated, challenges are coped with, new situations are approached and the way in which conflict is either avoided, initiated or sustained. The degree of success in making and maintaining mutually satisfying reciprocal relationships with those who can provide emotional safety and comfort depends on the factors contributing to individual attachment style. Therefore, the need to find appropriate measures robust enough to test these associations is critical.

The ASI is argued to be suitable for assessing adult attachment style in relation to a range of dysfunction, as well as in relation to social context. It also has the advantage of assessing along a continuum ranging from Secure to severely impaired Anxious, Avoidant and Disorganised categories which enables not only potential 'dose' effects to be explored, but also resilience at the lower levels of impairment. It also has the potential for predicting risks to aid with decision-making in service interventions including those partner and parent-related as well as for clinical disorder given the measure is easily operationalised.

The styles identified by the ASI fit with the ethnological origins of attachment theory in relation to fight, flight and other survival responses to danger. The styles thus relate to different strategies, for example Enmeshed to a clinging response, Fearful to flight, Angry-dismissive to fight, Withdrawn to hide and Dual/disorganised to either a freeze response or a chaotic lack of strategy. The Secure style could be seen as keeping close to the tribe or pack to gain safety from the group through support-access. Indeed, in a child version of the ASI currently under development animal characters of monkey, deer, bear, tortoise and family dog are used to represent these stress responses.

A major component of Insecure style as defined in the ASI is the inability to make and maintain relationships on an ongoing basis. There is substantial research to show that good close support is protective against a number of ills including psychological disorder. Conversely the presence of unsupportive relationships, particularly those where there is evidence of high conflict in itself increases risk of disorder. For those with Insecure attachment style both aspects are likely to be present, the absence of positive support leading sometimes to isolation, but also the presence of difficult, conflictful and sometimes dangerous relationships. These latter can generate crises and separations and thus add to stress as well as failing to support over stress.

The following chapters will focus on a range of roles and domains in turn to investigate research findings in the London studies of women and their offspring in relation to ASI-rated Insecure attachment style. The next chapter will look at stress, coping and disorder.

Note

1   The labels in brackets are those used throughout the review, to create some parity among different measures.

3 Adult attachment style, stress and disorder

3.0 Introduction

This chapter examines adult attachment style in relation to demographic characteristics, stress, coping and clinical disorder. The literature is reviewed and the analysis from the London women and their offspring outlined. Whilst the samples and details of the analysis can be found elsewhere (and with summaries in the appendices), new findings are presented on lifetime adversity, life events, coping and attachment style. For the adult women the focus is on major depression and anxiety disorder (Bifulco, Moran *et al.* 2002; Bifulco, Kwon *et al.* 2006). For the offspring, deliberate self-harm and substance abuse are examined (Bifulco 2008). Case examples from both generations are used to illustrate experience.

3.1 Prevalence of Insecure attachment style

Secure attachment style is highly prevalent in the population with 55%–60% of adults Secure in their attachment style (Shaver and Hazan 1993; Shaver and Clarke 1994). The National Comorbidity Survey (NCS) in the USA of 8,000 representative adults showed that 59% of individuals were Secure, 25% Avoidant and 11% Anxious with 5% 'unable to classify' using a self-report scale (Mickelson, Kessler *et al.* 1997). Secure attachment style was associated with being White, female, well-educated, middle class, married and middle aged. Those with Anxious attachment style were more likely to be under 25, previously married, Black or Hispanic, less well-educated and less well-off financially. Those with Avoidant style tended to be male, older, married or previously married, also to be from Black or other ethnic background (op cit). Another US study investigating ethnicity using a different self-report scale found White Americans were more likely to have Secure style, to be more educated, to be married and to have been raised in two-parent households compared with African-Americans (Montague, Magai *et al.* 2003). However, there was no association between being African-American and either Anxious or Avoidant styles. Regression analyses showed that associations between other social variables and attachment style were similar across the two ethnic groups.

The ASI was used to examine attachment style in the TCS-PND study. This involved 204 low-risk pregnant women, attending antenatal clinics in one US and eight European cities. Prevalence rates indicated that 45% were rated clearly Secure, 37% mildly Insecure and 18% 'markedly/moderately' Insecure (Bifulco, Figueirido *et al.* 2004). There were similar rates of Anxious (Enmeshed or Fearful, 28%) and Avoidant (Angry-dismissive or Withdrawn, 26%) styles. Individual styles were fairly equally distributed: Withdrawn (16%), Fearful (15%) and Enmeshed (13%). However, Angry-dismissive was least common at 10%. Insecure attachment style significantly related to economic factors (lower social class and unemployment), to single or cohabiting rather than married status, to having a mother living in the household, and lower contact with friends (op cit). To examine prevalence by gender, the ASI was used in a low-risk Portuguese study of couples expecting a baby (Condé, Figueirido *et al.* 2011). This showed that women had somewhat higher rates of Clearly Secure style (65%) than men (52%) but not at significant levels. Men were twice as likely to have an Insecure Avoidant style and women three times more likely to have an Insecure Anxious style. The NCS study similarly found 61% of females reported Secure style compared with 57% of males. It also showed Avoidant styles more common in males (28% vs 23%) but with Anxious rates similar across gender (12% and 11%) (Mickelson, Kessler *et al.* 1997).

There is broad consistency for the relationship of Insecure attachment style to ethnicity, gender and social class. But the specificity of Anxious or Avoidant style to different characteristics is less clear. This has been attributed to different measures used with different categorisation of attachment style and the use of self-report rather than more objective assessments (Stein, Koontz *et al.* 2002).

3.2 Insecure attachment style and emotional disorder

The relationship between Insecure attachment style and depression has been established both in terms of depressed symptoms assessed by checklist (Gerlsma and Luteijn 2000) and with clinical levels of disorder (Hammen, Burge *et al.* 1995; Mickelson, Kessler *et al.* 1997). However, while there is consistency in linking any Insecure attachment style with depression, there is little consistency in differentiating a specific type of style to disorder. Some studies show the predicted links between depressive symptoms and the more Anxious styles such as Enmeshed (Preoccupied) (Gerlsma and Luteijn 2000) and Fearful (Murphy and Bates 2000) but others have highlighted association with Avoidant styles (McCarthy 1999). The NCS study showed no differentiation between any Insecure style and depression (Mickelson, Kessler *et al.* 1997).

The TCS-PND study described earlier and undertaken in a European/US context involved the ASI and a clinical interview for depression (Bifulco, Figueirido *et al.* 2004). It found Insecure attachment style in the second trimester of pregnancy predicted major or minor postnatal depression as well as reflecting onset of depression in pregnancy. A 'dose-response' effect was observed for degree of insecurity and onset of disorder (22% among those with marked/moderate insecurity, 12% mildly Insecure and 6% Secure). Avoidant styles (Angry-dismissive or Withdrawn) were more common among women with depression during pregnancy whilst Anxious styles (Enmeshed or Fearful) more common in women having depression postnatally (Bifulco, Figueirido *et al.* 2004).

Fewer studies have examined anxiety disorder in relation to adult attachment style, but associated styles include those Anxious (Preoccupied) (Eng, Heimberg *et al.* 2001; Dozier, Stovall *et al.* 1999) and also 'Unresolved', equivalent to Disorganised classifications (Fonagy, Leigh *et al.* 1996). In a study of young adults with a range of anxiety symptoms lack of assertion, associated with Avoidance, and over-reliance on others associated with Anxious dependence, mediated the association between social anxiety and interpersonal stress (Davila and Sargent 2003). The fear and expectation of others' criticism and negative evaluations, were argued to be at the base of such responses (Rapee and Heimberg 1997).

Lack of consistency of findings for type of attachment style and emotional disorder may be due to studies small in scale, unrepresentative often utilising student populations (Bartholomew and Horowitz 1991) (Hammen, Burge *et al.* 1995), volunteers (Hazan and Shaver 1987) or small selected high-risk series (McCarthy 1999). Diagnostic interviews for disorder have been used infrequently, and yet the difference between these and self-report symptom checklists may be important. For example a study of high school leavers showed that whereas clinical interview-based symptoms reduced in relation to improved attachment cognitions this did not hold for self-reported depression changes on the Beck Depression Inventory (BDI) (Hammen, Burge *et al.* 1995). In addition there have been few prospective studies of attachment style with appropriate controls for the influence of symptoms on Insecure style ratings. Therefore methodological issues may in part account for inconsistency in patterning of type of style to disorder. The relationship of attachment style to other common disorders has been summarised by Dozier and colleagues (Dozier, Stovall-McClough *et al.* 2008). Only two substance abuse studies were included and showed association wtth Unresolved classifications of the AAI (Fonagy, Leigh *et al.* 1996) and to Avoidant (Dismissive) styles (Ward, Ramsay *et al.* 2001).

3.2.3 Insecure attachment style and experience of stress

Attachment theory argues that stressful life events trigger proximity seeking (support) and affect-regulation (soothing) and are thus highly relevant to understanding the attachment system. Mikulincer and Shaver's (2003) model of affect-regulation outlined in Chapter 1 examines behaviours in response to stressful experience as hyper-activating (Anxious) or deactivating (Avoidant) both of which reduce effective support-seeking and affect-regulation. Few intensive studies of stressful life events exist which also examine attachment style and support-seeking. Instead they focus either on daily hassles (Davila and Sargent 2003) or very high threat, trauma conditions (Mikulincer, Horesh *et al.* 1999). Insecure attachment style overall and Anxious attachment style in particular related to symptomatology in both sets of conditions, but only Avoidant attachment style related to psychopathology in trauma conditions. Thus level of threat of stressors may be important in relating type of attachment style to disorder outcome.

The critical role of severe life events in the triggering of depression has been well-documented since the 1970s (Brown and Harris 1978). The vulnerability-provoking agent model described earlier also includes the contribution of negative coping responses at the time of the crisis, for example inferred denial, pessimism and self-blame as further increasing depression risk (Bifulco and Brown 1996). This model has not previously been applied in the attachment field, in part because intensive measures of life events are required prospectively. The arguments put forward for intensive interview measure of life events rather than self-report checklists are still valid (Brown 1974) since checklists can only give a very approximate assessment of stressful experience and its timing (Uher and McGuffin 2008). The analysis described later uses intensive contextual measures to estimate the threat or unpleasantness of life events and difficulties. It is considered important not to underplay the objective severity of the stressor in favour of its psychological appraisal and the cognitive-emotional response – both are important in the final model. Events such as partner separation, offspring police involvement, housing evictions and loss of job are real external pressures which enforce major adjustments for individuals and families. These may escalate into trauma, for example, when domestic or neighbourhood violence is involved. The type of stressor individuals' experience and the way that those with Insecure attachment styles respond to them needs to be examined to illuminate underlying mechanisms in clinical disorder.

In the next section, results from the London studies using the ASI will be outlined giving prevalence of attachment styles, their relationship to demographic variables, stressful events and coping, and disorder. This data set includes data from intensive interviews including the ASI and clinical interviews of disorder, and interview assessments of life events and coping.

3.3 The London studies

(Details of the samples used in this analysis are outlined in the appendix. Also, see the prior research note over the abbreviated presentation of statistical analyses). The following analysis involves the midlife women studied.

3.3.1 Attachment Style prevalence in London women

In order to look at demographic characteristics of those with Insecure style, the degree of insecurity and also the type of style were examined first in the comparison subgroup of 80 women (sample 1C), who were consecutive responders to the original screening, and then in the high-risk remaining 222 women (sample 1A+B) who were all selected for having problem relationships or difficult childhood experiences. These were also utilised to determine prevalence. The comparison group rate should approximate to the population rates found in the research literature.

Prevalence of attachment styles are shown in Figures 3.1 and 3.2. To summarise:

- **Comparison women**: Nearly half (49%) were rated as clearly Secure, a further 32% mildly Insecure, 15% 'marked/moderately' Insecure and 4% Dual/disorganised.
- **High-risk women**: These had very different rates reflecting their risk status: 24% Secure, 21% mildly Insecure, 49% 'markedly/moderately' Insecure (three times the rate in the comparison women, $p<0.001$). Dual/disorganised rates at 6% were little different from the comparison group.
- **Fearful style** was the most common style and did not differ between groups (24% and 25%, respectively). Withdrawn styles were also similar in the two groups at 12% and 18% respectively.
- **Angry dismissive style** was three times higher in the high-risk women (18% vs 6%) with the Enmeshed rates also raised (15% and 9%, respectively).

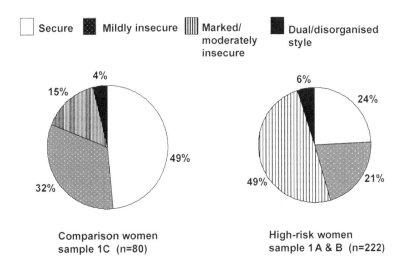

Figure 3.1 Prevalence of ASI attachment style in London women

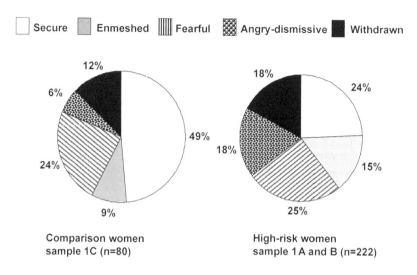

Figure 3.2 Prevalence of ASI attachment style in London women

3.3.2 Demographic factors

Attachment style was examined in relation to demographic factors. Whilst attachment style was not associated with age, the following associations were found:

- Insecure style (at marked/moderate levels) was significantly more common among those working class (58%) than middle class (38%, p<0.002). Anxious attachment styles (Enmeshed or Fearful) were more common among those working class.
- Insecure attachment style was related to financial hardship, with 80% found among those with financial hardship compared with 55% of those without (p<0.04). Financial hardship was most prominent in those with Angry-dismissive styles.
- Insecure style was significantly more common among parents (49%) than among women without children (36%, p<0.02), and amongst those cohabiting (49%) than single (36%, p<0.01).
- Insecure style was significantly more common among women from Black and Minority Ethnic (BME) communities (84%) than White (42%, p<0.0001). There was a non-significant trend for those from BME backgrounds to have more Avoidant (Angry-dismissive or Withdrawn) styles (47% vs 30%, p<0.09).

These findings are consistent with those reported in the research literature. The evident dual linkage between Insecure attachment styles and signs of deprivation (lower social class, financial hardship and minority ethnic status), as well as relationship factors (such as cohabiting and having children) illustrate the social adversity and interpersonal themes developed in this book.

3.3.2 Attachment Style Interview and adult lifetime adversity

For lifetime adult adversity the Adult Life Phase Interview (ALPHI) was used to measure objective levels of difficulty in five domains (partner, parenting, social, material and miscellaneous) across different settled life phases, as well as in the process of change between the phases, from age 17. 'Marked' or 'moderate' levels were considered indicative of severe levels of stress or adversity. More details can be found elsewhere (Bifulco, Bernazzani *et al.* 2000) and the measure has good reliability and validity.

A score of lifetime stress using the ALPHI was correlated with the overall attachment style scale. It showed the following:

- Insecurity of attachment style was significantly correlated with the lifetime adversity score (0.25, p<0.001). It was also significantly correlated with the number of adverse life changes between phases (0.20, p<0.001).
- Correlations with lifetime adversity were highest for Dual/disorganised style (0.22, p<0.003) and Fearful style (0.20, p<0.007) followed by Enmeshed style (0.12, p<0.001) with only a non-significant trend for those with Angry-dismissive style (0.10, p<0.06). The same associations held for a score of adverse change points between life phases.
- Those with Withdrawn style showed a trend to *less* lifetime adversity (−0.10, p<0.06).

3.3.3 Attachment Style Interview and severe life events

The Life Events and Difficulties Schedule (LEDS) interview was used as an intensive measure of 12-month stressors. The elements of the measure are outlined below.

Life Events and Difficulties Schedule (Brown and Harris 1978)

- A one-hour interview with questions about both acute events and ongoing difficulties of at least four weeks' duration, over the last twelve months before interview.
- It has good inter-rater reliability and shows good consistency of recall of events over the twelve months, and also over a longer five-year period.
- Events are questioned in detail to determine their date, context, duration of threat, focus (on self or other) and category.

- Only factual elements are used for final classification of events. Asessment of threat or severity is rated according to manualised examples based on the estimated degree of threat or unpleasantness to the average person in the same situation, for example, bereavements or marital separations.
- A severe event is one rated marked or moderate on threat or unpleasantness, present for at least 10 days after its inception, focused on the person excluding those attributable to a psychological disorder (e.g. admission to psychiatric hospital, or suicide attempt). Major difficulties are those of 'marked' or 'moderate' severity which had lasted two years continuously.
- A 'matching difficulty – D' event is a severe event arising from an ongoing difficulty of at least 6-months' duration. These are much more highly related to onset of major depression than other severe life events (Brown, Bifulco *et al.* 1987).
- In the 105 women measured in the London sample, these events were assessed in a 12-month follow-up period after the ASI had been measured at first contact.

Severe life events in the year of interview were examined in a subset of the London women with a focus on coping (sample 1A). Whilst the ASI was used at first contact, the LEDS interview was undertaken at twelve-month follow-up. Findings showed (see Figure 3.3):

- Those with Insecure attachment style showed a trend in being more likely to experience a severe life event at follow-up interview than those with Secure style (75% vs 65%). When those Withdrawn were excluded from the Insecure category, the finding reached significant levels (81% vs 62%, respectively, p<0.02).
- Significantly higher rates of housing and finance events were found for those with Insecure attachment styles (87% vs 13% amongst Secure, p<0.001) and relationship events (64% vs 36%, respectively, p<0.02).
- The toxic 'difficulty-matching' severe events were significantly more common in those with Insecure styles (72% vs 51%, p<0.02).
- Those with Enmeshed and Angry-dismissive style had highest rates of severe life events, and Angry-dismissive had highest rates of D-matching events.

3.3.4 Coping with adversity

A measure of coping with life events was added to the LEDS interview to ascertain responses to the events which occurred in the period (see box below). When coping responses to severe life events were examined in the

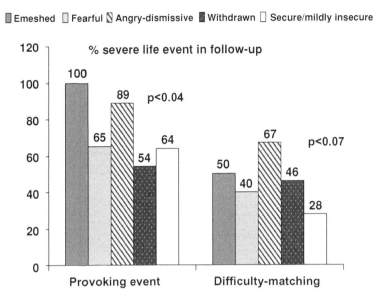

Figure 3.3 Attachment style and severe life events in 12 months

12 months after the ASI was measured, high helplessness was the most common negative response (61%), together with high anger (51%) and high sadness (53%). Blame of others was slightly less common (46%) but four times as common as self-blame (11%). Inferred denial was rated for a quarter (23%) of the sample and the related cognitive avoidance only for 15%. The difference between these two scales is one of degree. Those with inferred denial fail to recognise elements of the stressor and their actions show certain obliviousness to the extent of the problem whilst cognitive avoidance is more of an intentional strategy, putting off thinking about the difficulty in order to reduce distress.

The Crisis Coping Interview (Bifulco and Brown 1996)

- The Crisis Coping Interview was used in conjunction with the LEDS to encompass complexes of severe events and related difficulties.
- A series of questions were asked to find out the cognitive, emotional and behavioural response.
- This included both positive coping strategies (e.g. problem tackling, mastery, hope) and negative coping grouped into avoidant (cognitive avoidance, inferred denial) internalising (sadness, helplessness, self-blame) and externalising (blame of others and anger).

> • The measure has good inter-rater reliability and is tested prospectively in relation to onset of depression to overcome possible reporting bias.

Attachment style and coping findings are summarised in Figure 3.4 using Pearson's 'r' and showed:

- The dichotomous presence of any highly Insecure style was correlated with helplessness (0.28, p<0.001), inferred denial (0.27, p<0.005), sadness (0.28, p<0.005), anger (0.28, p<0.003) and blame (0.22, p<0.01).
- Enmeshed style was correlated with self-blame (0.18, p<0.05) but also with inferred denial (0.25, p<0.004).
- Fearful style was correlated with cognitive avoidance (0.26, p<0.007)
- Angry-dismissive style was correlated with anger (0.17, p<0.01), blame (0.23, p<0.003) and sadness (0.16, p<0.02).
- No pattern was differentiated for Dual/disorganised styles. They did not exhibit higher rates of negative coping than those with single Insecure styles.
- Withdrawn was not correlated with any negative coping strategy.
- Secure was inversely correlated with all the negative scales.

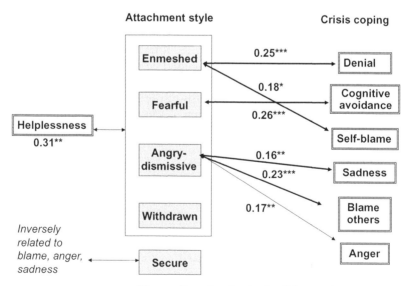

(No specific patterning for Dual/disorganised styles)

*p<0.05   **p<0.01   ***p<0.001

Figure 3.4 Summary of attachment styles and coping responses

Whilst some of these correlations are as expected in terms of internalising and externalising directions, for example Enmeshed and self-blame and Angry-dismissive with anger and blame, other findings were less expected. Thus both of the Anxious styles had associations with more avoidant coping strategies (Enmeshed with denial and Fearful with cognitive avoidance) and an Avoidant style with more emotional strategy e.g. Angry-dismissive with sadness. This suggests that these styles overlap in terms of their strategies at cognitive-emotional levels more than is suggested by the Anxious versus Avoidant dichotomy.

3.3.5 Attachment Style Interview and depression in the London women

The Structured Clinical Interview for the Diagnostic and Statistical Manual of Disorder (SCID) (DSM-IV) was used to establish clinical disorder in the recent 12-month period as well as over the lifetime. In this analysis major depression was examined, which involved depressed mood or loss of interest and further symptoms including poor appetite or sleep, poor concentration, tiredness, restlessness, suicidal thoughts and plans, being present almost daily for at least a month (First, Gibbon *et al.* 1996). In the adult comparison group there was a rate of 18% of major depression, similar to rates found in larger representative samples of women studied previously in the same area (Brown, Bifulco *et al.* 1990). For the high-risk London women studied the rate was double, affecting more than a third (35%) (Bifulco, Moran *et al.* 2002a).

Attachment style was examined in relation to a dichotomous scale of clinical depression. Significant associations were found (see Figure 3.5), namely:

- The rate of depression was similar across those with marked/moderate levels of three different styles, Enmeshed (52%) Fearful (47%) or Angry-dismissive (45%).
- Those with Withdrawn style had lower rates of depression (31%) similar to those Secure (24%).
- When 'mild' levels of any Insecure style were examined there was no increased rate of depression when compared with those Secure (20%–14% vs 24%). Mild levels of Withdrawn style had the lowest rate of depression (14%) of any group.
- When Dual/disorganised attachment style was examined rates were slightly lower than those with single Insecure styles at 32%. (Since there is no mild level for Dual/disorganised Figure 3.5 includes only single styles and the 'main' style for those dual.)
- In order to check for bias, the analysis was re-run with those with depression at time of interview excluded, and same findings held. In the half of the subsample (1A) examined prospectively, Insecure attachment style at first contact predicted new onset of depression (see Bifulco *et al.* 2002 for figures).

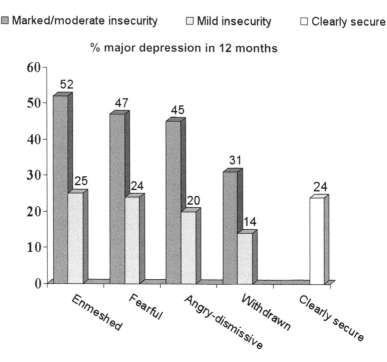

■ Marked/moderate insecurity   □ Mild insecurity   □ Clearly secure

Figure 3.5 Attachment style and major depression in London women

3.3.6 Lifetime depression

Attachment style was then examined in relation to *prior* lifetime chronic or recurrent episodes of disorder to see if it reflected a lifelong pattern and to preclude any bias from the current episode. This was confirmed.

• Nearly half (49%) of those with highly Insecure attachment style at interview had recurrent or chronic lifetime depression compared with 25% of remaining women (p<0.0001).
• The same held for teenage depressions: 24% of those with highly Insecure attachment styles at interview had a teenage depression compared with 9% of other women (p<0.0001).

This suggests a robust relationship of Insecure attachment style to depression at different life stages. Statistical modelling showed that Insecure attachment style predicted depression outcome when controls were made for social class and ethnicity.

3.3.7 Attachment Style Interview and new onset of emotional disorder

The relationship of ASI to disorder was re-examined in a three-year follow-up of the London women (Sample 2), to new onsets of both depression and anxiety states (Bifulco, Kwon *et al.* 2006). Over half (55%) of the women were shown to have at least one clinical level disorder at follow-up, including major depression, social phobia, Generalised Anxiety Disorder (GAD) or panic and/or agoraphobia (First, Gibbon *et al.* 1996). The following findings are shown for the follow-up disorder:

- Highly ('marked or moderate') Insecure attachment style combined was significantly related to new onset of depression or anxiety (50% vs 28% of those Secure/mildly Insecure, p<0.003).
- Highest rates of anxiety were for Fearful style (51% vs 30% of other styles, p<0.01) and Angry Dismissive style (69% vs 31%, respectively, p<0.004).
- When type of anxious disorder was examined, Fearful style was significantly associated with Social Phobia (20% vs 7% of other styles, p<0.02).
- Angry-dismissive style was significantly related to GAD (50% vs 16% of other styles, p<0.004).
- Those with Dual/disorganised styles were no more likely to have a disorder at follow-up than those with single Insecure styles.

The relationship of Insecure styles to new episode of depression was therefore confirmed, and extended to anxiety disorders, with the beginnings of some specificity of style uncovered. Case examples from the research will be used to illustrate these findings.

3.4 Case examples

The following case examples illustrate the findings in this chapter concerning demographic characteristics, adversity and disorder. We present four from the midlife sample of women and will look briefly at attachment and disorder in the young offspring sample with a further two illustrative cases.

3.4.1 Ellie – Moderately Enmeshed style and onset depression

Ellie, aged 40 at first interview, was a single divorced parent with two teenage children. Her moderately Enmeshed attachment style was described in the last chapter. She was beginning a relationship with her boyfriend Lester (a man 10 years younger), and was experiencing problems with her possessive ex-partner. She only had one close confidant, so she had only 'some' ability to relate and 'moderate' level of attachment insecurity. Ellie showed high need for company from various friends (*'It's important to have friends because I'm very nosy, very inquisitive, I love a good laugh and if you haven't got friends you can't do that'*) and fear of separation ('*I hate it when people leave me, I hate being on my own'*). When followed-up for interview three years later, she describes the recent breakdown of the relationship with Lester. This, together with chronic financial difficulties had provoked a new onset of major depression.

Life events and adversity: Ellie had a very high score of 11 separate adversities in different domains over her lifetime. She left home age 16 having been fostered, and started an affair with a married man from age 15. She subsequently had two children with him, the first given up for adoption. Her partner left her after 10 years and she managed as a single parent briefly before marrying Graham, a man who had numerous affairs during their marriage and became violent. They had one daughter and divorced after 13 years, with Ellie again left alone with her children. She has had more than one episode of clinical depression in the past. At first interview Ellie's life events and difficulties revolved around her adverse relationship with her ex-husband Graham, and her serious financial difficulties. At follow-up she also had difficulties with her partner Lester who was dependent on her for money. Her depression was triggered by her separation from Lester.

Coping: At follow-up interview, Ellie's negative coping included inferred denial of her financial difficulties. Whilst she did tackle some aspects, for example by pawning her wedding ring, cutting down on meals and borrowing essential items from a neighbour, the delay in recognising and confronting the issue led to greater problems: '*Sometimes I know of a situation for quite a while before I actually manage to tackle it or even assimilate into my system. That is how I am. I definitely put off doing anything about it.*' When asked how, with Lester not working, her financial difficulties might be resolved, she said: '*I know that Lester will help me if he's got the money. This afternoon I'm taking him to see a job. I think even if he doesn't help me, if he's got some money we can go out. I think that's very essential, that we do go out because with money as it is we can't go out . . . and being in here and being on top of one another.*'

Her illogical reasoning was taken to demonstrate her denial, given that Lester was broke, unemployed and dependent on her for money and yet she looked to him to save her financially. When asked if there was anything else she could do practically to help the situation she said: '*No. I don't think I have any treats, I don't go anywhere'* immediately followed by the statement: '*I am determined I will go away for a week with Lester. I don't know where my bit of money will come from – maybe on my credit card, but we will go.*' She exhibited helplessness about her money situation and its cause: '*It's generally the recession. Food prices have gone up. I don't go shopping in the same way I did. You do have to shop around. And yeah, I blame the materialist world. I am materialistic, I love buying underwear and records. I don't buy these things now, but I don't like stale underwear, I like pretty underwear and I'm not buying it. It's depressing. And I love buying records. Because I'm depressed I can't even play my music.'*

Ellie's split with Lester followed a long period of negative interaction. She finally asked him to leave when he threatened her son, but she remained in contact. Her account of the separation was inconsistent, oscillating between saying how it made her depressed but how she was hopeful of a reconciliation: '*I wasn't upset, because I thought it isn't finished, because I'm not going to allow it to finish, because on the one hand we've had this relationship of getting to know each other, then all of a sudden you're [Lester] in my house. You're here all day with my son, which I don't think was ever very healthy. So, on the one hand I wanted him out of the house because I think there are things to deal with to make our situation better. I can't do it with him, and I need to sort out my money. I see all the positive sides, Lester doesn't.*' This also shows some contradictoriness in her description – there is confusion over whether she wants Lester to go or stay and whether she has recognised that he has left.

Disorder at follow-up: Ellie described her depression: '*Every day, day and night I was upset and on the brink of tears. I couldn't be cheered up, I was very, very low. I'd even wake up crying.*' She felt hopeless at times: '*I was in despair and could not see a future. I didn't enjoy anything. I didn't want to read or listen to music as usual. I also stopped my writing. It was like that every day.*' She lost weight, was unable to sleep, was agitated and unable to concentrate: '*I couldn't have a conversation on the phone. I couldn't make decisions. I was like that all the time.*' Her depression lasted for nine months.

Comment: Ellie had a high degree of stress in both finances and relationships during the follow-up period but her coping was both helpless and involved denial. Her 'rose-tinted' view of her difficulties showed she had little grasp of the reality of the separation, she had muddled thinking about its cause and solution and poor practical coping to prevent escalation. Her partner's leaving, whilst initiated in part by her, provoked her depression possibly by tapping into her fundamental fear of separation, a basic underpinning of Enmeshed style. Her dependency and fear of being alone, as in her previous partnership, led her to persevere with an inadequate relationship due to her fear of loss and being able to cope alone.

3.4.2 Fiona – Moderately Fearful – onset depression and anxiety

Fiona, aged 43, was married to Terry, with four children of whom the younger two teenagers still lived at home. She worked in a nursery and her husband worked in the media. Her moderately Fearful attachment style was described in the last chapter. Fiona was unable to confide in her husband and had only one friend, Martha, in whom she could confide and was therefore rated only 'some' ability to make and maintain relationships and therefore moderately Insecure. She described her mistrust around others spreading gossip, acknowledged that she kept to herself too much and expressed fear of being let down: '*Underneath I am afraid of being let down. If they knew the sort of person I was they wouldn't like me. They would make fun of my worries and laugh behind my back. It stops me getting close.*' She thus expressed a Fearful attachment profile.

Life events and adversity: Fiona's recent life events included her sister's diagnosis with thyroid cancer and the loss of her own job at the nursery. At three-year follow-up interview Fiona had suffered further stressors, involving violent attacks on her family, which triggered the onset of her depression and anxiety. Her son was stabbed on his way home from work which left him partially disabled. Soon after it happened, whilst she and her husband knew he was not in danger of dying, his considerable blood loss made them concerned about his hospital recovery. She also feared for his safety in case of further attack by gangs in the area.

Fiona's coping response included feelings of helplessness and anger. She also felt upset and guilty that she had been out with a friend when her son was assaulted. It was on her mind constantly although she tended to hide her feelings about it: '*I suppose I felt quite helpless, because when he was in hospital for a week there was nothing I could do.*' She felt angry at the person who stabbed him, but not angry at herself. She remained worried because her son was subsequently unable to work and became withdrawn and cautious about going out. A few weeks after her son's attack, his close friend was also stabbed and killed in the same area, and this made her feel more upset, helpless and pessimistic.

A second event and ensuing difficulty followed when a neighbour assaulted her friend's daughter who was visiting her home. The neighbour was drunk and threw a plate at the child who had to be taken to the emergency hospital department with cuts. In retaliation, Fiona's husband Terry pulled the neighbour over the fence and hit him. Both men were charged by the police, her husband with actual bodily harm (ABH) and the neighbour with ABH on a minor. Fiona and her husband received a letter from the housing authority threatening them with eviction in the event that Terry should be found guilty. They also had to pay £1,500 towards legal costs. Living next door to hostile neighbours was an ongoing daily stressor, as was Terry's lasting symptoms from the injuries sustained.

Coping: Fiona showed good practical coping with the attack on her husband and the associated adversity: '*We've been to court twice, we took out a private summons against the neighbour and Terry has taken one out against next door's wife because she came out with a cosh and started hitting Terry. We've been to Scotland Yard Police Complaints Department because the police didn't listen to anyone in my house.*' She is supportive of her husband and accompanies him to court and has made savings to pay the legal costs. Despite her evident mastery, she did express feelings of helplessness: '*I just feel helpless because it's* *just waiting now. It's just hanging over me. I just feel like we'll pay the money, hope that we win and I'll get the money back. It's very hard to say how optimistic I am.'* She relied on cognitive avoidance by minimising the problem and keeping her feelings to herself: *'I suppose I hide a lot, I mean I am really worried, but I think I've got to be supportive of my husband and so can't show how I feel. I try to put it out of my mind. Sometimes it works.'* Keeping the problem out of mind, however, meant that she did not approach her friend Martha to tell her how she felt.

Disorder: When her son was stabbed Fiona fell into a depression: *'I was crying then and felt very low. I felt very down all the time. I would cry to myself when the others were out. I didn't go out. I didn't want to meet anyone else, didn't take any interest in anything. I just wanted to sit on my own inside.'* Her concentration was poor: *'I couldn't seem to read a newspaper or my books. I couldn't tell you what happened on any TV programme I watched. I couldn't seem to think straight, I couldn't make decisions. I just kept thinking "He could have been killed".'* It affected her sleep: *'I couldn't get to sleep, it would take more than two hours, sometimes late into the night, and then I woke up much earlier than needed. I was tired all the time. I couldn't eat and lost 5 or 6 lbs in weight – I just lost my appetite. It also affected my confidence, I felt really bad about myself, I felt I was worthless, I felt I couldn't even protect my family. I was also irritable – snapping at the children, getting angry at anything.'* It went on for about three months.

Fiona also experienced anxiety, developing social phobia after her son's attack. She described feeling fearful in company: *'I just couldn't face other people. If I had to meet someone new, or go to one of the legal meetings, I just used to get churning in my stomach, I would get sweaty and go hot all over and get a fast heart beat. I dreaded having to meet people. I also stopped seeing friends, I felt I just couldn't face the contact – I would get anxious about even seeing people I knew quite well. I couldn't eat in front of people I didn't know, so I wouldn't go out to restaurants.'*

Comment: Fiona experienced two traumatic events within a relatively short period. These resulted in the onset of both depression and anxiety. Fearful style involves an anxious mistrust about others being rejecting or harmful, and having both her son and her husband attacked confirmed her worst fears. Nevertheless, she showed certain good coping skills but also used cognitive avoidance of the problem, common among those with Fearful style, to reduce the emotional distress. This also effectively limited her ability to seek support and thus provide outside help with emotion-regulation. The events also reduced her self-esteem and belief in the future, thus further consolidating her Fearful style.

3.4.3 Alexa: Markedly Angry dismissive with Generalised Anxiety Disorder

Alexa has already been described in Chapter 2 as having a markedly Angry-dismissive style. Aged 32 at first interview, she was living with her two young children in social housing and was not working. Alexa had a non-live-in partner, from Zimbabwe, who was the father of her children and she was aware that he was involved with another woman.

At first interview she had no support either from her partner or from any other friend. Her style was characterised by angry-mistrust and highly self-reliant ratings. For example she said: '*I'll let people be close to me but I find it hard to be close to them. I've not known really what it is to trust. I wouldn't say I had ever trusted anyone.*' She also said: '*I realised in adolescence and early years that I was on my own – doing things for myself. I was very self-sufficient. I am self-contained.*' She was also very angry, for example: '*I still can't forgive my mother for how she treated me. I get angry when we meet up, and we often row... I still feel very angry about it. I'm reminded of it each time I see her.*'

Life events and adversity: Alexa had experienced a high level of adversity in her adult life. During each of three life phases investigated she was rated for severe adversity in seven different domains and phases. Her most adverse change point followed the break-up of a previous cohabiting relationship when her partner left her for someone else and she felt suicidal and had recurrent depressive episodes. During the study period she experienced difficulties in her relationship with her boyfriend, increasing rows and arguments, culminating in him returning to his wife and separating from Alexa for six months. She also had financial problems, with high credit card debt due to spending on foreign holidays. Another life event involved her flat being burgled and the loss of considerable cash and jewellery for which she was not insured. At follow-up yet another difficulty reported was a time of 'hell' when she had a difficult relationship with a childminder whom she had hunted down and harassed.

Coping: Alexa blamed others for her difficulties, for example she blamed her boyfriend's wife for the ending of the relationship with him, despite being aware that as a married man he might give her up in favour of his wife: '*We were arguing a lot. But that was because she was putting pressure on him. We could have carried on like before. There was no reason for him to leave. He has been in touch with me again and we are getting back together.*' She also directed a lot of anger to the childminder who had let her down on one occasion and with whom she now had ongoing conflict: '*Other people just seem to mess things up for me.*' Alexa also felt a lot of upset, sadness and helplessness regarding her problems: '*I don't see what else I can do. It's always important for me to be in control, but right now I don't seem to be able to be.*' She had no capacity for minimising problems and felt unable to take her mind off her worries. She also felt pessimistic about things improving.

Disorder: Alexa previously had chronic GAD. She was preoccupied with worry most days which she couldn't control: '*I don't allow myself to worry about a specific thing. I try to suppress them all. I spend endless time worrying or* *trying to stop worrying. I never get any housework done.'* Her generalised anxiety was accompanied by being easily fatigued (*'I fall asleep during the day'*), irritability (*'I snap at the children and smack them more'*), muscle tension (*'in my neck, in my back and feet'*) and sleep disturbance (*'I was shaking I was so tired, and falling asleep during the day'*). She also had autonomic anxiety symptoms of trembling, palpitations, sweating, feeling dizzy and nervous tension with exaggerated startle responses. *'This happens when I worry, I felt extremely anxious.'* Her condition had lasted for seven months.

Comment: Alexa dealt with her stressful relationships with anger and blame and lacked practical coping strategies that might have improved her situation. In addition to poor problem tackling, she was unable to see herself as needing help and thus did not seek crisis support. Many of her difficulties seemed to arise as a result of her maladaptive coping and her anger with others. Her attachment profile, involving anger and blame as coping responses, was typical of those with Angry-dismissive style.

3.4.4 Deirdre's Dual (Angry-dismissive and Enmeshed style) and her anxiety disorder

Deirdre's dual attachment style was described in the last chapter. She was a 36-year-old married woman with two children aged 11 and 13. Deirdre and her husband had lost a son, who died in an accident. She was distant but hostile to her husband and had only one confiding relationship with Mary, a friend seen weekly. Her attitudes, characterised by high mistrust and anger, were consistent with Angry-dismissive style but her contradictory comments on self-reliance and desire for company, together with her high fear of separation confirmed a subsidiary Enmeshed style in relation to her children. Her fear of separating from the children coexisted with her high negative interaction with her daughter, indicating a level of ambivalence. She described her daughter as being rude and cheeky since the bereavement and felt angry towards her. When her daughter went to counselling, Deirdre thought she was telling lies about the family to her therapist. She found it difficult to show her any affection and felt angry with her much of the time.

Life events and adversity: The couple had a son who had died three years ago at the age of 12 when he fell through the roof of the school whilst playing out one evening. Deirdre had never really got over his death. She herself was in hospital at the time of the accident and had left her husband and brother in charge of the children and had felt resentful towards them both since. The relationship with her husband was now distant. Before her son's death she had considered leaving him and had had an affair some time prior to this. The only reason she stayed in the relationship was for the sake of her other two children. She would feel too guilty if she left them.

She was seeing a clinical psychologist to help her get over her son's death, but she decided to stop going because she just got more upset each time she went.

Coping: Deirdre's symptoms became exacerbated in the follow-up period by a memorial event which had been held for her son, by his school. She had never felt able to make use of any practical ways of coming to terms with her son's death: '*No, the only thing I've always said is if I could have my son back [I would get better], but I couldn't. I know now I can't have him back.*' She gave up on therapy soon after starting it and was still in denial at some level about the fact that he would not be coming back. She felt helpless: '*I haven't got my son anymore, and that I can't handle. I'm not in control anymore and I do like to be in control. It makes me feel helpless.*' She felt pessimistic: '*Anniversaries get to me, I don't know why. People say it gets better but I don't know, I think it gets worse. I don't think it gets better. People say eventually it gets better – but I don't think time heals – it just makes it more of a reality.*' She tried to avoid thinking about her son: '*But it doesn't work well.*' She blamed her husband and brother for letting it happen on their watch and blamed the school for holding the memorial event which she resented. Whilst she did have a close friend Mary she could go to, she did not want to talk to her at the time of the memorial service and did not seek out any support.

Disorder: Deirdre experienced panic attacks after her son's death and developed GAD, with depression emerging at the follow-up interview after the memorial event. The worry about her children was constant and difficult to control. '*Problems with my daughter growing up, her boyfriends, cars, getting home at the weekend, I'm on tenterhooks. I make her phone when she gets where she's going and when she is due to come back. I worry about my husband. If anything happened to him then I don't think my children would cope. I worry that I might drop dead, then how would my children survive? I'm not in control – I feel completely out of it.*' She also brooded on things: '*If I have something on my mind it will be on my mind for days. I'll sit around instead of doing things – like house-work. I can get nauseous – I can be sick if a really bad anxious attack comes on. I get shaky, my heart pounds, muscles ache, can't breathe, get sweaty.*' She could not get to sleep and then could not get up in the mornings. She took tranquillisers and had been offered counselling which she refused.

Comment: Deirdre was unable to come to terms with her son's death, causing her to fall out with both her partner and her daughter. Additionally her daughter's increasing independence may have been experienced as a further threat of separation. Clearly her loss remained unresolved, and her coping, whilst understandably poor given the highly traumatic circumstances, was particularly characteristic of Angry-dismissive coping style (anger, sadness, blame and helplessness). However, Enmeshed characteristics influenced her level of denial and coloured her interactions with her daughter and her already increased fear of future loss and abandonment was further complicated by her anxiety and depression. The recent memorial service for her son had activated additional grief, and thereby her depression, yet she refused help from psychological services, possibly due to the self-reliant and mistrustful Angry-dismissive part of her style.

The chapter will conclude with examining briefly two more disorders related to attachment style as investigated in the young Offspring study, involving substance abuse and deliberate self-harm (DSH) behaviour. This involves the 146 adolescent and young adult children of the women in the midlife sample. Further details are given in Appendix 1.4 (sample 4).

3.5 Attachment Style Interview and disorder in the London offspring

Whilst space precludes a detailed outline of attachment style and disorder in the 146 mixed gender offspring of the women studied, more details can be found in Bifulco (2008); Schimmenti and Bifulco (2008).

Summary prevalence findings are:

- Four out of 10 of the young people who were the offspring of the high-risk women studied, had a clinical disorder in the year, with equal levels of emotional disorder (depression or anxiety) or substance abuse. DSH in the form of suicidal behaviour or behaviours involving self-cutting, biting or burning or head-banging occurred in a fifth of the young people. Rather more girls than boys had a disorder and there was more emotional disorder and DSH in girls, but no difference in substance abuse rates by gender.
- Nearly half (47%) of the young people had marked or moderate levels of insecurity, a further 23% mild levels of insecurity and 30% were clearly Secure. This is similar to the high-risk mothers. Of the highly Insecure, Fearful was the most common style (14%) the other styles ranging from 7%–10% and Dual/disorganised style 7%.

Figure 3.6 shows the relationship of marked or moderate level of Insecure attachment styles to emotional disorder (depression or anxiety) or substance abuse. It shows:

- Dual/disorganised has equally high rates of both disorders (60%).
- Fearful (60%) and Enmeshed (30%) have highest rate of emotional disorder (p<0.0001) after Dual/disorganised.
- Enmeshed (39%) and Angry-dismissive (30%) have somewhat raised rates of substance abuse, but with Dual/disorganised much the highest rate (p<0.01).
- Dual/disorganised style also related to having more than one disorder concurrently (50% vs 4% in other styles, p<0.0001).

- DSH was highest in those with Angry-dismissive style (50%) followed by Fearful (45%) and Dual/disorganised (40%), this compared with 13% in other styles, p<0.01).

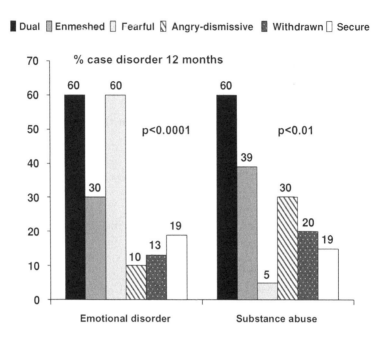

Figure 3.6 Attachment style and disorder in the Offspring sample

Two cases will serve to highlight such links: Felicity with a Fearful style, who had a history of deliberate self-harm behaviour as well as depression, and Dean with a Dual/disorganised style, who had substance abuse.

3.6.1 Felicity's moderately Fearful attachment style and depression with self-harm

Felicity is a 19-year-old young woman living with a friend and working as a telephonist having left school with no qualifications.

Life events: Her very adverse childhood is described in later chapters, and it culminated in running away from home with a violent and criminal boyfriend at age 14, followed by a rape, pregnancy and termination. This left a legacy of emotional and eating disorder. Life events in the last 12 months included her ending her cohabiting relationship following her drug-addicted boyfriend's overdose. This coincided with her brother's suicide attempt in prison. More positive events include Felicity's moving in with her close friend and starting a new job.

Disorder: In addition to episodes of depression from age 13–16, Felicity exhibited deliberate self-harm as a teenager, making three suicide attempts. '*I tried taking tablets once to kill myself, when I was 16. I was at home, took mum's tablets and dad's tablets. I ate loads of them and I was sick. I didn't go to hospital and my parents never knew. A couple of times I tried to slash my wrists, age 15, and twice I tried taking loads of pills. I was not depressed at the time, it was a real spur of the moment thing, really childish. Compared to now I had nothing to worry about.*' Felicity was subsequently referred to a hospital for counselling. She reports depression at interview.

Felicity's moderately Fearful attachment style: Felicity had little support in her ongoing relationships. Her boyfriend was a drug addict, which caused conflict and problems in their relationship. She was unable to confide in him and he was not supportive. She had a friend Carole whom she labelled 'very close', but didn't confide in her. '*We don't see much of each other at the moment – I miss her but I'm pretty independent of her. We get on well – we don't argue.*' She also named Ben, a father of a friend as very close: '*He is away at the moment, so I don't see him. He let me use his flat, he's like a father figure. I do confide in him, although I don't open up completely, but I have talked to him about my depression. I do hold back though. He is supportive. He lets me use his flat when I want a break from my boyfriend, and he lends me money. I could cope without him, but I'd miss him. Sometimes we argue – but he tells me he worries about me.*'

Having only one support figure (Ben) she was rated as having 'some' ability to make and maintain relationships, leading to a 'moderately' Insecure attachment style rating. She had a moderately Fearful attachment style, characterised by mistrust, constraints on closeness and fear of rejection: '*I am suspicious of people. People are out for themselves, they use you. I am cautious of people – you see what they are like. I have been let down by my Mum, by my brother, by my partner and by Carole . . . I try to cope on my own, but sometimes I will ask for help. I feel uncomfortable being close to my partner because he can change his mind so easily. I trust my friends to a certain extent, but I won't let them be as close as him. A lot of the time I can't talk about my feelings of depression. I hold things back from everybody, I'm quite evasive.*' She also reported fear of rejection: '*I can't trust because I have been let down so often. I'm afraid of getting close in case I get hurt. I'm really wary about men. I'm weird – I feel horrible if someone whistles at me. If someone says I'm pretty, it's threatening. Sometimes I can't go near my boyfriend – I can't face him. He gets to me – I can't see why he wants to be with me. I want to be by myself.*'

Comment: Felicity's traumatic teenage experience was reflected in her various emotional disorders. Unstable elements in her life included involvement with a drug-addict partner and criminal brother, which made it more likely that she would experience severe life events such as those in the last year. Her Fearful attachment style might have been the result of the rape and termination in teenage years, but may also go back to earlier maltreatment from parents (described in Chapter 6). It has made her intensely mistrustful, this expressed as fear of others, rather than anger. Her coping style was self-blaming. She tried to get her life back on track through her work, through leaving her drug-addict boyfriend and distancing herself from her family. This was helped by her friend Ben who helped her with support and accommodation. She had very low self-esteem as indicated in the description above.

The next case study looks at stress and substance abuse in a young man who was also in the London Offspring study.

3.6.2 Dean's Dual/disorganised style and substance abuse

Dean is aged 29, unemployed and lives alone, surviving on benefits and criminal activity. He has recently split up with his girlfriend. He had two children by previous girlfriends but has had no contact with his children or previous partners. His childhood is described in later chapters.

Disorder: Dean had a history of substance abuse from the age of 12 when he began drinking heavily, using cannabis and abusing solvents. By age 15 he was using heroin and crack cocaine. His substance abuse worsened in the recent period after his girlfriend left. He took cannabis, cocaine, magic mushrooms, ecstasy and speed for over three weeks and spent over £1,000: '*Drink and drugs, drink and drugs, going to work, going to the pub, having a few pints, take a little bit of speed, then something else . . . I spent a month drinking. I didn't avoid friends, I drank with them. It made me tired all the time, but I did sleep. I didn't have to drink a lot more for the same effect. I felt in control. If I didn't want to drink I wouldn't, so if I didn't enjoy it I wouldn't do it.*' He reported no withdrawal symptoms, no seizures or no shakes. He was restless, however: '*I'm always hyperactive, everything I've done I've done with a little bit of extra pace. I'm not really that susceptible to drugs. I've never really had any withdrawal symptoms. Cannabis does not get me high. It calms me and stops me from having serious road rages when I'm driving.*'

Attachment Style Interview support: Dean had no close confidants and only one friend: '*We were glue sniffing partners, partners in crime, fighting partners . . . but I never ever told him anything*'. He never confided in his girlfriend when they were together and was possessive and aggressive towards her. He was rated very low on ability to make and maintain relationships with a 'markedly' Insecure attachment style. His profile showed both Angry-dismissive and Enmeshed aspects, and hence Dual/disorganised style.

Dean's Angry-dismissive and Enmeshed Attachment attitudes: Dean's Angry-dismissive style involved high mistrust of others: '*I am suspicious and find it hard to trust anyone. I only listen to 50 per cent of what somebody tells me and I won't* *even believe that unless I hear it from the horse's mouth.'* He also had high constraints on closeness: '*I never go to a friend with problems. If I'm down I do it on my own. I just go and get drunk! I've been in the most extreme positions and not asked anyone for help. Sometimes having someone close is important and sometimes it can be a pain in the neck. I like having someone around at first and then I don't like it as much as when they weren't around.'* His self-reliance was rated as high: '*I haven't relied on anyone since childhood.'* He felt in control of his life: '*Yeah, very much so, even though I'm not.'* He had high anger: '*I'm a very paranoid person. I do get into arguments, I can't help it. I'm not argumentative on the whole but sometimes people will say things to me that touch me the wrong way, or they will say something and sometimes it will head to a fight, with people in the pub or at home. If I've got something to say I'll say it. I wouldn't sit back and not say anything . . . the odd time when the police have been involved I said it was nothing to do with me. It was not because I'd been drinking. My girlfriend didn't like my drinking. It didn't cause a problem for me and I said to her "if it is causing a problem with you, then don't be there when I have a drink. You don't have to come out and drink with me".'* He was very hostile to his stepmother and had been violent to her as well as to his girlfriend and had 'road rage' when out driving.

However, Dean also had anxious elements to his profile, categorised as Enmeshed involving a high need for company and high fear of separation. His desire for company was considered 'contradictory' having both high and low elements. He described himself as sociable and 'enjoys being with friends'. However, he also liked spending time alone and it could be a nuisance having somebody around all the time. He didn't want to see friends more often. He also commented: '*I do get very jealous and worry about girlfriends going off. I don't allow them to have friends – particularly men friends. It's always in the back of my mind that something might be going on.'* His desire for company was rated as 'contradictory', both craving company and also being irritated by it. His fear of separation was high: '*Yeah, I do worry if someone is back late. If it's pre-arranged then I'm not so bad but if not then I start asking questions and worry about them, yeah. If my girlfriend hadn't called when she said, or if she was late, I would start getting angry. I'd want to know where she was. If she did turn up here safe I'd want to know where she had been and who she had been with if she hadn't called . . . I start getting angry. I want to know where she is and start getting the hump. If she did turn up here safe I want to know why!'*

Comment: Dean's very poor ability to make supportive relationships denote a 'markedly' Insecure attachment style and his attitudes show a mixed pattern of Dual/disorganised style. The anger showed itself in early teenage years and was accompanied by conduct disorder. He was violent to his stepmother and as a result was put into residential care, and had been violent to more than one girlfriend. The pattern of disorganised attachment style thus links to violent behaviour as described in the research literature. Consistent with the analysis in this chapter, such style is also associated with substance abuse.

The findings presented in this chapter are summarised below:

Summary of Attachment Style Interview prevalence and demographics

- In the adult sample of women, Secure attachment style was found for nearly half (49%) the comparison women, another third had mildly Insecure style and 19% marked/moderately Insecure styles with 4% Dual/disorganised styles. In high-risk women rates of Insecure style were more or less double.
- Angry-dismissive style was three times more common in high-risk women and Enmeshed nearly twice as common. Fearful was the most common style affecting a quarter of women in both groups.
- Insecure styles were higher among those working class, among mothers and those from BME backgrounds. Anxious styles were more common among working class and those married/cohabiting with Avoidant more common among BME women.

Attachment Style Interview, adversity and life events

- In sample 1A (the 105 women studied to examine Coping) those with Insecure attachment styles had higher rates of prior adult life adversity. The effects were strongest for those with Fearful, Enmeshed and Dual/disorganised styles.
- Those with Withdrawn style and those Secure or mildly Insecure had low rates of prior adversity.
- Those with Insecure attachment style had an increased risk of experiencing a severe life event in the 12 month follow-up. Those with Enmeshed or Angry-dismissive styles were most at risk. Finance/housing, or relationships were most common events in those Insecure.
- Those with Insecure attachment style more likely to have a 'matching difficulty' severe event, known to be much more highly linked to onset of depression. This was particularly prominent in those with Angry-dismissive styles.

Attachment Style Interview and coping

- When coping with crises was examined at follow-up, Insecure attachment style at first interview was significantly correlated with negative coping strategies including inferred denial, cognitive avoidance, helplessness, blame of others, anger and sadness.
- Predicted associations included Anxious styles and self-blame, helplessness; and Angry-dismissive styles and anger and blame.

- Unexpected findings were the association of Anxious styles (Fearful and Enmeshed) to cognitive avoidance and denial, respectively. Also Angry-dismissive style to high levels of sadness. Dual/disorganised styles showed no particular patterning.
- Withdrawn style was unrelated to any negative coping, as was Secure or mildly Insecure style.

The findings in relation to clinical disorder are also summarised:

Summary of attachment style and clinical disorder

- Insecure attachment style was significantly related to 12-month depression. The more Insecure the style the higher the rate of depression, showing a dose-response effect. The rate among those with marked or moderate level insecurity had double the rate of those with mildly Insecure or Secure style.
- All Insecure styles apart from Withdrawn had high rates of depression (38%–41%). Women with Withdrawn styles were not significantly different from those Secure.
- Women with highly Insecure styles had double the rate of lifetime chronic or recurrent depression and teenage depression than women with mildly Insecure or Secure styles.
- When controls were applied for ethnicity and class, the relationship between Insecure attachment style and depression was unchanged.
- The relationship between Insecure attachment style and depression held prospectively for those followed-up an average three years later. It also related to onset of case anxiety, particularly GAD and social phobia.
- A significant relationship was found between Fearful style and social phobia and Angry-dismissive style and GAD.
- No particular patterning of depression or anxiety was found for those adults with Dual/disorganised styles.
- In young people, Dual/disorganised and Anxious attachment styles (Enmeshed or Fearful) related to emotional disorder (depression or anxiety).
- Dual/disorganised was most strongly related to substance abuse. It also related to comorbid or dual disorders.
- DSH was highest in those Angry-dismissive as well as Fearful and Dual/disorganised.

3.7 Discussion

This chapter has considered adult attachment style in terms of its prevalence, demographic correlates and its association with stress and psychological disorder. Findings are consistent with those in the research literature – whilst half the unselected groups studied had Secure style, an additional third had mildly Insecure style and nearly a fifth the more problematic 'marked-moderate' insecurity of style. This echoes rates found in the TCS-PND project. Such Insecure style relates to markers of disadvantage such as lower social class, BME status, financial hardship as well as higher lifetime adversity and more frequent recent severe life events. Such events involved both relationships and finance. Thus those with Insecure attachment style are shown to experience more stressors. They also coped poorly with such events, with helpless, avoiding, blame attribution and negative emotional responses evident. Insecure attachment style (with the exception of Withdrawn style) was highly related to emotional disorder, both depression and anxiety.

The analysis has served to highlight some of the associations anticipated in the stress model as summarised in Figure 3.7. Whilst much of the patterning of coping style with attachment style was consistent with profiles, the relationship of avoidant strategies (cognitive avoidance or inferred denial) with Anxious attachment styles (Enmeshed or Fearful) is of interest. This is because usually Anxious styles are considered hyperactivating and Avoidant styles deactivating. This is the pattern observed with relationship approach and avoidance. But underlying this, the Anxious styles appear to be deactivating in their appraisal of stress in order to reduce their emotional responses. This is consistent with the fact that all the Insecure styles have poor support-seeking. Failure to confide about problems allows avoidant cognitive strategies to remain in place. Confiding involves recognition and communication of stress and need.

The Anxious styles of Enmeshed and Fearful style related to depression, with Fearful style also relating to social phobia in both adult and offspring samples. Perhaps surprisingly, the Avoidant style of Angry-dismissive was highly related both to depression and to anxiety (GAD), but only in the adult women. Dual/disorganised attachment style related to emotional disorder, but with no higher rate than in the single Insecure styles. In the young sample the Anxious styles (Enmeshed and Fearful) and Angry-dismissive related to lifetime deliberate self-harm, with Dual/disorganised style relating to substance abuse, as well as multiple disorder concurrently.

Withdrawn style showed indications of being a more resilient style with lower rate of stressors, better coping and less disorder in the London women. Similarly, 'mild' levels of Insecure styles were unrelated to disorder and as with Secure style, may confer resilience. This also held in the Offspring sample. Thus the distinctions made in categorising Avoidant styles in the ASI, has proved critical, and the conflating of Angry-dismissive

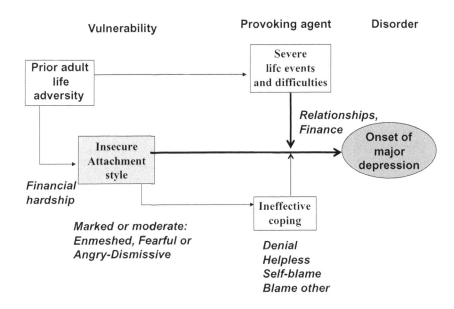

Figure 3.7 Attachment style and stress model

and Withdrawn in other measures may account for inconsistencies in the research literature. This is because all the styles apart from Withdrawn relate to stressors or disorder. In the adults, Angry-dismissive style was highly related both to depression and anxiety, and in the young sample it related to deliberate self-harm. In contrast Withdrawn style was unrelated to any disorder. Both these styles have high self-reliance and low need for closeness, the difference lies in the mistrust and anger of the former. Unlike Withdrawn style, Angry-dismissive style is a highly emotional style where the argumentative involvement with others exists with overly high self-sufficiency. Individuals with Angry-dismissive style have high levels of recent stressors, and their crisis coping not only includes anger and blame of others, but also sadness and helplessness. It can be speculated that such anger is a defence against anxiety, which shows itself in GAD. When attachment has been examined in relation to conflict resolution, anger is argued to underpin helplessness and guilt in close relationships (Rholes, Simpson *et al.* 1998). Such anger is thought to spring from resentment towards childhood attachment figures that resurfaces in close adult relationships. Bowlby describes two types of anger in this context: 'functional' anger expressed to maintain the bond when the close other has been neglectful or inattentive, and 'dysfunctional' anger, the principle aim of which is malice or revenge. This latter becomes so intense and persistent that it alienates the close other (Bowlby 1973). Thus dysfunctional anger may well characterise that found in very markedly Angry-dismissive styles, but also in Dual/disorganised styles such as in Dean's case. His anger and violence fuelled by his substance abuse, but was not fully recognised by him, indicating some possible dissociation linked with this style. Withdrawn style has a completely opposite profile, with high self-reliance but none of the anger and with no associated poor coping strategies. Clearly differentiating these two styles is critical to research investigations and clinical practice.

The origins of 'mild' levels of Insecure attachment style also needs to be considered. At these levels there is no association with disorder, stress or poor coping. One possible interpretation is that insecurity at higher levels may be activated and maintained by chronic interpersonal stressors. The samples reported here had particularly high rates of interpersonal difficulties both lifetime and recent. Thus expression of attachment style may involve a more dynamic relationship to an adverse social environment than is generally acknowledged or documented. Conversely if those with Insecure attachment style find themselves in more benign settings with sympathetic support figures then their levels of insecurity may reduce as their confiding behaviour increases. Clearly complex and dynamic models are implied.

The next chapter will look more closely at partner and support relationships and self-esteem as additional elements in the attachment-style profiles.

4   Relationships and self-esteem

4.0 Introduction

This chapter will focus on investigating the quality of adult relationships and the association between attachment styles, support and features of problem relationships involving conflict or apathy. A primary focus will be on the partner relationship as the likely main attachment figure in adulthood, including past partner relationships, and those involving domestic violence. Reference will also be made to other supportive relationships, which can include both family members or friends. A self-esteem measure will be used to determine whether Insecure attachment styles relate to negative views of the self and how this contributes to risk of disorder. Details of the analysis can be found elsewhere (Bifulco, Moran *et al.* 2002b), but new analyses of domestic violence are presented.

4.1 Background

A key precept of attachment theory, as already outlined in introductory chapters, is that an Insecure style will impede the ability to make supportive close relationships in adult life. Indeed, this aspect of attachment theory has underpinned the construction of the ASI, in which security is predicated on being able to form close adult attachments. Attachment style has implications for the success of partner relationships, close friendships and family relationships as well as for family stability and a caring parenting context, explored in the following chapters. Distortions of the internal working models developed from childhood inform expectations of mistrust, rejection, hostility or unreliability of other people and these in turn affect how an individual will relate to those expected to be close. The manner of relating (for example whether involving anxious, hostile or detached elements) will vary depending on the particular distortions to the cognitive-affective templates determining insecurity of style. These will have influenced the choice of partner or friend and the attitudes and behaviours brought to the interaction. As a result, some close relationships will involve conflict, others indifference or apathy, and in some instances individuals will avoid relationships altogether and be socially isolated. These aspects are all argued to be associated with Insecure attachment styles but patterns involving particular styles to particular relating patterns and experiences will be sought.

In parallel with internal working models influencing perceptions of others, exist internal working models of the self which influence the extent of self-acceptance and feelings of self-worth. Bowlby (1973) identified two key facets in the development of Secure attachment – that the self is perceived as worthy of love and attention, and that others are viewed as warm and responsive. The two develop together with children developing representations of attachment that allow them to predict and interpret the behaviour of attachment figures and view themselves in relation to others. Such working models serve as templates for the interpretation of later relationships throughout the lifespan as well as attitudes towards the self. Thus early relationships with parents and key others in childhood exert long-term impact on subsequent relationships and the self by affecting the nature and development of cognitive models.

The seeking of support from close and trusted others at time of threat or danger is argued to regulate negative emotions and increase feelings of security and keep a level of equilibrium and wellbeing. At times of threat, stress, pain or illness attachment behaviour in the child is aimed at seeking and maintaining proximity to the caregiver (Bowlby 1973). This provides the 'safe haven' function of attachment relationships. In adulthood the same need exists for proximity seeking to those who we look to for support and care. Absent or unpredictable support or angry critical response reduces feelings of security and thus can predispose to emotional disorder (Bowlby 1977; Holmes 1993). In adults the behaviour is similar, although support figures or partners are those first approached to provide the emotional help needed.

Given that this book focuses on a psychosocial model of attachment, as well as the psychological elements involved in relationships, we need to also consider the social environment and the barriers which limit the choice of close relationships. Environments too have trajectories, and a child forced out of a hostile or neglectful home may find scant support in his or her hostile or barren surroundings, only to find attachment with similarly damaged people, with the resulting relationship patterns dictated by others' psychopathology and lack of material resources. Thus meeting the first partner in teenage years in a hostel, or choosing friends among those socially excluded, for example from drug subcultures, can have long-term effects on the life course.

4.2 Support

Any real or perceived obstacle to proximity-maintenance is argued in attachment theory to result in anxiety which in turn triggers attachment behaviours designed to re-establish proximity. The establishment and maintenance of proximity engender feelings of security and love, whereas disruptions in the relationship cause anxiety or anger and sadness (Hazan and Shaver 1994). As long as an individual experiences felt security, the attachment system is acquiescent and emotions are regulated. Unlike infants, adults do not require daily contact for their relationships to confer security. The secure adult can hold the other in mind, with the knowledge that the other will respond when needed. But when assessing support from adults, it is important to determine the frequency of contact to differentiate those relationships idealised with a fantasy level of closeness and confiding despite little actual contact. Behavioural evidence can help differentiate these from truly supportive relationships. Establishing actual contact, as well as actual confiding and positive interaction can attempt to base such experiences in reality.

Individuals' with Insecure attachment styles report poor marital functioning, communication and problem-solving (Kobak and Hazan 1991), low flexibility and reciprocity in confiding (Mikulincer and Nachshon 1991) and low support-seeking in situations where anxiety increases (Simpson, Rholes *et al.* 1992). Insecure styles are associated with low self-esteem (McCarthy 1999; Murphy and Bates 2000) supporting the model of negative attitudes to self as a central feature of attachment classification (Griffin and Bartholomew 1994). Among women with adverse childhood experience, Insecure attachment style relates not only to poorer functioning in partner relationships but also to the presence of a 'deviant' partner with antisocial or problem behaviour (McCarthy 1999).

Few would doubt that having a close and supportive relationship with a partner will increase wellbeing and reduce the likelihood of severe stress responses. Yet many couples experience relationships without such support and many have little stability in interaction, and are at risk of separation. There can be numerous social reasons for problems in relationships including those emanating from the partner's behaviour (such as psychiatric disorder) or partner's stressors (such as unemployment) or stressors common to both (teenage child's antisocial behaviour). The resulting difficulties are not necessarily due to partner's Insecure attachment style. However, the presence of such a style is more likely to escalate stress through lack of mutual support, poor emotion-regulation and poor coping strategies.

Of course not all support comes from partner relationships. Adults also form close relationships with peers as well as retaining support from adult family or friends has attracted rather less focus. Reciprocal supportive relationships can ideally be formed although the function of close attachments to adult family or friends and this area has attracted rather less focus in attachment style research. However, one study of 100 adults grouped by the presence or absence of a romantic relationship examined peer-orientation in both proximity seeking and safe-haven behaviours (Zeifman and Hazan

2008). Most reported a preference for spending time with and seeking emotional support from their friends as well as partners. Other studies have focused on peer friendships and attachment style in young adults finding significant correlations between the young people's attachment relationships with family and with peers (Bartholomew and Horowitz 1991).

Poor support from partner or other close persons is well-documented as a vulnerability factor for onset of major depression (Brown and Bifulco 1985; Bifulco, Brown *et al.* 1988; Brown, Bifulco *et al.* 1990c). The vulnerability/provoking agent model of depression described earlier shows that deficiencies in support from close relationships gives reduced resistance to the impact of major stressors and hastens episodes of disorder. This is seen to work through two routes: first the longer-term erosion of self-esteem through the chronic lack of close supportive others, and second through the acute lack of support at the time of crises, which is correlated with reduced coping opportunities (Bifulco and Brown 1996).

Previous findings, in a representative sample of 400 London women (Brown and Bifulco 1985; Brown, Andrews *et al.* 1986) using the same support scales to assess VCO as in the ASI, found that whilst 44% of women had a VCO who was also a confidant; remaining women either had no one identified as VC (21%) or their VCO was not a confidant (35%). VCOs were equally likely to be relatives or friends, but most were female. Lacking a confiding VCO was predictive of future depression for single mothers. For married/cohabiting women a partner relationship that lacked confiding was more predictive. Nearly three-quarters (71%) of women had a close supportive relationship with their partners but a quarter (28%) described highly negative interactions (Brown, Andrews *et al.* 1986). Amongst those with problem partner relationships half reported high levels of negative interaction and half reported indifferent or apathetic relationships. Negative interaction with partner proved a potent vulnerability factor for new onset of depression studied prospectively (Brown, Bifulco *et al.* 1990c). In the same sample, domestic violence was experienced by 25% of the women over a lifetime (Andrews and Brown 1988). This was related to prior teenage pregnancy and childhood neglect (rather than abuse). These factors were also associated with a longer period in the violent partner relationships. Women experiencing marital violence were more likely to have had clinical depression and to have low self-esteem when interviewed.

A study of London couples using the same measures of marital and support relationships as used in the ASI, showed similar findings for men and women. Thus 68% of husbands had good supportive relationships with their wives and 62% of the women reported good relationships with their husbands (Edwards, Nazroo *et al.* 1998). For both men and women, around 30% with poor support had an onset of depression compared with the 10% norm, the increased effect on disorder being higher in men. For women with a good partner relationship who did not receive the expected crisis support from the partner at the time of a severe life event, risk of depression was increased. In terms of gender difference, women expressed more need for emotional support than men and were more likely to seek support from family or friends outside the marriage which also served to protect against depression (op cit).

Similar findings on support were shown in a Portuguese study of couples expecting a baby using the same support measures from the ASI (Condé, Figueirido *et al.* 2011). Equal rates of poor support were found for women (24%) and men (25%) but with 60% of pairs having good support rated by both partners. Poor support for one of the partners was found in a third of couples with 10% having poor support in both members. In this sample it was only in men that poor support was associated with self-reported depression or anxiety symptoms (Condé, Figueirido *et al.* 2011).

Whilst it could be argued that supportive relationships are in many ways alike, those unsupportive show different characteristics. The degree of unsupportiveness where there is low level confiding, can be categorised on the basis of apathy and lack of felt closeness or conflict and negative interaction. Feelings of attachment can be rated independently of actual support received and may be high even when the relationship is poor. Individuals may feel a need to stay in a violent or empty relationship due to a strong emotional dependence on their partner and may report feeling lost without such an unreliable and even dangerous other. Such dependency needs may be based on an idealised evaluation of what the relationship offers, or a pessimistic view of other options, which may keep the individual in a relationship when little objective pleasure or support, or safety, is gained from remaining together. Felt Attachment is thus subjective and often reflects the individual's high need for attachment even when there is evidence that the relationship described is unrewarding, uncaring or hostile.

Another route than that provided by poor support, occurs from crises which arise from the difficult relationships themselves. It is now well-established that a high proportion of the severe life events which provoke episodes of depression involve crises in close relationships (Brown, Bifulco *et al.* 1987). Women who are vulnerable to such events are those with low self-esteem who additionally have conflict with partner or lack any outside support (Brown, Bifulco *et al.* 1990c). Such interpersonal vulnerabilities can be seen as potentially a result of insecurity of attachment. The links between conflict and poor support in relationships common to depression models therefore need to be examined in terms of type of attachment style to see if these follow predictable patterns of hostile and distant relating.

4.3 Domestic violence

Given the importance of partner relationships in attachment security, the issue of domestic violence needs to be examined in an attachment context.

Violence from a partner is common, affecting one in four women during their lifetime, 8% in any one year (Andrews and Brown 1988), and accounting for 18% of all violent incidents reported to the police in the UK (Dobash and Dobash 1992). The health consequences for victims are considerable: high proportions incur physical injury and chronic health difficulties and substantial long-term mental health problems including suicide. Risks to children are also high. Yet reporting of domestic violence is notoriously low with the British Crime Survey (2000) describing it as a largely hidden crime, significantly under-reported and with only 5% of reported cases resulting in conviction. Barriers to reporting to services can be due to fear of retaliation or abandonment, feelings of loyalty, dissociative amnesia for the abusive episodes, stigma and a number of other social or psychological constraints. Understanding the attachment underpinnings of such relationships will help inform interventions in this area. Yet research on victims of domestic violence and attachment theory is still relatively undeveloped (Henderson, Bartholomew *et al.* 1997; Morgan and Shaver 1999).

One of Bowlby's key observations was that the strength of an attachment bond is unrelated to the quality of the attachment relationship. As in childhood where an abused child can retain a strong attachment and need for proximity to an abusing parent, so in adult abusive relationships the victim can be strongly attached to the abusive partner. This is in part because threat and fear activate the attachment system and this can serve to strengthen the bond, even when the attachment figure is the source of threat. Feelings of abandonment may emerge even in leaving a threatening partner. Also, the partner may also be idealised and the violence incorrectly associated with strength, and thus security. Leaving abusive partnerships can be hampered by an expectation of similar bad treatment in other relationships, particularly if the victim feels to blame for the abuse.

In terms of the perpetrators attachment needs, Bowlby viewed interpersonal anger as arising from frustrated attachment needs and functioning as a form of protest directed at maintaining or regaining contact with the attachment figure (Bowlby 1982; Bartholomew, Henderson *et al.* 2001). Such protest can range from verbal abuse of the attachment figure, to control over their behaviour or to violence. In attachment terms such abusive behaviour is likely to be precipitated by real or imagined threats of rejection, separation or abandonment by the partner. In individuals with problematic early attachment experience, perception of ambiguous behaviour by the partner as rejecting or unsupportive can make for dangerous partnerships. There is a large body of literature suggesting physically abusive men are Insecure, overly dependent on their partners and that jealousy and fear of separation are common triggers of abusive episodes (Dutton 1995; Bartholomew, Henderson *et al.* 2001). Women too can perpetrate violence although less often than males, and more often in situations where both partners are violent. There is, however, less research on the typology of women perpetrators than males.

Physical aggression among cohabiting and married partners tends to be predicted by an interaction between the perpetrator's Anxious attachment and the partner's Avoidance. Anxiety is argued to be linked to aggression only if the partner is Avoidant, establishing a pattern of fear of abandonment in one partner and fear of intimacy in the other (Roberts and Noller 1998). Anxious style is linked to more severe long-term effects on the victim (e.g. loss of confidence and self-esteem) with Avoidant style linked to more severe long-term effects on the relationship (distrust and dislike of partner) and weakening of the bond (Feeney, 2007). A study of attachment style in 41 couples presenting to clinics due to marital discord issues (Bond and Bond 2004) showed the combination of Anxious styles in females and Avoidant (dismissive) styles in males was a potent predictor of violence. The longer duration of the marriage and poor problem-solving communication added power to the prediction. Marital interaction, influenced by couples' attachment styles and problem-solving communication, is thus a significant factor in marital partners experiencing and perpetuating physical violence.

Another study examined self-identified reasons for women returning to abusive relationships among women living in a refuge (Griffing, Ragin *et al.* 2002). The results indicated that participants appeared to underestimate their likelihood of returning to the violent relationship. Participants with a history of past separations were significantly more likely to indicate that they might return to the abuser because of their continued attachment. Those who considered returning because of their emotional attachment to the abuser were significantly more likely to have done so for this reason in the past.

4.4 Self-esteem

The relationship of self-esteem to attachment style has been outlined in the introductory chapter. As already described, the perception of the self is also viewed as an internal working model and one directly connected to that governing attachment style and perception of others. The most developed approach is that by Kim Bartholomew and colleagues identifying the styles most related to positive or negative view of self or other (Bartholomew and Horowitz 1991). In this scheme, Fearful is the style which has negative perception of both self and other; with Anxious (Enmeshed) a negative view of self alone and Avoidant (Dismissive) a negative view of others alone. Secure involves having a positive view of self and others. (Disorganised style was not identified as a category). Related to this is the investigation of mentalising, of which self-reflective function is the inward-looking ability to identify mental states. Here Disorganised style is highlighted to reflect the introjection of an identified 'alien' malignant self derived from the abusive parent (Allen and Fonagy 2006). If this is also expressed as negative self-evaluation, then high rates would be expected amongst those with Disorganised style.

Negative evaluation of self is highly related to onset of depression when measured prospectively (Brown, Andrews *et al.* 1986) and highly related to an index of problem relationships (poor support, negative interaction with partner or child) (Brown, Bifulco *et al.* 1990c). These together were shown to provide the best vulnerability predictors of new onsets of depression (Brown, Andrews *et al.* 1990). The expectation in the following analysis is that negative evaluation of self will relate to poorer quality of relationships and to Insecure attachment styles, particularly those Anxious or Disorganised.

Issues of partner and support relationships as well as domestic violence and self-esteem will now be examined in the London midlife sample of women (sample 1).

4.5 The London study findings

The women were questioned about their partner and other supportive relationships. Of course, given that the ASI includes partner and VCO relationships in its profiling of Insecure attachment style, there is a danger of circularity in showing those Insecure have worse relationships. However, the aim is to compare across styles to see the nature of the problem relationships, and whether these involve conflict or apathy in the expected directions as well as to see if these extend to prior partner relationships not part of the ongoing ASI assessment.

4.5.1 Very Close Other support

The supportive context of the women studied was examined in terms of close confidant support. Just over a quarter of the women (29%) had *no* close confidant seen at least monthly. See Figure 4.1 for VCO support characteristics. Findings are summarised here:

- Overall attachment style was correlated with the lack of any one confiding VCO (0.38, p<0.001). Of those with 'marked' or 'moderate' level Insecure attachment style 72% had no confiding VCO vs 13% of those Secure/mildly Insecure, (p<0.0001).
- Highest rates for lack of a confiding VCO were found among those Withdrawn (69%) closely followed by Dual/disorganised (60%), then Fearful (57%) and then Angry-dismissive (54%). Those with Enmeshed style had much lower rates of poor VCO support (29%) but still double the rate amongst those Secure (13%, p<0.0001).
- However lacking a confiding VCO did not relate to depression, although a trend was evident in single mothers where 35% lacking a confiding VCO became depressed vs 25% of the remainder (p<0.09).

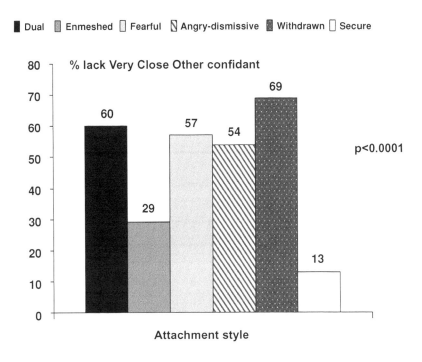

Figure 4.1 Very Close Other support and attachment style

4.5.2 Partner relationships

Examining partner relationships in the adult sample showed:

- Half of the women studied (52%) had been separated from a cohabiting partner at some point in the past.
- Insecure attachment style was significantly more common in those who were single mothers (27%) than those in partnerships or single without children (15%, p<0.005).
- Half of those with a partner reported poor partner support and 35% reported high negative interaction in the relationship.

The relationship of marital status to individual attachment styles can be seen in Figure 4.2. To summarise:

- Those with Enmeshed or Angry-dismissive styles were most likely to have a live-in partner (71% and 73%, respectively).

- Women with Fearful styles were least likely to have a live-in partner (42%, p<0.07), but most likely to be single parents (38%) (more than double the rate among other women, p<0.001).
- Those women with a Dual/disorganised style were most likely to have been separated (72%) from a partner compared with 49% of others (p<0.05) and those with Withdrawn style the least likely (41%) to be separated from a partner.

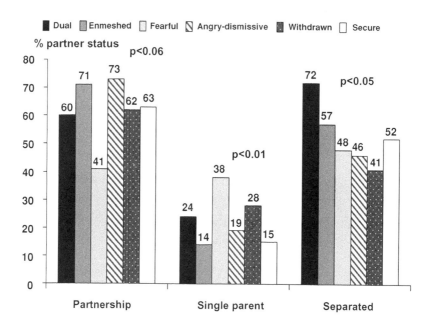

Figure 4.2 Marital status and attachment style

Of adult women in this sample who were in a partnership, just under half (44%) had poor partner support as denoted by lack of confiding and active emotional response. Poor partner support (see Figure 4.3) was related to:

- Any highly Insecure attachment style of the woman (75% Insecure had poor partner support compared with 46% of those with Secure/mildly Insecure style, p<0.001).
- Dual/disorganised (80%), Enmeshed (90%) and Withdrawn (83%) styles.
- Partner conflict was highest in those with Enmeshed (70%) and Angry-dismissive (53%) styles.

- Lowest partner conflict was for those with Withdrawn (33%) or Secure (23%) styles (p<0.001).
- For 'indifferent' or apathetic partner relationships, Withdrawn style had the highest rate (50% compared with 22% for remaining women, p<0.025).

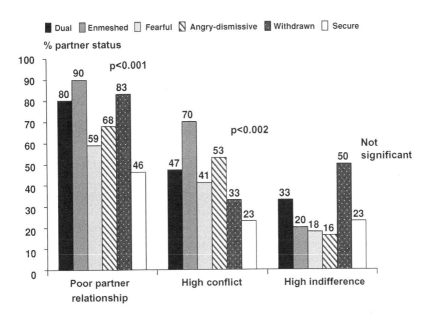

Figure 4.3 Partner support and attachment style

When ethnicity was examined it was apparent that those from BME backgrounds were more likely to be single parents (53% vs. 18%, p<0.001) and generally less likely to be cohabiting (32% vs 63%, p<0.007) but no more likely to be separated/divorced. However, when in a partner relationship, women from BME backgrounds were less likely to have poor support (26% vs 36% of other women, p<0.017) or partner conflict (11% vs 21% of other women, p<0.05).

4.5.3 Problem partners

A history of previous partnerships of at least 6 months' duration was collected with the ALPHI measure of adversity to look at incidence of domestic violence. The ALPHI marital domain questions about domestic violence with additional questions about the level of force used, the nature of the attacks and their frequency. The scale of violence was rated and only severe level of attack was included in the following analysis (e.g. threat to life, serious attack with possibility of multiple injuries or repeated assault with an implement or kicked or punched) with 20% of women reporting violence at such levels. Of these, 15% experienced violence from more than one partner. In addition, partners' probable antisocial behaviour was assessed (score of three or more of impulsiveness, recklessness, lack of remorse, deceitfulness, consistent irresponsibility, failure to conform to social norms and aggression). Again, a fifth of women reported at least one partner with such characteristics. Women were also asked about their partner's treated psychiatric disorder (including substance abuse), and convicted criminal record with 21% reported. Partner violence was significantly correlated with partner antisocial behaviour (0.45, p<0.0001) and his treated psychiatric disorder or convicted criminal behaviour (0.32, p<0.0001).

The following findings emerged for prior domestic violence:

- Partner violence was more common among those working class (27% vs 15% in other women (p<0.02).
- It was more common among women who were single mothers at interview (41% vs 14% among other women, p<0.0001).
- There was a somewhat raised rate among BME women (32% vs 19% of other women) but this was not statistically significant.
- Having had a partner who was violent did not relate to the woman's depression in the 12-month period but did relate to chronic or recurrent lifetime depression (48% vs 35% amongst those with no violence, p<0.05). Also the number of violent partners correlated with the number of lifetime cases of depression (0.12, p<0.03).
- The presence of a violent partner related to lifetime suicide plans or suicide attempts (31% vs 18% of women with no violent partner, p<0.02). The rate of suicidal behaviour increased with the number of violent partners (18%, 26%, 50% and 67% for 0, 1, 2, or 3 violent partners, respectively, p<0.03).

Domestic violence and attachment style were related (see Figure 4.4). The findings showed:

- Women with Insecure attachment style had twice the rate of current or prior partner violence (28% vs 13% in other women, p<0.001) and five times the rate of partner with antisocial behaviour (21% vs 5%, p<0.001). However, they were not significantly more likely to have had a partner with clinical disorder or criminal behaviour (24% vs 18%).
- Violence from a partner was highest amongst those women with an Enmeshed style (43%) but there were raised rates among all Insecure styles except Withdrawn (p<0.009).

- Having a partner with antisocial behaviour was highest among those with Dual/disorganised style (36%) followed by those Angry-dismissive (27%).
- Having had a partner with psychiatric disorder or criminal record were found most often amongst those with Dual/disorganised (36%) or Fearful (31%) style.

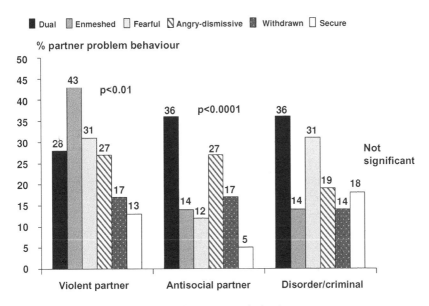

Figure 4.4 Attachment style by problem partner behaviour

4.5.4 Negative Evaluation of Self

Low self-esteem was measured by means of an index of three scales measuring negative evaluation of personal attributes (such as intelligence, attractiveness), negative evaluation of role competencies (e.g. in partner, parent or work role) or overall lack of self-acceptance. These 4-point scales were dichotomised into high (marked or moderate) and low (some, little/none) and then the presence of any high level in any one of the three scales taken to denote NES. This is consistent with prior analyses described elsewhere (Brown, Andrews *et al.* 1990).

Among the midlife London women half scored on the NES index. NES related to lower social class: 42% working class had NES compared with 31% of middle class (p<0.02). It was also associated with a higher lifetime adversity score: 57% of those with prior high adversity had NES compared with 47% with low adversity scores (p<0.05). However, there were no differences in rates of NES by ethnicity. NES was highly related to 12-month depression: 42% with NES were depressed compared with 16% without (p<0.0001). The same findings held for those women studied prospectively. NES also related to previous depression: 48% with NES had lifetime repeated or chronic disorder compared with 27% with no NES (p<0.0001).

In terms of NES and close relationships findings showed:

- NES related to the lack of a confiding VCO (63% vs 46% with a confiding VCO, p<0.003),
- NES was related to poor quality of partner relationship (62% of those in poor partner relationships had NES compared with 47% of those in good partner relationships, p<0.02).
- There was no association between prior partner violence and NES (23% with NES had partner violence compared to 17% without NES).

The relationship of NES to attachment style is summarised (see Figure 4.5):

- NES was highly correlated with the overall attachment style scale (0.36, p<0.0001). NES was also significantly related to the presence of any highly Insecure style: 71% of those Insecure had NES compared with 36% of those Secure (p<0.001).
- Highest rates of NES occurred for those with Fearful (86%), Dual/disorganised (76%) and Angry-dismissive (69%) styles. Enmeshed was marginally lower at 57% as was Withdrawn (52%). Rates for Secure/mildly Insecure were 36% (p<0.001).

The surprising result here is that Angry-dismissive, identified as an Avoidant style presents with low self-esteem, whereas Enmeshed, identified as Anxious had low self-esteem only marginally more often than those Withdrawn. The expected patterning of denigrating of self or others was not as expected from predicted models.

When looking at the most parsimonious model for depression, a binary logistic regression showed that each of the highly Insecure styles (apart from Withdrawn) and NES together provided the best model. Poor support and ethnicity did not add to the model.

Figure 4.6 provides a quick eyeball summary of the relationship of different Insecure styles to relationship and self-esteem variables.

4.6 Case examples

The cases already outlined in the previous two chapters have illustrated both unsupportive and supportive relationships with partners or VCOs. Therefore the cases outlined here will involve those partner relationships involving domestic violence among those with different attachment styles.

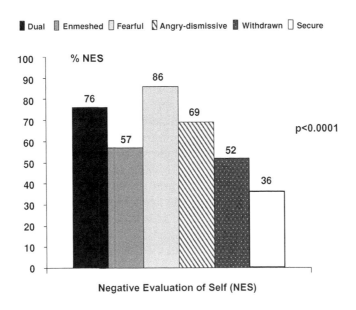

Figure 4.5 Attachment style and Negative Evaluation of Self

ASI style (Marked/ Moderate)	NES	Current relationships			Past relationships	
		Lack confiding VCO	Poor partner support	Conflict with partner	Prior partner violence	Partner disorder/ criminal
Dual/ disorganised	√	√	√		√	√
Enmeshed	(√)		√	√	√√	
Fearful	√√	√			√	√
Angry-Dismissive	√	√		√	√	
Withdrawn		√√	√			
Secure/ Mildly insecure						

√ or √√ indicates significant relationships; (√) at p<0.10.
ASI = Attachment Style Interview; NES = Negative Evaluation of Self;
VCO = Very Close Other.

Figure 4.6 Summary of relationships and attachment style

Description of the individual's self-esteem will also be included to illustrate how this is collected.

4.6.1 Alma's Moderately Angry-dismissive style

Alma is a 37-year-old woman who lives with her second husband and two youngest sons. She has an older son and daughter (Felicity, described in the last chapter) from a previous marriage, and both have left home. She and her husband are currently unemployed and have money difficulties, with her husband collecting sickness benefit. In terms of clinical disorder, Alma had one chronic episode of depression after her father died in her early thirties, and has had GAD for a number of years. She also had a brief episode of depression during the study period when her daughter Felicity ran away from home.

Previous partner violence: After a very difficult and abusive childhood (described in the next chapter) Alma left home to marry James when she was 17 years old, having become pregnant by him at 16. Her relationship with James was unsupportive and conflictful from early on. He was frequently violent and drunk as well as unreliable with money. The problems escalated after her second pregnancy and James' father's death. Alma had no social life as, once married, they had moved away from her family and friends. When she gave birth to her daughter Felicity, her husband did not visit her in hospital for two days, and when he did he was drunk. Once discharged Alma came home to find her husband in bed with another woman. She packed her bags and left with the two children to visit her mother in Scotland.

Alma describes the relationship which lasted only two years: '*Everything seemed wonderful, we put down a deposit on a house and we started renovating, the first baby was on its way and we thought everything was going to be wonderful, for a while anyway. But within a few months, with my first child being born, James's father died in Ireland and he went back for the funeral and to sort out his family estate and I never saw him for three months. He stayed there and constantly drank. When he came back, he was a different man . . . he just became an alcoholic. He used to get very violent and angry with me if I complained about the housekeeping money or that I had had a really bad night with the baby. And then I'd get really angry and shout and scream at him and say things to him and then he started to hit me. The alcohol made him very violent. One time I had to call the police in the middle of the night and they had to take him away. I was lying on the floor with my mouth pouring blood, and, I think, seven months pregnant with Felicity at that time. He had given me a terrible kicking and they thought I might lose the baby. I knew then that the marriage was over and I knew there was no way for the safety of my children that I could allow him to be within a few miles of us. That's when I started making plans to move on.*'

Alma's support and Angry-dismissive attachment style: When seen at interview Alma had low support from her current husband. She could not confide in him, he was not emotionally supportive and they had frequent arguments fuelled by spending a large part of each day together. She named a friend Jane as VCO, who was supportive and in whom she could confide, and her mother as second VCO, with whom she had a highly conflictful relationship. She confided nothing in her mother, who was critical, and when her mother visited they would start arguing within a day or two.

Alma had a moderately Angry-dismissive style. She had high mistrust: '*I think having someone close is important to me, but I've never been able to trust anyone enough. If I think I'm saying something to the wrong person and it might get back to somebody else that I don't want it to get back to, then I'm very cautious. I've never been inclined to pour out my heart instantly. I don't tell anybody anything I don't think they need to know. I don't tell them anything personal in case it gets around. That is one of my main fears. If I do tell anybody it will be those close, trusted few. I can be trusting until someone tells me there is something wrong. It's one of my fears that people will take something tragic and then gossip about it. That would make me really unhappy and so I tend to bottle up a lot of the emotional things. I've always found it difficult to get close. I've never really had anyone to get close to. I'll only tell what I need to because I don't want to be hurt, vulnerable or left open to criticism. That's basically how I feel inside and probably why I never tell anybody anything.*'

She also had high self-reliance: '*I don't think I've ever relied on anybody's help in making decisions – I've always been a one-man band. I've been self-sufficient for years and always have been able to be in charge. I just manage without others. I don't like being undermined. I like to be independent and know what I say, goes. I cope better than most people.*' She also had moderately high anger in relationships and was resentful of her husband and children '*What did I ever do to deserve this? Someone up there hates me. I think everyone takes you for granted. People see kindness as weakness. You have to be tough sometimes – I'm not a mug so don't treat me like one. My mum let me down when I was a child – she made me grow up with a chip on my shoulder. I still get angry about my childhood. I felt deprived of love – my home life was so bloody hellish.*'

Self-esteem: Unlike other women with Angry-dismissive styles, Alma had good self-esteem: '*Basically I'm just a pretty happy-go-lucky person. I'm a strong believer in saying what you have to say and getting it off your chest. I'm a hard, strong-willed, forceful type of woman that fights for the best for her family and for herself, and deep down there is a real decent-type motherly figure that tries to do the best for everyone that she can. I'm concerned about other people's health and welfare. I do voluntary work. I'm just an ordinary type of person. I don't think I've got any real bad qualities apart from being... I can be quite vindictive... but it's all words. I haven't got a bad personality. I'm quite strong-willed and I can be quite aggressive if there is something I need to do – I think ruthless would be quite a good word.*'

Thus, despite using words like vindictive and ruthless, she felt basically positive about herself.

Comment: At a young age Alma got involved with a partner who was violent and alcohol abusing and they married because of an unplanned pregnancy. Although her experience was traumatic and isolating, she did have the courage to leave him with two young babies. Since leaving that relationship, however, she had not been involved again in a violent relationship. Whilst her attachment style was Angry-dismissive and she projected her anger at a range of others (including her children, partner and mother), there was no escalation into violence with her partner – although her daughter's account of her parenting discussed in Chapter 6 shows she has used violence. Alma's negativity in relationships was not mirrored in her self-perception which was in her terms positive, seeing herself as hard, strong and self-sufficient. She shows strength and toughness in surviving. This may have been at the expense of sensitivity, particularly as a parent. Alma saw herself as a victim who had become a fighter to combat a hostile world. The literature on domestic violence emphasises how having an Avoidant style impacts on the relationship rather than on the self. A Fearful person in this situation is likely to have had their self-esteem shattered; the Angry-dismissive person fights back, which in some situations preserves self-esteem.

4.6.2 Ellie's moderately Enmeshed style

Ellie was described in the last chapter where her Enmeshed attachment style and poor support from boyfriend Lester was outlined. She has had two previous partners before Lester. Her first partner was a married man whom she met when she was 15 and who left her after ten years. Her first child by him was adopted but she kept the second child. The relationship was poor and unsupportive but never violent. He was very unreliable with money and had many affairs when they were together. She then met her second partner Graham who already had two ex-wives and 14 children from these marriages and from various affairs. She also had a child with Graham who lived with her.

The relationship with Graham was poor from the beginning. When they married he was already having an affair with a younger woman and then went to live in South America, leaving Ellie behind. She acknowledged how bad the relationship was after a year of marriage. Graham was possessive and jealous and would not allow her to have friends. He was frequently violent during rows although she reports never having sustained severe injuries. He provided no financial support, would accuse Ellie of having affairs and even of poisoning him. He was also involved in criminal behaviour and drug selling, and was rated as having antisocial behaviour. Ellie did eventually separate from him but did not terminate the relationship. At interview she described him, without apparent irony, as 'charming and lovely'. She also described how he was 'courting' her by phoning three times a day and sending her red roses. She did express her determination not to have him back because of his unreasonable behaviour but still welcomed his attention.

Self-esteem: About her self-acceptance Ellie said: *'I like myself, I like my own company, but I do like to be in a relationship. I do like 'me'. I'm very vain. I love my fingernails at the moment! [Laughs] I like me, yeah. I've had to work at it since my divorce. I've hated myself in the past. I do look younger now than I did when I was having a really hard time in my marriage. People who maybe haven't seen me since then would probably not recognise me at all. I like treating myself and I like a lot of attention. I think I may find it hard in a sexual relationship, because I do think I deserve to be spoilt, not just with material things but emotionally, because I know I'm capable of giving a lot and if I don't get that back, there is something wrong.'*

When asked about her positive attributes she said: *'I suppose I like to think I'm funny. I'm very clean. I'm prejudiced against crude people, I don't like crudeness. I think I'm too sympathetic. I can be efficient but I can also muddle through. I'd like to think that I was more efficient than muddling... I was a total doormat to Graham and never, ever will be again. I like a lot of attention.'* When asked if she felt she was attractive: *'Don't forget, I'm 40 now, so there are some sags and some lines. I've got to learn to like them [laughs] because they are there. But I'm confident, yeah. I think when people first meet me they are in awe of me. I don't know why. I'm very bolshy, I'm very blunt. People tend to think I'm quite severe, but when they do get to know me, they know I'm actually having fun. When they see the sense of humour I've got I think they appreciate it.'*

Comment: Ellie's Enmeshed style shows that she did not have a realistic view of adversity in her relationships, and since she hated being alone and could not handle separations easily she did not finally terminate her problematic and dangerous earlier relationship. Despite two problematic relationships with men, the earliest from age 15, she did not have negative self-evaluation and saw herself in a positive light and as special. However, her reference to having 'hated herself' indicates some oscillation in her self-view. As with Alma, she recognised that others found her blunt and severe, but this, in her view, was mitigated by her sense of fun.

4.6.3 Donna's Dual/disorganised attachment style

Donna is a 24-year-old woman from the young Offspring sample (daughter of Wendy described in Chapter 6) who is involved in a violent relationship and has been in the past. She had a Dual/disorganised attachment style. She lives with her two-year-old daughter and her partner James lives with her some of the time, despite an injunction to keep away. Donna felt very isolated and only sees her sisters and her mother Wendy. She has lost contact with her friends, whom she no longer trusted.

Donna had been suffering from postnatal depression since her daughter was born, and started to experience panic attacks in the last year during the period of the injunction against her partner. She had also suffered from agoraphobia for some years and was socially phobic. She found it hard to leave the house and got her mother to do her shopping. She had become dependent on alcohol since leaving home age 16 and also had a substance-abuse diagnosis.

Partner relationship: Donna moved in with her first partner Nick whilst living in a hostel age 16. She started her relationship with James whilst also living with Nick. She remained in a relationship with the two men for some years. James had stayed with her on and off for four years since she got her flat. She had his child a year later. The already argumentative relationship with James became violent when she told him she was still seeing her previous partner Nick, and has remained violent ever since. However, Donna said that she also caused the violence and hit James when she got angry. She had also threatened him with a knife. She had taken out the injunction against him seeing their daughter six months before interview when he had threatened to take their daughter away. However, Donna allowed James to come back and live with her. She felt she should leave James and end the relationship but admitted that the chances of her doing so were slim.

Support and Attachment style: As well as her problematic and unsupportive partner relationship, Donna has a history of poor relationships with friends and family with whom she frequently falls out. She did have a close relationship with her mother Wendy who helped her out financially and with childcare but she did not confide in her mother because she knew her mother wanted her to end her relationship with James. With no support figure, her ability to make and maintain relationships was rated as 'little/none' and her attachment insecurity as 'marked'.

Donna had high mistrust and constraints on closeness and her self-reliance was rated as contradictory. Given her high anger and mistrust she was rated as markedly Angry-dismissive style. '*I can't be bothered with any friends because they all try to backstab me. Any relationship I'm in, they try and break me up. I have fallen out with a lot of friends through trust. If things don't go the way I want them to I just explode. With James, I'm the violent one. If he does something I don't like I just switch and become violent. He gets scratches and a few little bruises. It is me who is throwing things and banging and thrashing about.*' About her daughter she said: '*I do get angry with her, I have to control myself. I really don't like smacking her. If she does not listen to me or she is cheeky I'll give her a little smack and leave her. I do take my anger out on her.*'

Donna also had high fear of rejection which led to an additional Fearful style rating: '*Because I'm so sociable I'm a friendly person, I'm easily led and I get too friendly too quick, and then they become my enemy – I say 'hello' to people but that is as far as it is going to go. At certain times I'm scared, I don't know what to say to people, I am afraid they might repeat it. I feel stupid telling other people how I feel. When I know I'm going to open up fully I back down because I'm scared. In the relationship I had before with Nick I was hurt badly. I was faithful and he was messing about having affairs. I find it too hard to fall in love and trust someone else. That is why I have to be in control.'* When asked if she felt afraid of being let down by her partner James she said: '*Yeah, every day I do. I trust him 100 per cent but I don't know what it is I'm scared of but I am scared. I'm scared of getting hurt I suppose, everyone is. I just wish that I could feel like I did about Nick towards James.'* It was noted how contradictory her account was, for example switching between saying she trusted James and that she was scared of him.

Self-esteem: Donna also presented a mixed picture of her self-evaluation with both positive and negative aspects rated highly. She had good self-acceptance: '*I'm happy within myself. I wouldn't want to change places with anyone.*' However, if someone criticised her, she would take it to heart and it would affect her for the rest of the day: '*But it wouldn't make me feel worse about myself.*' She was also self-critical: '*I would like to be a bit more strong-minded and for people to take me a bit more seriously. I'm not altogether happy with myself the way I am.*' She thought herself 'very' attractive as well as intelligent: '*Yes, but not perfect.*' She also thought she was sociable: '*Yes, very, I'm not shy. I'm easy to get on with and a very good friend.*' Her best qualities: '*I'm a good listener, I like sitting down and talking. I'm warm and caring.*' Her worst quality: '*Not being able to speak my mind and having to write everything down because I get confused.*' She felt positive about her roles and thought she was 'too good' as a partner and 'excellent' as a parent.

Comment: Donna's profile had many inconsistent features, reflected in her Dual/disorganised style as well as her self-perception. She presented as very angry, and this seemed to be impulsive anger where she lashed out. Such anger and violence is typical of Dual/disorganised styles and may have some dissociated aspects. Her problematic relationships and poor relating style do not impact consistently on her view of herself which was both positive and negative. Her mother's practical support was the one positive relationship in her situation, but Donna's psychological barriers prevented her from confiding or accessing support from her mother. Her mixed attachment picture ran parallel with a number of mixed psychological disorders, as well as the substance abuse common amongst those with Dual/disorganised styles in this analysis.

The next case study is of a young man Eric, aged 23, and is included to examine support in a young male, as well as describing his Anxious style, often thought to be less common in men. In the London Offspring study, equal rates of supportive relationships were found for the young men and women, and there was no gender difference in attachment styles. The example also illustrates that for young people still living in the parental home and without partners, the mother can still be an important attachment figure and is routinely questioned about as first support figure in the ASI. This case is an example of a young man with an Enmeshed style who reports violence from his girlfriend but also describes his own aggressive behaviour. He is half-brother to Dean, described in the last chapter, who also had Enmeshed style but in combination with Angry-dismissive features.

4.6.4 Eric's moderately Enmeshed style

Eric is 23 years old, living at home with his mother and working as a security guard. He has recently left his partner Rose, a volatile relationship, after seven months' cohabiting. He described her as violent – on one occasion she burst his eardrum and on another she threatened him with a knife. During this time they had left each other several times. Towards the end of the relationship she became pregnant and had a termination, not consulting him in this. He walked out and returned to live with his mother. He had held down the job as a security guard for nearly two years. Eric has no history of depression or anxiety. However, like his half-brother Dean he has a history of substance abuse (cannabis) and alcohol abuse.

Support: Eric described his relationship with his mother '*as almost being in a relationship but without sex*'. He described being able to confide in her and having '*talked to her about everything really*', but when probed for examples of confiding, there were numerous crises about which he had not confided, for example his relationship with Rose, his break-up, his drug taking and the violent attacks. Therefore, this relationship was not rated as confiding or supportive. His felt attachment was very high: '*She loves me more than life itself. If she left the country I would probably go with her. I would be distraught if I lost her. She has always been there, to lose that would be devastating in all ways.*' They spent at least a couple of hours together each day and the atmosphere was '*brilliant*'. But they also argued – they would bicker about the rent, about bills and about household chores such as washing the dishes. They had been arguing a lot recently and she had been in tears: '*We argue for about an hour or so and then we try and sort things out.*' The relationship was rated as 'inadequate support with discord'.

Eric named two VCO support figures, both males his own age. He described confiding in his first friend Ryan: '*There's nothing I cannot confide. I cried on his shoulder when I broke up with my girlfriend. First thing I did when I broke up was to pack my stuff and go straight round to his place to have a shoulder to cry on.*' Ryan listens and does give support. Eric sees him once a month and speaks on the phone for hours as often as three or four times a week: '*If he wasn't there I would feel the same as if I'd lost a brother. It would hurt but I would get over it, but not quickly.*' The atmosphere when together was good and they didn't argue or fight. This relationship was rated as 'good-average support, no discord'.

His other VCO was his friend Sam, with whom he also had good inter-action but without confiding. They spent time together going to the pub. The relationship was rated as 'inadequate support, no discord'. With only one effective support figure, Eric was rated as having 'some' ability to make and maintain relationships and therefore as moderately Insecure. He acknowledged his shortcomings in making relationships: *'Every relationship I've had has been disastrous with girlfriends. They've always been argumentative girls and I've always been an argumentative type. We've always conflicted. I argue my side of things and they don't want me to, they storm out crying and kick doors.'* But in terms of other relationships: *'Quite good with everything else.'*

Eric's Enmeshed Attachment style: Eric's attachment attitudes showed a high need for company and fear of separation typical of Enmeshed style: *'That's my problem, I don't back off. If I'm getting too close to someone I just don't walk away. I'm quite a trusting person. I've always been an emotional person, I've never been one to hold back my feelings.'* He gets close easily: *'I'm a very talkative person so I can talk to anyone in the pub or at work. It's very easy to make relation-ships. But I'm a very possessive person. When my girlfriend was dancing with someone else I started a fight and threw something at a mirror. My girlfriends do always let me down.'* He would like to see more of his other male friends: *'Sometimes it would be nice to go out clubbing with them more often, but it's not always convenient. I get close to women quite a lot because I've lived with my mum all my life. A lot of people say I have very feminine attributes. I feel like I can talk to women and I tend not to get too close to men. There are a few men I can get close to but only a select few.'*

His fear of separation was high, and particularly linked to his mother: *'I would miss just the fact that she wasn't there, just not to be able to see her and give her a hug at the end of the day. When I was away at boarding school aged 11 it almost made me ill at the beginning missing my mum. But I spoke to her every day.'* Aged 17 he moved out of the family house for a few months but then moved back: *'I didn't like being away from my mum.'*

Eric had high levels of anger: *'Most of the time it's arguments in the pub, some-times physical fights. It happens about twice a month but last time was three months ago. Me and my brother Dean walked past a pub and we were tanked up with drink and these blokes said something to us. One went for my brother, I stood up for myself, then I picked up the other one and dragged him off down the street and hit him.'*

Eric described himself as argumentative: *'Yes. I've always got a point to make. Once I've had a drink I'm the most argumentative person. Not everyone has the same idea of fun as me. There are friends I've upset and they want to have a fight over it, but most of the time I'll let them swing their punch and then forget it. On the odd occasion you can't back down so you have to knock them over and hope they stay down.'* He described attacking someone: *'I hit one bloke across his face. The bone in his nose came out and you could see it. I just saw red!'*

Self-esteem: Eric had high self-esteem and high self-acceptance: *'I think I am brilliant in everything that I do. I'm kind, passionate, caring, easy-going,* *good-looking – an all-round nice bloke! I've never had any complaints about the way I am.'* He was generally happy about himself. His acknowledged worst characteristics were: *'I drink too much, I'm lazy. People are better than me at some things, but I'm better with people than others. I put my mum first and I come second. She's number one and I come second and family come after that.'* About his partner role, he said: *'I like to think I am good. I like to think I give my girlfriends everything they want.'* However, at work he was *'mediocre. I want to see the easy side of life'*, but at sports, *'I'm one of the best footballers I know.'*

Comment: Eric was a sociable individual, very close to his mother with close friends and a positive view of himself. However, this belies an underlying vulnerability. His dependence on his mother is much higher than average for his life stage and there is evidence that he has never 'individuated' or truly left home. His actual confiding in others was very limited and by his own admission his relationships with girlfriends were very poor. He described violence experienced from his girlfriend, but also described his own violence in other settings. It was not clear whether he and his girlfriend were both violent and whether he was underplaying his violence in the relationship. He described himself as having female attributes due to being close to his mother and getting on well with girlfriends, perhaps seeing his Enmeshed style as more typically female. Whilst his Enmeshed style (with its jealousy and anger) is shared by his half-brother, he did not have the mistrust and self-sufficiency of Dean, hence no dual style. His idealised perception of himself as kind, caring and easy-going was at odds with the violent and possessive behaviour he described.

Summary of findings

Support and partner relationships

- Those with Insecure styles were more likely to lack at least one close confiding support figure. This was highest among those Withdrawn, followed by those with Dual/disorganised styles.
- Individuals were more likely to have a partner if they had Enmeshed or Angry-dismissive styles. Those Fearful were least likely to have a partner, highlighting avoidant aspects, despite the Anxious elements of the style. Fearful individuals were more likely to be single parents, perhaps due to stressful separations from previous partners adding to the fear of rejection involved. Those with Dual/disorganised were most likely to be separated from a partner.
- Poor support form partner was highest in those Enmeshed and those Withdrawn. However, patterning by partner conflict showed Enmeshed to have most conflict and Withdrawn most 'indifference' in relationships. Given Withdrawn have lower rates of stress, poor coping and depression as outlined in the last

chapter, it is clear they are not totally devoid of risk, specifically around the lack of good support.

- Current or previous partner problem behaviour was most highly associated with Dual/disorganised styles in terms of either antisocial behaviour or psychiatric/criminal behaviour. Violence from a partner was most common in those with Enmeshed style, although also higher in all Insecure styles (apart from Withdrawn), at around double the rate of those Secure.

Self-esteem
- Negative evaluation of self was highly related to Insecure attachment style with highest rates for those Fearful, followed by Angry-dismissive and Dual/disorganised. The high rate among Angry-dismissive is surprising but the other associations were expected from the literature review. Also surprising is that Enmeshed style is not associated with greater negative evaluation of self.
- A statistical model of depression showed all the Insecure styles apart from Withdrawn contributed significantly, as did Negative Evaluation of Self. Poor support or ethnicity did not add to the model.

4.7 Discussion

The ability to make close supportive relationships in adult life is a critical task of attachment. This involves partner relationships, but also friendships and adult relationships with family of origin. Support from someone close in terms of a high level of confiding and active emotional support is crucial for wellbeing. Lack of such support increases risk of depression. Understanding adult relationships, particularly partnerships, involves substantial complexity. This is because of the admix of two attachment styles and sets of emotional needs, the pressure from joint stressors, including those financial as well as those relational, two sets of psychopathology as well as the dynamic progression in relationships and the circumstances of break up can create complex patterning. Poor relationships can have different characteristics. In ASI terms these all include lack of confiding and support from partner or close other, but some involve conflict, whether from frequent arguments, or physical aggression and others apathy and indifference. Some of these characteristics correlate with attachment styles, with those with Withdrawn styles having more distant indifferent relationships and those Enmeshed or Angry-dismissive having more conflict. However, having a problem relationship is not synonymous with Insecure attachment style. It is when a range of relationships are negative that Insecure attachment style is invoked.

Different patterning is associated with different attachment style profiles, particularly around Anxious-avoidance (Fearful) or detachment (Withdrawn), and conflict (Enmeshed, Angry-dismissive and Dual/disorganised). Thus dual themes are apparent. First, for those Fearful or Withdrawn the theme is isolation where there is lack of support during crises and lack of practice at developing new support figures in the event of loss. Second, conflict can escalate to domestic violence levels when partners have psychopathology and this interacts with the individual's own fear or anger patterns. Both patterns seem to involve negative evaluation of self. Here the distorted internal working model of others seen as untrustworthy and rejecting is paralleled by the distorted internal model of the self (as unlovable). Thus there is only partial support for the model proposed by Bartholomew and Horowitz (1991) about the relationship of poor self-esteem and attachment style. Their view of Fearful attachment style having negative view of self and others is borne out as is their view of Secure style as involving positive view of self and other. However, there is inconsistency in the other styles. Those Enmeshed tend to have rather mixed views of self, any negativity mixed with some idealisation in reporting and sometimes feelings of specialness. So while they see others in a rosily positive light, their view of themselves is bound up in their use of denial and contradictory emotional reporting. Also surprising is the high rate of NES among those with Angry-dismissive styles. The prediction would be for high self-esteem and denigration of others. Whilst the latter is there this seems to mask a more anxious persona than is immediately evident, with negative views of self perhaps related to fear of loss of control. This is consistent with their high rates of anxiety states as described in the last chapter. This seems very different from a typically avoidant pattern, tending more towards an ambivalent style.

The role of partners and close support figures is to increase feelings of safety, providing a 'safe haven' and regulating negative emotion at times of stress. When these relationships are absent there is no such safety mechanism and no mechanism for external regulation of emotion. However, there are added risks. Negative relationships themselves can create the stressors, for example through conflict, violence, infidelities or separations, which provide the doubled vulnerability of both creating problems and failing in supportive provision. This is one reason why a range of support figures (or at least a minimum of two supportive) are needed and why attachment style in the ASI is based on the concept of being unable to generate support from more than one source. For those Secure, a problematic relationship with partner or family member can also occur for myriad reasons, but here other support figures can then provide the affect-regulation and safe-haven opportunities to preserve wellbeing. For those Insecure, there is no such safety net.

The issue of attachment style and domestic violence is an important one which needs further investigation in attachment research and greater dissemination to services. Violence is seriously under-reported to services and some of these barriers may come from Insecure attachment styles where psychological barriers include a dread of abandonment from impending separation from the dangerous partner, or a level of denial and minimising of violent incidents. Examples are also shown of females being violent in partner relationships and the association with Insecure attachment styles needs further elucidation in specifically designed projects. In order to understand how victims come to be significantly under-treated in services more extensive research on the attachment style of either partner and domestic violence needs to be pursued. The nature of couple relationships and how stresses within these impact on childcare will be explored further in the clinical examples provided in later chapters.

The next chapter will examine the role of childhood experience in Insecure adult attachment style.

5 Attachment style and childhood experience

5.0 Introduction

At the very heart of attachment theory is the principle that interactions with parents or caregivers from the earliest point in life are critical to the development of Secure attachment behaviour. As already described, the continuity of attachment styles from childhood to adult life occurs through the mechanism of the 'internal working model' or emotional-cognitive template which holds in place the beliefs and expectations of others and the self. Thus a great deal hangs on the quality of the early bonding experiences with parents and main carers: the ability to form primary close relationships necessary for survival, the development of the self, the capacity for regulating emotions and understanding the meaning of close relationships. This chapter will provide findings on the childhood experiences of the women and young people studied in the London samples in relation to adult attachment style. In particular it will search for the specificity of different experiences to different attachment styles, as well as these in relation to clinical disorder.

Research has provided understanding of the way in which child and adolescent behaviours and disorders reflect aspects of poor family functioning, relational failures and the process by which attachment strategies might have developed and the function they may serve in the child's life (Cassidy 1994; Crittenden 1995). The relationship dynamics revealed in the child's internalising (minimising-avoidance and blocking of distress), externalising (hyper-activating anxious-ambivalence or intensifying distress) or frozen and disorientated disorganisation (inability to mobilise a strategy to cope with distress) indicate the way in which the child–parent relationship has contributed to the child's inability to resolve difficulties within dyadic relationships critical for subsequent attachment style.

Each of the strategies hold risks for childhoods in which there is little trust in the provision of care, or belief that the child is worthy of attention. Survival in such situations may require inhibition of need, pandering to critical or violent parents or caring for those parenting adults who may otherwise emotionally disintegrate. Each of these short-term protective strategies has important implications for development. The need for mobil-ising such strategies, and the intensity or type of affects displayed in maintaining them contributes to changes in neurobiology and impacts the organisation of processes underlying abnormal development.

For insecurely attached children the corresponding representation of the self is of being unlovable and unworthy, and often at the receiving end of anger and hostility or parental fear and helplessness, each of which involve self-experiences that erode trust in the availability of care from the caregiver (Bowlby 1969; Bowlby 1973; Bowlby 1980; Bretherton 1985). Research has sought to confirm such associations and to look for pattern-ing of children's negative experience and the coping style employed to deal with the specific anticipated caregiver's response (Buchsbaum, Toth *et al.* 1992; Bretherton, Ridgway *et al.* 1990).

The effect of the mother/carer–infant relationship is fundamental for understanding the development of emotional-regulation and mentalisation skills (Fonagy and Target 1997; Fonagy, Gergely *et al.* 2002). The failure of the primary care relationship, when lacking awareness and insight into the child's mental states, may lead to a deficit in the child's reflective function, the ability to envision mental states in both the self and others, to integrate the functions of experience and observation and to generate connection between thoughts and affects. This results in similar deficits in later life, for example in the recognition that one's own and others' thoughts and actions are driven by emotions, beliefs and desires (Fonagy, Gergely *et al.* 2008). Maltreatment is viewed as responsible for disorganising the attachment system and disrupting mentalisation (Cicchetti and Valentino 2006). Research shows that young maltreated children fail to show empathy when witnessing distress, have poorer emotional regulation, make fewer refer-ences to internal states, struggle to understand facial expressions, misattribute anger and show developmental delay.

In normal development, the mother or main carer interacts with the child's pre-verbal cues and can attune her responses and behaviours to the child's communications, and thus modulate the baby's emotional state. This aids the infant's understanding of its own emotions and cognitions (Winnicott 1965). By mirroring the mother's emotions and observing her facial and vocal responses the child learns to differentiate between the physiological stimulation activated internally, and that activated from the environment (Gergely and Watson 1996). By internalising the mother's behaviours and reactions, slowly the child generates a mind representation of emotional states which is linked to attachment figures. Gradually this representational system starts to function independently of the mother as a self-regulator of emotional and cognitive states and as a basis for further attachment representations and behaviour.

However, if the mother (or main carer) has excessive personal conflicts or psychological difficulties, perhaps as a response to her own stressful and hostile environment, she can be overwhelmed by the child's negative displays of emotions and react by displaying markedly negative emotion in response. The perception of this negativity in the mother can lead to a traumatising escalation in the child's state of arousal leading to either projecting or dissociating the emotions (Schimmenti and Caretti 2010). Thus, the failures in the system of mirroring with the mother may generate in the child deficiencies in self-perception and in regulation of emotion, as well as difficulty in understanding his/her own internal states and in identifying and communicating emotions (Taylor, Bagby *et al.* 1997).

5.1 Maltreatment and trauma in childhood

When considering adverse experience in childhood, a wide range of experiences can be included. These are variously termed as neglect/abuse or maltreatment or interpersonal trauma. Whilst most are intra-familial they can also reflect experiences with non-parent perpetrators, most notably sexual abuse from strangers or acquaintances, or indeed bullying from unrelated peers. However, most maltreatment reflects the quality of the relationship with a parent or substitute parent and includes neglectful or hostile behaviour to the child through a range of negative interactions. Other distortions include over-protectiveness or role-reversing (where the parent becomes dependent on the child) or sexual abuse with its boundary violation. Physical abuse extends the hostile interaction, and psychological abuse the controlling aspect. The experience of witnessing conflict or abuse (between parents, or towards siblings) is also at times included as a form of maltreatment.

Neglect is often underestimated as a childhood maltreatment because it reflects deficits in parenting and care rather than hostile acts, and is chronic rather than acute. However, neglect is highly related to a range of adult disorders, and is thought to have a particular link to problems in the development of self- and other-perception, with the absence of the parental 'looking-glass' function of reflecting back to the child a validation of their emotions and perceptions. It is thus hypothesised as a factor in the failure of self-formation common to depression (Brown, Bifulco *et al.* 1990b) but also to personality disorder (Fonagy, Gergely *et al.* 2008).

Trauma is defined as 'threat to personal safety or integrity' or as 'unmanageable stress' and provides an extreme and more dangerous level of stress or adversity usually linked with abuse. Complex trauma (multiple and/or chronic experience) can interfere with neurobiological development and the capacity to integrate sensory, emotional and cognitive information into a cohesive whole (van der Kolk and Fisler 1994; van der Kolk 2005). Such developmental trauma sets the stage for unfocused responses to subsequent stress leading to psychological disorders, including post-traumatic stress disorder and other problems. Specifically it leads to lack of a continuous sense of self, poorly modulated affect and impulse control including aggression against self and others and uncertainty about the reliability and predictability of others. This is often linked to Disorganised attachment style in children and externalising disorders.

Varieties of childhood neglect, physical, emotional and sexual abuse are well-established as risk factors for adult psychopathology in general (Cohen 1996; Bifulco and Moran 1998; Hill, Davis *et al.* 2000; Harkness and Wildes 2002; Fergusson, Boden *et al.* 2008). Cumulative trauma is also encompassed through multiple incidents of abuse, which increase risk of disorder in a 'dose' effect (Bifulco, Moran *et al.* 2003). When such multiple threats occur from different perpetrators, it reduces the possibility of the child finding relief in Secure relationships or support figures and sources of resilience. This can be overwhelming and result in 'developmental trauma disorder' (van der Kolk 2005). This defines the worst outcome of such adversities in childhood with neurological damage resulting in modifications of the HPA axis and noradrenergic system with failure of regulation of physiological arousal and emotion by either the self or others (Shore 2003; van der Kolk 2003). The child becomes entrapped in a pattern of dysfunctional responses to traumatic cues, experiencing confusion, dissociation, somatic symptoms and traumatic re-enactment, together with a persistent negative evaluation of self-attribution, characterised by self-hate and shame, and absence of trust in the protectiveness of others (Schimmenti and Bifulco 2008).

5.2 Researching childhood experience

Differentiating neglect characterised by absence of necessary care, and abuses characterised by excessive anger, harshness or control are likely to be critical for developing different attachment styles (Goldberg 2000).The emotional dynamics of the two sets of experience are different in important ways, suggestive of different parental states, with neglect involving parental disengagement, through withdrawal, helplessness and emotionless contact, and abuse indicating high involvement but of a malevolent type. The simplest interpretation is that these two parental approaches lead to Anxious or Avoidant styles, the demands for closeness and clinging deriving from distant or intermittent parenting and the detachment arising from distancing from the hostile parenting. However, when fear and anger are added to the attachment mix the responses are likely to be more complex. Also, since neglect and abuse commonly co-occur over the course of a childhood from the same or different parent figures, and because some maltreatments are not clearly neglect or abuse, differentiating patterns becomes extremely difficult. For example, sexual abuse and psychological abuse can involve distortions of apparent care as well as hostile control. For all of these reasons a clear differentiation between these childhood experiences and adult styles has been difficult to determine, with a lack of specificity in empirical models of attachment (Hill, Young *et al.* 1994; Booth, Rubin *et al.* 1998; Belsky 2002).

However, there is increasing evidence that the style most often associated with abuse and multiples of maltreatment is that of Disorganised style (Crittenden 1997). Main and Solomon found rates of 80% Disorganised attachment in maltreated infants compared with 20% in non-maltreated (Main and Solomon 1986) with stability of style found over a four-year period in preschool children (Cicchetti and Barnett 1991). This is also found in adolescents in residential care with high levels of prior neglect and abuse as well as parental separation, with Disorganised styles the most common, along with Avoidant styles (Wallis and Steele 2001; Zegers, Schuengel *et al.* 2008).

Linking childhood experience to adult attachment style can be a difficult hypothesis to test empirically. The ideal study would be one where childhood maltreatment could be carefully documented in infancy, in middle childhood and adolescence in high-risk samples, and then the individual followed-up into adulthood with attachment style measured at regular intervals. No such comprehensive study exists. Large-scale prospective population cohorts on the whole do not include attachment measures (e.g. the Christchurch and Dunedin samples in New Zealand) and the prospective attachment studies rarely extend from childhood to adulthood, or where they do, have not assessed childhood neglect/abuse (Sroufe 2005). This aim is further complicated by the lack of comparable measures of attachment styles for different developmental periods, with few teams having rating competence in all. Thus, although the SST exists for infancy and Story Stems for preschool there has not yet been sufficient mainstream research for measures such as the Child Attachment Interview (Target, Fonagy *et al.* 2003) or Crittenden's School-age Assessment of Attachment (SAA).

There is also difficulty collecting accurate information about neglect and abuse in childhood for developmental, ethical and social reasons. Children are not always able to describe their experience of maltreatment for reasons of conflicting loyalties, misunderstanding of its nature or fear of reprisal or family disruption. Often it is more productive for adults to reconstruct from memory from the vantage of having survived the experience and with adult cognitions to help them to both formulate the memory of experience and place it in a time frame. In selecting such a sample, it might be supposed that approaching adults with childhood contact with social services would be best, but historically this would only represent a portion of those with maltreatment and may preclude children or families who are more resilient despite adverse experience. A community-based sample of adults recalling their childhood experience can remove biases in such selection, as used in the studies described here.

It is therefore more feasible to study the childhood experience of adults or young adults retrospectively as long as due care is taken over the quality of the childhood information collected. For this reason, the studies outlined with the ASI have utilised high-risk community samples (in order to ensure sufficient numbers with experiences of childhood neglect or abuse who may or may not be in contact with services) and with childhood experience measured using standardised procedures to maximise objective and factual accounts of early life experience. In addition to finding an association between childhood adversity and adult or adolescent attachment style, testing its role as a causal linking factor (or mediator) is also needed to confirm attachment theory hypotheses. The mediating role is important in understanding the perpetuation of risk for adult outcomes (Cummings and Cicchetti 1990; Whiffen, Judd *et al.* 1999). Mediation is best tested in a prospective design where the reporting and time order of attachment style, and disorder, are separated. This can overcome any biases in potential attachment style reporting by ongoing symptoms. Therefore mediation will also be examined in the prospective part of the London studies.

5.3 Measuring childhood experience: The Childhood Experience of Care and Abuse Interview (CECA)

Measuring experience retrospectively can create methodological difficulties. Individuals with vulnerability or disorder may report earlier experience in biased ways – either over-stating adverse experience in an 'effort after meaning' for their disorder or to state their need for redress – or minimising early difficulties as a means of controlling their negative emotions about such experience. Methods are therefore needed which can collect information in a systematic way, emphasising factual aspects of early life, rather than opinions, attitudes or emotions, and providing a classification which can differentiate types of early experiences and record whether they are more or less severe. The CECA interview fulfils this function (Bifulco, Brown *et al.* 1994). It questions in chronological detail about childhood and early adolescent experience during different household arrangements and from earliest years to the end of the 16th year. It asks about relationships with each parent figure or substitute parent figure during that time, reflecting antipathy or hostile parenting, neglect and role reversal (parentification or young carer experience). It also questions about a range of abuses: physical, sexual or psychological. The latter is defined in terms of sadistic control of the child, utilising techniques such as terrorising, humiliation, depriving of basic needs or valued objects, etc. Whilst physical and psychological abuse are assessed from parent figures, sexual abuse is assessed from any older peer or adult. Key scales are summarised below.

The Childhood Experience of Care and Abuse scales

All care scales are measured for each change in household arrangement with different caretakers, and for each parent figure. Abuse is rated for each one from different perpetrators. Scales are 4-point (marked, moderate, some, little/none) and the top two points are used in dichotomised analysis to denote severe neglect or abuse.

Lack of Care

- **Antipathy:** Cold, hostile, critical or angry behaviour from parent to child. Intensity and pervasiveness determine severity. Evidence of verbal interaction and behaviour required.
- **Neglect:** Parental indifference to child's health and wellbeing, including material care, medical care, socialisation, schooling and indifference to child's distress.
- **Role reversal:** Pressure placed upon child to take on an adult role in both providing for the family (household responsibilities and sibling care) as well as providing care for the parents (e.g. acting as confidant or advisor). The number of domains of such role reversal (e.g. both behavioural and psychological) and pervasiveness determine severity.

Abuse

- **Physical abuse:** Physically attacking the child, usually with an implement, but also punching or kicking, sufficient for potential injuries. Severity determined by intensity and frequency.
- **Sexual abuse:** Sexual approaches to the child, usually involving physical contact from any older peer or adult. Instance of forced witnessing of sexual activity also included. Severity determined by the intrusiveness of the abuse, relationship to perpetrator, age and frequency. Worst cases tend to be intra-familial or from authority figures.
- **Psychological abuse:** Sadistic forms of coercion used to control and subjugate the child. Many categories of behaviour, including: terrorising, humiliating, depriving of basic needs or valued objects, cognitive disorientation, exploitation. More severe instances involve more than one category of sadistic control and more pervasive use of the abuse. It often co-occurs with other abuses, particularly sexual abuse.

Estimating the severity of negative experiences is determined by use of carefully specified definitions and benchmark ratings for what constitutes 'marked, moderate, mild/some or little/no severity of experience'. These are outlined in manuals and in training, with consensus ratings with other researchers blind to key outcome variables can help improve reliability of rating. Inter-rater reliability is good when formally tested (agreement 0.75 and above).

In order to validate these retrospective accounts part of the London sample included sister pairs interviewed independently to get corroboration on early life experience (Bifulco, Brown *et al.* 1997; Brown, Craig *et al.* 2007). This showed significant levels of agreement between them for the presence and severity of particular experiences. Highest agreement was for neglect (0.70), mid-range for physical abuse (0.63) but lower for sexual abuse (0.40). The latter was due to the secrecy of the experience and the fact that only one of the sisters had experienced it. When sexual abuse by family member was looked at, agreement between sisters was higher (0.56). Professor Peter Fonagy and his team at the Menninger Clinic in the USA undertook a further test on 70 young adults interviewed with the CECA. These individuals had attended the Menninger clinic as children, and so comparison of CECA adversity and clinical notes was possible. Good agreement was found with 59% agreeing on the presence of adversity and 75% agreeing on its absence. In addition, 25% were reported only in case files and potentially 'missed' by the CECA, but 41% reported adversity not reflected in the notes (Fonagy, Stein, Allen; personal communication).

Previous analyses with the CECA have shown that an index reflecting the presence of severe neglect, physical or sexual abuse in childhood raises the risk of adult depression three-fold (Bifulco and Moran 1998; Kaess, Parzer *et al.* 2011), and raises adolescent risk of a range of disorders (depression, anxiety, substance abuse or conduct disorder) five-fold (Bifulco, Moran *et al.* 2002; Bifulco 2008). This finding has been replicated by other researchers (Hill, Davis *et al.* 2000; Harkness and Wildes 2002) and internationally (Gianonne, Schimenti A *et al.* 2011; Kaess, Parzer *et al.* 2011). It has also been extended to other disorders, more recently to psychosis (Fisher, Jones *et al.* 2010).

Specific links between type of attachment insecurity and type of childhood experience as well as with the different parents involved may all influence attachment style in later life. These research questions are examined in the London midlife women, followed by the offspring data sets.

5.4 Findings of the London studies

A high rate of neglect or abuse in childhood was expected given the selection of the London women for vulnerability. Thus half the women (56%) were found to have at least one experience of severe neglect, physical or sexual abuse before age 17, significantly higher than the 20% or so expected in the community at large (Bifulco and Moran, 1998; Cawson, Wattam *et al.* 2000).

This index of neglect or abuse was highly related to Insecure adult attachment style in the women studied. This showed:

- Of those with neglect or abuse, 58% had a highly Insecure style compared with 29% of those without neglect or abuse.
- As well as the presence of an Insecure attachment style, it was possible to look at degree of insecurity of attachment to check for a 'dose' effect. This was confirmed with childhood neglect/abuse occurring for 83% in those markedly Insecure, 68% in those moderately Insecure, 47% in those mildly Insecure and 35% in those clearly Secure (p<0.0001).

Figure 5.1 shows the proportion with different Insecure attachment styles among those with childhood neglect/abuse compared to those without. This shows:

- The most common Insecure style amongst those with neglect/abuse was Fearful (19%) followed by Dual/disorganised (13%) and then Angry-dismissive (12%).
- Only 5% of those with neglect or abuse had Enmeshed style and 10% Withdrawn style.
- The rates among those with no neglect or abuse ranged from 9% (Withdrawn) to 3% (Dual/disorganised).
- All the Insecure styles were significantly related to childhood neglect/abuse apart from Withdrawn. This latter finding is consistent with earlier chapters where Withdrawn style showed little association with disorder or stress.

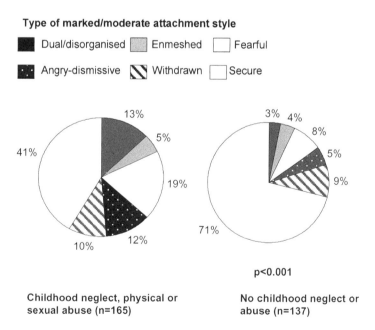

Figure 5.1 Rate of attachment style among those with childhood neglect/abuse

5.4.1 Type of childhood adversity and attachment style

The next step was to examine the different types of childhood adverse experience from the CECA, in relation to the different attachment styles at interview. This showed (see Figure 5.2 for the correlations):

- None of the negative childhood experiences were associated with Withdrawn styles.
- Enmeshed style related only to antipathy from parents.
- Fearful style was associated with neglect, role reversal, physical abuse and sexual abuse.
- Angry-dismissive style was correlated with parental antipathy, physical and psychological abuse.
- All the negative childhood experiences were associated with Dual/disorganised style.

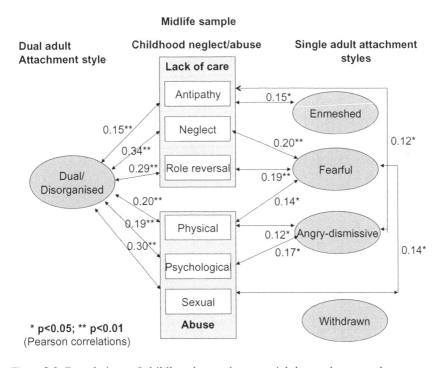

Figure 5.2 Correlations of childhood experience to Adult attachment style

In order to simplify the number of categories the childhood experiences were grouped in to indices of Lack of Care (neglect, antipathy or role reversal) or Severe Abuse (physical, sexual or psychological) and these examined in logistic regression to different style outcomes. (Enmeshed and Fearful were combined into Anxious style because of low numbers with Enmeshed style). Lack of Care alone proved the best fit for such Anxious attachment styles. For Angry-dismissive style Severe Abuse was the only significant predictive factor. Disorganised attachment was predicted best by Lack of Care, Severe Abuse did not add. This is shown schematically in Figure 5.3 with the regression odds-ratios given. Again, neither index predicted Withdrawn style. Therefore some patterning of poor care to Anxious style and Dual/disorganised and abuse to Angry-dismissive style was evident as predicted in the research literature.

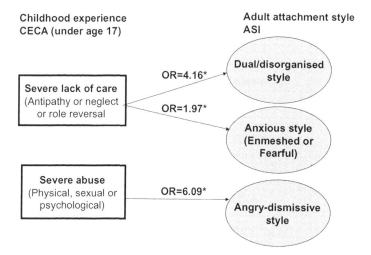

Odds ratio (OR) = significant ORs taken from binary logistic regression analyses. *p<0.05
ASI = Attachment Style Interview; CECA = Childhood Experience of Care and Abuse.

Figure 5.3 Summarised regression analysis – childhood experience and attachment styles

5.4.2 Mediation analysis

The relationship of childhood experience to attachment style was re-examined in sample 2 (154 women) followed-up for an average three years (Bifulco, Kwon *et al.* 2006). This examined new onset of disorder prospectively, which enabled an analysis of mediation to be undertaken. This to see if Insecure attachment style fulfilled conditions as a causal factor linking childhood experience to adult disorder. As in earlier chapters, major depression and clinical anxiety onset in follow-up were combined in this analysis. Just over half the sample (55%) had at least one new disorder in the follow-up period. As described in earlier chapters, highly Insecure attachment style, apart from Withdrawn was significantly related to both Major Depression and Anxiety outcomes at follow-up and these associations remained after controlling for disorder at point of first interview. Overall attachment style was significantly associated with childhood neglect or abuse in the subsample followed-up (0.30, p<0.0001).

Tests for a mediating role of Insecure attachment style (excluding Withdrawn style) were undertaken using the accepted three-step method (Baron and Kenny 1986), with the requirement that all three elements are significantly related. Thus logistic regression analysis showed a relationship between childhood neglect/abuse as the predictor variable and highly Insecure attachment style as the potential mediator variable (a=4.34, p<0.0001) and for Insecure attachment style and emotional disorder as the criterion variable (b=4.95, p<0.001) as well as childhood neglect relating to Insecure attachment style (c=2.09, p<0.02). When both childhood and Insecure attachment were examined in relation to emotional disorder, the childhood variable no longer added to the model (c=1.46). This shows that childhood experience no longer exerts a statistical effect once the mediating Insecure attachment style is utilised.

Figure 5.4 shows the significant path analysis coefficients between childhood adversity highly Insecure attachment style (excluding Withdrawn) and onset of depression or anxiety at follow-up, indicating the mediating relationship.

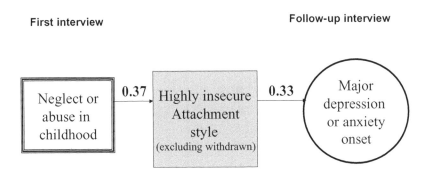

Figure 5.4 Childhood adversity and emotional disorder mediated by Insecure attachment style

---

Summary of childhood findings in adult women

- Childhood neglect and abuse occurred for half the high-risk women studied.
- An index of childhood neglect, physical or sexual abuse was highly related to Insecure attachment style. A dose effect was shown with the higher the insecurity of attachment, the higher the rate of childhood neglect or abuse associated.
- When individual styles were examined, all correlated with childhood neglect/abuse apart from Withdrawn style. Nearly three-quarters of those with Insecure attachment style had childhood neglect or abuse. Only 42% of those Secure had similar neglect or abuse. Nearly all (90%) of those with Dual/disorganised style had childhood neglect or abuse.
- When type of experience was examined in relation to type of attachment style; Fearful style related to a wide range of Lack of Care and Abuse scales; Enmeshed style related solely to antipathy from parents, Angry-dismissive related to physical, psychological abuse and antipathy. Dual/disorganised style related to all the lack of care and abuse scales.
- Using combined childhood scales and attachment style outcomes in logistic regression analysis, the index of Lack of Care experience (neglect, antipathy or role reversal) predicted Anxious (Enmeshed or Fearful) attachment styles. An index of Severe abuse (physical, sexual or psychological) solely predicted Angry-dismissive style. Lack of care also predicted Dual/disorganised attachment style.
- Having prospective data on the sample allowed for investigation of attachment style as a mediating factor for new onset of disorder. Statistical analysis showed that Insecure attachment style (excluding Withdrawn) mediated between childhood experience and onset of emotional disorder thus a key linking experience.

5.5 Case examples – adult women

The following case examples illustrate the linkages between childhood experience and attachment style in adult women.

5.5.1 Eloise's moderate Enmeshed style and Lack of Care from mother

Eloise is a 43-year-old divorcée, living with her second husband of nine years and her two children, a son aged 14 and a daughter aged 11. She works part-time as an assistant at a junior school and her partner is a self-employed builder. Her partner has children from a previous relationship whom he sees at weekends. Her first marriage was to a violent man. She has no history of clinical level disorder.

Support and Enmeshed attachment style: Eloise had poor support from her partner and stated that the relationship was very unsatisfying as she could not confide in him, nor rely on him in any way except financially. They argued constantly and he had recently been threatening, saying: *'If you were a man I'd smack you.'* The relationship was considered 'inadequate support with discord'. At first contact Eloise had already asked her partner to leave and he moved to the flat upstairs which they also own. She named two VCOs who were friends seen weekly as support figures. She did confide in one of these, Cathy (rated 'good-average support, no discord'), but did not talk about important issues to Sarah (rated 'insufficient support, no discord'). She was rated as having 'some' ability to make and maintain relationships and therefore moderately Insecure. She had an Enmeshed style. Eloise had some ambivalence in her description of trust and ability to get close. Whilst she says of her friends *'These are all people I can just turn up on their doorsteps with and it doesn't really matter, they will help',* she indicated constraints on getting close: *'I don't know. I don't know – I think I'm quite selective. I feel as close as I can get. I don't think that I am a particularly... I let other people get close to me but I don't seem to be able to get that close to them. I don't know if that makes sense to you?'* She had a high need for being with people and a fear of separation: *'Being alone in the house – sometimes I get very scared – it sort of depends how I'm feeling – when I do get scared, I do get scared and I think, you know, I have to make sure the windows are all locked and double check things and it doesn't feel very nice.'* She worried when her partner was away: *'The thing that I'd feel anxious about was that he'd have a motorbike crash or something like that, that he'd get beaten up or have a crash or something. So I was anxious that something would happen to him.'* It is therefore interesting that when she tells him to leave, it is only to go to live upstairs in the same building.

Eloise felt she needed her friends around her all the time. She was also quite possessive with her son and felt anxious when he was out. *'It's actually quite difficult standing back and allowing a child you've been totally responsible for to take up their own space rather than yours.'* She also had a lot of anger in relationships. Her partner relationship was very stormy. In addition she rowed with her son and had threatened to *'beat him up'*. She also had arguments and rows at work. She referred throughout the interview to her resentment of her mother who was critical and unsupportive. *'She will never ever, and never has ever, said a word in support of me. ever. I find that very hard to understand. She has always, always done it.'* Eloise's style therefore fitted the moderately Enmeshed angry profile.

Self-esteem: Eloise had a mixed view of herself, on the one hand negative and critical, but also having a feeling of specialness. She was self-blaming about finding herself again in a relationship with an aggressive man. She thought she was *'dumb'*. She also said *'I don't have an intellectual bone in my body'*, but prized herself on having intuition. She sometimes felt attractive, but felt bad about the weight she had put on. She was self-critical of her parenting: *'It wears me out being a mother'*, and described herself as a *'wreck'*. When asked if she was sympathetic or hard, she said *'I am both. I can be quite hard if I want to but it's not a ruthless kind of hard. It is a bit cruel to be kind.'* When asked if she was difficult to live with she said *'everyone will tell you I'm difficult to live with but I think that is partly because I've never lived with people who are the same as me. I've always been odd.'*

She described her feeling of being different: *'I've always felt completely different, even to people that I've got on very well with. The main thing I feel at the moment is in a certain way, a very wicked and earthly sense of superiority. I think one of the things is learning to love the person I really am and not the person you see sitting here, but the "me" that I really am. If you look in the mirror, look at yourself but look behind the person you see there and start loving yourself for all your faults and for all your needs and wants and things like that, it's a very difficult thing to do and I think that that is beginning to work. I'm beginning to allow myself to love myself.'* Thus, while she gave some contradictory responses, her self-esteem was not considered low.

Childhood experience: Her childhood experience revolved around her mother's antipathy towards her. She describes rejection from her mother, but being her father's favourite, although he was not demonstrative in his care. *'I couldn't say I felt rejected but I always felt left out. My mother would always ridicule me, she'd use me as this battering ram. She'd use the other children to consolidate her position in the family and made very sure in her own way that I was left out. I have no memories of her ever being caring and physically affectionate or even verbally affectionate at all, very strange. Yet she was to the others. She was always changeable like that.'* Eloise said she was isolated, that her mother 'ganged up' with her siblings against her and stated that her mother was doing the same with her children now in setting them against her. *'I remember many years ago there was a woman in the street where we lived and she actually came to see my mother and told her that she ought to do more to support me and look after me and I remember my mother telling me this years later and laughing. She is very cruel. There was no support. There was nobody to come home and tell if something awful had happened to you. My aunt says my mother has no understanding at all, absolutely none... In childhood she would ridicule me all the time. She probably didn't dislike me, and she probably loved me and she probably still does. Because I'm very different to the others I probably was more difficult because I was a much stronger person than any of them, and I have strengths that she could probably always see but she could never compete with. I think I always did feel embarrassed about walking into a room where my mother and sisters were, so I must have had the feeling that it was odd in some way. She would threaten to send me away. My mother was always saying that my father said that I ought to go to boarding school. She* *always used to say that, always, always, because she said I was so difficult, awkward and unpleasant. Now that I think about it she used to say that all the time. My father never said anything like that to me directly. But the other side of it is that she said she was the one who wouldn't let him do it – to make her seem like the good guy.'*

Her parents got on badly: *'My mother couldn't cope with my father. They had no communication at all. She isolated him and then she isolated me, but I don't know why. It is only in recent years that I've seen that that is what she did, because she has tried to do it between me and my children. She used the children as a weapon against my dad and influenced us all greatly against him. It wasn't till I was an adult that I actually realised it. I used to side with my mother in arguments against my father. I don't remember any arguments between me and my parents as a teenager, but it was a very stormy household in some ways. There was always an air of argument about even if there wasn't one going on.'*

Comment: Eloise had the typical characteristics of Enmeshed style – combining both dependency and anger in her relationships and with very frequent reference to other people's opinions rather than her own. She traced this to her childhood experience of antipathy, her mother's dislike of her and her mother's use of power play against her father. Eloise did not have insight into how she might be repeating this with her son – she was both passionately close but also hostile and threatening to him and unable to accept that he was growing into an autonomous teenager. She similarly had little insight into her friendships and believed them to be many and close, but when questioned closely only one was available for support. She still seemed 'enmeshed' in her relationship with her mother, who she saw often and who still had the power to upset her with her criticisms. In interview she would slip from childhood to present-day descriptions of her mother's behaviour, seemingly unaware of the disparity between herself as a child subject to mother's critical tongue and herself in midlife perpetuating the dynamic.

5.5.2 Faye's moderately Fearful attachment style and childhood lack of care and physical abuse

Faye is a 24-year-old secretary who lives alone. She is very involved with her job and has taken up further training encouraged by her employer. She has few social contacts and only one close relationship with a man that she had ended recently because he wanted more closeness and commitment from her than she was prepared to give.

Disorder: She had a history of various types of disorder. She had depression and bulimia from age 17 related to a big row with her parents which led to her leaving home. She became depressed again age 22, this time with alcohol abuse following a miscarriage, which was the result of a rape by a family friend. Aged 27 she developed GAD and a year later developed depression, panic disorder and alcohol dependence following splitting up with her boyfriend.

Support and attachment style: Faye had markedly Fearful attachment style. She was very close to an older friend Jill who had been a mentor since childhood and with whom she spoke daily. But she did not confide fully in Jill because of trust issues: '*Although I'd talk to her, after I'd said something I'd regret saying it because she might be laughing at me. I might tell her four or five weeks later and she'll say "why didn't you phone me at the time"– I'll say "you've got your own life . . . I'm not your responsibility".*' Faye did not socialise and found it difficult to mix: '*I find it difficult to meet new people . . . I'm a little bit shy and I feel a bit inferior to them. Once I get over that step I'm okay. Going to college was a real effort, but it's surprising how friendly people out there are. I'm too nervous to make the first attempt so the initiative normally comes from somebody else, unless it's in work and then I'm better.*' She was not close to her family and had no other close friends or confidants. She went to see her birth mother for the first time just over two years ago. They did not become close: '*I had to go to just see what she looked like – I won't go again. She was thick, fat, lazy, and how many people do you know who can't spell the name that she gave you when you were born?*'

Faye was very mistrustful: '*It takes me time to get close. Over the past four years I've improved in that field, because before then I didn't trust a person, not a single person, not even Jill. But now, since I've been working here and after going to the therapist for so long – I find it easier now . . . I can decide who to trust and who not to trust. I still don't talk to anybody about personal things, so if I'm having trouble with a guy I don't discuss it with anybody – it's between me and him. I can't stand it when people want to know too much. Close as I am with my boss, I only told him anything personal after one and a half years. The people who should be here for me, I won't allow to be because I just can't stand it.*'

She had high fear of rejection: '*With the way we've been brought up, I'm not one for physical contact at all with people. I'm frightened of men! It's true – older men, not boys my age. Why live with a man when you've got your own place? I know that once people I've been out with start getting a bit too close, I start to push them away again. I'll hurt the people that love me way before they'll ever hurt me. It's not that I intend to, it's just what happens. People who know me can see the 'wall' going up, slowly but surely. One day hopefully the right person will come along and take the wall away and then it will never go up again.*'

Faye felt lonely at times, but preferred to be alone: '*Life is good, but you can be as happy as anything one moment and then all of a sudden it just hits you like a ton of bricks – the feeling of being alone. I've always had a real yearning for a mother and a mother is something I will never have . . . something you really regret missing out on. People like Jill don't make up for it – no matter how close you are, eventually they have their own family and, whilst they're real people, it's hardly the same . . . I enjoy living on my own, it's so much nicer. I am a little bit of a loner perhaps.*'

Self-esteem: Faye had negative self-evaluation: '*I know I underestimate myself. When I'm with people who are better educated, I feel inferior because I don't have the same vocabulary. I realise it's stupid, because if somebody says something that you don't know, you should just ask. My confidence is improving – I'm beginning to enjoy situations that I used to avoid, like going out with clients and my boss for a meal in a restaurant... I don't like myself sometimes because sometimes I can come over to others as very forceful. I feel that's not very nice. You shouldn't be like that to people. And I've got no patience with certain people at work. But I am equal to other people... I'm a pretty private person on the whole. I'm reserved – I'm a softie, although people think I'm quite hard. I've got a lot of patience, except when people can't follow my instructions after being shown five times! I'll tolerate a lot, being pushed and pushed for quite a long time, because it's in my nature to be that way. But once I snap I completely snap. I'm impatient. I say what I think. I'm afraid it gets me into a lot of trouble. I give way to other people too much.*'

Childhood experience: Faye's early life was spent in residential care, having been abandoned by her mother at age three when she and her sisters were left without warning at the social services office. Their mother told them she would be back in half an hour but wasn't seen again until Faye was aged 22 and sought her out. Her father remarried when Faye was age nine and took the children back to live with him and his new wife who was much younger than himself. Neither he nor his new wife were capable of coping with Faye and her two sisters, and the children were neglected and physically abused. The atmosphere was generally very tense and hostile. Faye's role in the household involved a great deal of responsibility for both the younger children and for doing the household washing and cleaning. To her parents she felt she was just a skivvy.

About her father she said: '*I just think he saw us as an inconvenience – but he likes having little maids about and there were plenty of us, we were all girls. He name-called all of us. My stepmother wasn't affectionate – I was at the wrong age for her. If you're a baby she'll love you. She doesn't have the patience for children. She just couldn't cope.*' Whilst her stepmother would slap the children, her father would physically abuse them by beating them regularly throughout their childhood. '*A good hiding... either slipper or a hand or a leather belt or whatever, and depending what sort of mood he was in... wherever he could use to reach you... We all went to school with the odd black eye and bruises. Dad's got a very hard hand... Oh, he'd be in an absolutely terrible mood, screaming and swearing. I mean, he'd knock you off every wall... with the force of the blow, with his slap or his punch... All of us got hit. Hit with buckle end of the belt sometimes.*' Her father told them not to tell anyone: '*You didn't even tell your best friend that your dad beat you, it was kept within the home. We'd become a little bit wise, you get one hit, you cry and don't get too many more after that. When I was age 15 he hit me with the brush on my hand and I just looked him straight in the face as if to say "You can hit me as much as you like – I'm not going to cry for you" and he just kept on hitting me until the brush broke in half and he never ever struck me after that.*'

There was also neglect in the household – Faye's stepmother was help-less and unable to cope with the basic care of the children. This led to the role reversal where Faye herself had to provide care for the family: *'I was never allowed to go out in the evening – I had to help with the housework and look after the younger sisters. It was the same at the weekend ... I had to be up at the crack of dawn with dad, doing the hand-washing which included sheets – and help with the housework and go out to do the shopping. I was just a skivvy. I resented it. No child minds helping out ... but to force a child to have no life outside the home – you've got to resent it. My stepmother couldn't cope, particularly when we got evicted and had to live in a bed and breakfast hostel.'* Faye did, however, recall feeling upset and responsible for her father when he had to go into hospital: *'I don't know why I was upset but nonetheless I was. He went into intensive care because of his breathing difficulty ... It was not because I loved him but because I was a bit concerned as to where I'd end up if anything happened to him.'* Faye felt great responsibility and concern for her younger siblings and half-siblings and this prevented her from leaving home earlier.

This sense of responsibility also affected her adult life. Once she left home she was afraid for sisters. *'Even though I'd moved away from home I still went to make sure everything was OK. I still said to my dad if you ever hurt Cathy I'm going to take her away from you. My half-sister Liz was being very rebellious, she did try to commit suicide and that's why I went back home. Later when she came to stay with me I wouldn't let her go back to dad's, because I couldn't bear the thought of her doing anything to herself again. She stayed with me for quite a while.'*

Comment: Faye's Fearful attachment can be traced back to harsh physical abuse, neglect and role reversal from a young stepmother who was unable to cope with the demands of parenthood and a father who was controlling and saw the children as an inconvenience. This re-emphasised her experi-ence of having been rejected by her birth mother in infancy. The experience of physical harm from those who are meant to be close is clearly a theme that emerges in Fearful attachment style – the anticipation of rejection, criticism or attack from others that leads to fear and avoidance of closeness. This has in turn damaged Faye's self-esteem. Role reversal has other negative effects, in part related to an impoverished school and social life due to working in the home. One aspect that aided Faye's survival was meeting her older friend Jill in early teenage years. Jill helped teach her life skills, offered support and helped her to eventually stand up to her father. She was also being helped in her work to further her education and to learn greater confidence and this aided by her ongoing psychotherapy.

5.5.3 Alma's moderately Angry-dismissive style and childhood psychological abuse

Alma is a 37-year-old mother living with her second husband and two younger children, described in Chapter 4 in relation to her previous violent partnership. Her only source of support was a friend she went to bingo with. Her partner relationship was unsupportive and conflictful. Her attachment style was moderately Angry-dismissive: she had a high need for control in relationships, high self-reliance and had high anger in her partner relationship, with her older children and with her mother. Her self-esteem was high and she saw herself as a strong and capable person, able to withstand challenges. She was still very hostile to her stepfather who was abusive to her in childhood and to her mother who failed to protect her.

Childhood experience: Alma had a very difficult childhood characterised both by lack of care and by severe abuse. Her mother took her and her two siblings away from home, leaving their father when Alma was aged eight. Her father drank heavily and was unreliable with money but Alma was his favourite and they were very close. From age eight to 14 Alma lived with her mother and stepfather during which time she suffered extreme abuse and neglect. Her parents failed to provide basic care for the children. The stepfather was very controlling, although this did alternate with periods when the children were just left unsupervised, for instance when the parents went on holiday leaving the quite young children alone in the house unsupervised. Alma's stepfather disliked her intensely, and physically and psychologically abused her. She was badly beaten by him: '*It got to the stage I would want to commit suicide to get away from the horrendous beatings. It wouldn't be one or two it would be seven or eight, until you were physically marked, with a leather belt.*' This was often because she was found talking about her birth father to her sisters. '*I would be hurt, quite badly, slapped or thrown upstairs. I got punched, literally.*' She would, however, fight back. She also told her teacher about the abuse and social workers were informed, but ultimately took no action.

Her stepfather became less physically and more psychologically abusive after she disclosed to her teacher. He was extremely controlling: '*We were all his little soldiers . . . we were lined up along the couch in the evening watching TV and if we stopped for a moment to glance, "You're not watching TV? Right, fine, go to bed" is what you got shouted at you, because he happened to notice that you weren't fixed on the TV screen. You'd be halfway through watching your favourite programme and he'd say: "Right, I want you to go and polish all the shoes for school tomorrow. Get in the kitchen, set the newspaper down, polish all the shoes for school tomorrow . . . and I want to see my face in them when you've finished".*'

Alma's stepfather also deprived her of basic needs, a marker of psychological abuse. She would be locked in a room with no light bulb, no curtains on the windows, no blankets on the bed for weeks at a time during school holidays and was only allowed to come downstairs once a day to eat over a period of weeks. '*It was to make you feel as if you didn't exist . . . And he almost got me to believe in it for a while, and then one day something just snapped and I just thought "No, you're not going to win this battle. I just can't let you, for my own self-respect will just go if I do that." And so I would sit there and let him think that I didn't care. When he looked in the door and expected me to lay crying, I'd sit and smile at him, and I began to give him back what he did to me and make out it wasn't getting to me. But it did, believe me. I still carry the scars from that. It took me a long time to beat his games, his sort of mental torture and his attempt to make you feel totally degraded and useless. And for quite a while he succeeded in making me feel like that, and then just something inside me snapped, and I just had this feeling that I had to survive him, that I had to wait until I was old enough to walk away.'*

Comment: Growing up in a household governed by fear, in anticipation of both physical and psychological harm, Alma toughened herself in order to survive. The experience of telling her teacher of the abuse only to have social workers disbelieve her, convinced her that she could only rely on herself and no one else to get out of the situation. Her current high self-reliance was thus forged early in her childhood. She also acknowledged that she used some of the same psychological abuse back to her stepfather – she would smile to let him know it wasn't affecting her, and psychologically she argued back with him, accusing him of not being her 'real' father. This made him very jealous and she knew it made him angry. She did finally run away from home to get out of the situation and was returned home by the police only to leave again on her sixteenth birthday when she was legally allowed to choose where to live. Her problem first marriage was violent as described in Chapter 4, but she had little parental guidance and her partner choice was determined by her teenage pregnancy. Whilst her second marriage started supportively it also deteriorated in terms of support, but was not violent. Her Angry-dismissive style involves harbouring resentment to both her mother and stepfather, although she voices it more towards her mother whom she feels should have protected the children (and who she identifies as her VCO, but from whom she gets no support). In many ways she has adopted her stepfather's view of the world: her mistrust, over self-reliance and blame of others mirrors some of his attitudes. She does, however, profess concern and protectiveness of those close, but with little actual sensitivity to their needs, and this has severely hampered her parenting skills (described in the next chapter). Alma refuses to express any neediness herself, instead seeing herself as providing resources for other people's need, and this was accompanied by her need to control those around her.

The next section will look at childhood experience in the Offspring sample. Since this sample is younger (average age 20) this will allow for an exploration of attachment style closer to the childhood experience, and to compare maltreatment from mothers or fathers. It will also be able to look across gender and to examine peer and school relationships and self-esteem to add to the developing model.

5.6 Childhood experience in young people

Neglect, physical or sexual abuse was reported by as many as 41% of the young people. Most had been brought up by their birth mothers also in the study but over half (59%) had been separated from their birth fathers and had a single mother upbringing for at least part of their childhood or early adolescence. Around a third (32%) of young people experienced Lack of Care (neglect, antipathy or role reversal) and the same proportion Severe Abuse (physical, sexual or psychological). However, rates of sexual abuse (4%) and psychological abuse (6%) were particularly low in this sample, so physical abuse was the main component of the latter index. There was no difference in rates of Lack of Care or Severe Abuse by gender.

Various associations between different neglect and abuse experiences were examined with some replication of the adult sample for Anxious styles. Thus significant correlations were found consistently for Fearful style, relating to nearly all experiences with correlations of 0.16 to 0.34 (p<0.05 to p<0.001). As with the adults, Enmeshed style related solely to antipathy (0.18, p<0.01). However, in this sample Angry-dismissive style was only associated with antipathy (0.18, p<0.05) not abuse.

Since the analysis is a preliminary to the test of intergenerational transmission through the behaviour of mothers explored in the next chapter, the childhood scales were differentiated by parent. Significant associations held between mothers' problem parenting and the Anxious (Fearful and Enmeshed) styles (see summary in Figure 5.5). Dual/disorganised style showed less association than in the adult sample but did relate to physical abuse from mother and neglect from father. A gender difference was found for Angry-dismissive style which related to maternal and paternal neglect only for girls.

Therefore, in this sample of young people, it was mothers' poor parenting that related most consistently to Anxious attachment style in the young people. This held across gender. Fathers parenting had less association but then mainly with Angry-dismissive or Dual attachment styles.

5.6.1 Self-esteem

Negative evaluation of self has been examined in earlier chapters as one of the psychological factors related to poor support, attachment style and depression. In the young people the following relationships were found (see summary Figure 5.6):

- NES was highly related to Anxious attachment style (0.36, p,0.0001) and to Dual/disorganised style (0.27, p<0.001) but was unrelated to Angry-dismissive style (0.04).
- NES was associated with mothers' problem parenting (0.22, p<0.008) but not fathers (0.04).

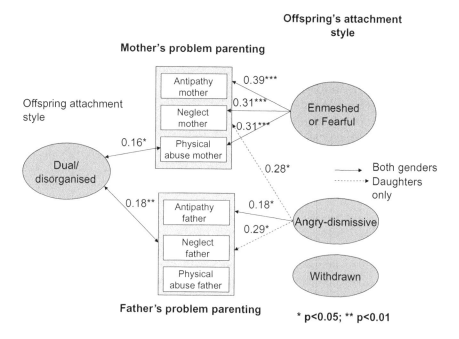

Figure 5.5 Correlations between childhood experience and attachment style

- NES was related to emotional disorder in the 12-month period (0.19, p<0.02) but not to substance abuse in the year (0.11).

5.6.2 Teenage peer group

Various peer experiences as recalled at age 16 were examined to see if they related to attachment style at interview. An index combining reports of isolation, problem peer group, lack of confidant or being a victim of bullying occurred for as many as 73% with 32% having two or more indicators. The research literature generally finds that problem peer group relates to behavioural disorder. This was examined in relation to attachment style and disorder. Findings showed (see summary Figure 5.6):

- Problem peer index related to Angry-dismissive attachment style (0.16, p<0.04) and Dual/disorganised (0.16, p<0.04) but not to Anxious styles (0.05).
- It related to mothers' problem parenting (0.21, p<0.01) but not fathers (0.01).
- It related to substance abuse (0.27, p<0.001) but not emotional disorder (0.14).
- Problem peer group related to NES (0.19, p<0.02).

Risk factor in offspring sample	Negative Evaluation of Self	Peer problems
Dual/disorganised attachment style	√	√
Anxious (Enmeshed or Fearful) attachment style	√	—
Angry-dismissive attachment style	—	√
Mother problem parenting (Neglect, Antipathy or Physical Abuse)	√	√
Father problem parenting (Neglect, Antipathy or Physical Abuse)	—	—
Peer problems	√	N/A
Substance abuse in 12 months	—	√
Emotional disorder (Depression or anxiety) in 12 months	√	—

√ indicates significant relationships

Figure 5.6 Summary of risk factors related to NES and peer problems

Two models were explored, using logistic regression for emotional disorder and substance abuse. This showed:

- Anxious attachment style was found to be the best predictor of emotional disorder with mothers' poor parenting. NES and peer problems did not contribute.
- Fathers' poor parenting and peer problems were the best predictors of substance abuse. Neither type of attachment style nor NES added to the model.

Finally the risk factors for emotional disorder were examined in terms of a structural equation model, and significant pathways shown for mothers' problem parenting, anxious attachment style, NES and emotional disorder (see Figure 5.6). This held for both genders and across ethnicity. (More details can be found in (Bifulco 2008; Schimmenti and Bifulco 2008). The models were unchanged when examined by gender or ethnicity.

Partial model of interrelationships — structural equation model

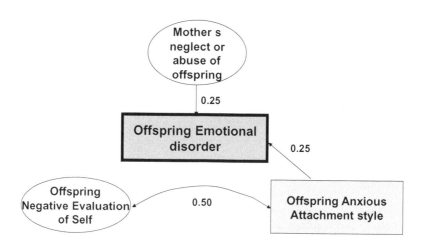

Figure 5.7 Mothers' poor parenting and offspring anxious attachment style

5.7 Case examples – Offspring sample

Only one example is given here from the Offspring sample, but the child-hood experience of Felicity and of Donna, both described in earlier chapters is outlined in the next chapter on parenting.

5.7.1 Dean's Dual/disorganised attachment style, and childhood Lack of Care and Abuse

Dean, a 29-year-old man who lived alone, was described in Chapter 3 in relation to his attachment style, his violence to his partner and his substance abuse. His Angry-dismissiveness is typified by high mistrust and a confrontational style with both peers and his girlfriend, to whom he has been violent. However, he is also possessive in his partner relationships, and has contradictory needs for closeness which contribute to his Enmeshed profile.

Self-esteem: His self-esteem was in the medium range, neither high nor low: *'I like to be poetical. Make people laugh. Usually I can be very serious, but I override it when I'm in company. I would say I was hard rather than sympathetic, I would like to be more sympathetic. I don't think I'm handsome but I don't really care*

– *people find me how they want. I'm not unhappy with my looks. I'm not academically [intelligent] but pretty logical with common sense. Sometimes I do think long and hard enough about things.'* As a boyfriend: *'I'm selfish. I want to do what I want to do, but I'm no worse than she was. I did treat her with respect. I am a good listener. I'm loyal to the hilt.'*

Childhood experience: Throughout his childhood, Dean's father was in and out of prison for fraud convictions. At 18 months old Dean was diagnosed as having coeliac disease and was sent away from his parents to a care home until he was three as his mother couldn't cope. He remembered no closeness to his birth mother. Dean went to live with his father and his father's new partner who was also his aunt (his mother's sister) and who at the time was only 17 years old. Dean's relationship with his aunt was turbulent and after her own son was born (Eric, described in Chapter 4), she favoured her own son and scapegoated Dean. When Dean was 10 his father finally left home and Dean stayed with his stepmother and younger half brother. His conduct disorder started to become evident at around 11 years old and his aggressive interactions with his stepmother deteriorated further. She placed him in residential care aged 15.

Antipathy from his stepmother was inconsistent but increased when his father left: *'Once dad was gone I always felt like an outcast. She didn't want me around. She would say "you are not my son". But then again, she would always back me up to the hilt with outsiders, then when the door was closed she would be critical. She was always telling everyone what a good kid I was even though I wasn't. But it was her actions that made me feel that she didn't want me.'* There was moderately high neglect: *'If she had time we would have breakfast, but that was not regular. If I was sick she would worry and I would get special treatment. If I was hungry I would get chips from the chip shop myself. She did try to make me go to school – I'd get a good hiding if didn't go to school. She always tried her best to get us what we wanted. Tried her hardest.'* Dean was allowed to roam the housing estate from a young age until quite late into the night without supervision. Discipline was variable as he was allowed to come home at whatever time he chose, but would be beaten over small things he did wrong. His stepmother would hit him with anything to hand, and typical injuries from the beatings would be bruises. On one occasion she threw a vacuum cleaner at him and he got concussion. On another occasion she punched a couple of his teeth out after he was caught stealing money from her friend's purse.

Dean's father was not involved at all in his upbringing and was in prison during most of Dean's childhood. Even when he was around he showed very little interest in Dean's care. Childhood risk factors therefore include separation from mother when he was very young, and from father later in childhood, and poor parenting from his aunt/stepmother who raised him. Other risk factors were neglect, lax supervision, antipathy and physical abuse. Dean also had a problem peer group, got involved in fights and had delinquent friends. This escalated once he was in residential care. He did not do well at school, truanted frequently and did not get any qualifications.

Comment: Dean's childhood shows no early attachment to his birth parents through separations and then poor mothering from his aunt/stepmother who was physically abusive and neglectful, and a father who was absent and often in prison. This culminated in Dean's conduct disorder which then led to him to go into residential care as a teenager. His Angry-dismissive style can be readily linked to the physical abuse he experienced and his Enmeshed style to the antipathy from his mother figure and his early separations. He made ambivalent comments about his stepmother's care, stating the negatives but also trying to make positives. The multiples of negative experiences can be seen to link to his Dual style, expressed in his very aggressive behaviour in residential care and confounded perhaps by his early substance abuse. Having a Dual/disorganised style is common among youth in residential care, perhaps linked to early separations preceded or accompanied by antipathy, physical abuse and lack of care, as described in Chapter 9.

Summary findings in the Offspring sample

- Among young people in the Offspring sample 41% had childhood neglect/abuse. However, they had low rates of sexual and psychological abuse.
- Under a third of the sample had Lack of Care experience and the same rate of Severe Abuse was rated.
- There were significant associations of attachment style to childhood adversity scales. Fearful had the highest association with a range of neglect or abuse experiences.
- When maltreatment from different parents was examined, an equal rate of mothers' problem parenting (neglect, antipathy or physical abuse) or fathers' was found (27%).
- Anxious attachment style (Enmeshed or Fearful) related to mothers' poor parenting but not fathers'.
- NES was related to Anxious or Dual/disorganised attachment style, to mothers' problem parenting and to emotional disorder.
- Problem peer group was associated with Angry-dismissive or Dual/disorganised style, mothers' problem parenting and substance abuse.
- A model was developed showing NES, poor parenting from mother and Anxious attachment style relating to emotional disorder.
- Fathers' poor parenting and problem peer group was related to substance abuse, but neither attachment style nor NES contributed.

- There were only a few gender differences in the sample in relation to attachment style or childhood experience but this did not
  affect the overall models produced.

5.8 Discussion

The basic premise that attachment style in adolescence or adulthood
relates to adverse childhood experience was confirmed. The likelihood of
having a highly Insecure attachment style was doubled in those with
adverse early experience, and for those with Insecure attachment style
nearly three-quarters had early life neglect or abuse. In looking for differentiation in experience and style there was some patterning found in the
adult women for different styles with poor care relating to Anxious styles
and abuse to Angry-dismissive style. However, this was only an approxima-
tion, with Fearful styles in particular experiencing both lack of care and
abuse, together with those Dual/disorganised. Among the young offspring
sample, the parent providing the poor care or abuse was a better predictor
of disorder, with maternal parenting problems predicting Anxious styles as
well as negative evaluation of self and emotional disorder. Fathers' problem
parenting contributed to substance abuse disorders, but not through
offspring attachment style. We do not know whether this is because in this
samples many fathers were absent and therefore had less opportunity to
influence attachment style, or whether this pattern would be repeated in
other samples.

There is thus support for the main underpinning of attachment theory:
that very adverse childhood experience relates to the developing adolescent and then adult attachment styles in a way that increases vulnerability
to clinical disorder. Whilst this study was not able to measure aspects in the
youth such as capacity for mentalising, this is likely to be a correlate of
negative evaluation of self, and also underpins some of the attitudes seen
in the different attachment styles. In the next chapter the childhood theme
will be continued, but this time in relation to characteristics of the mother's
in the study, their parenting and intergenerational transmission of risk.

6   Parenting and attachment style

6.0 Introduction

Attachment theory holds that parents or carers transmit to their children when young, distinct modes of coping, communicating, interacting and regulating emotion, and this can aid or impede the development of the child in ways that affect attachment capacity. When parents have poor functioning in these areas it shows itself in the parenting practices directed at the child. This can range in intensity from levels of insensitivity and lack of psychological attunement, to overt neglect or abuse. Whilst emphasis is usually placed on the mother's behaviour as the primary caregiver, transmission can occur from others with significant childcare responsibility, including fathers or alternative caregivers. Thus the influence and behaviour of mothers, fathers and others responsible for the child needs to be examined to determine their impact on the child's developing attachment capacity. This chapter will use the London intergenerational data to show how a mother's Insecure attachment style transmits risk to her children, but only through her actual parenting behaviour, and dependent upon her partner's behaviour. This relates to her neglect/abuse of her children which increases their risk of emotional disorder as already described.

Ainsworth's insightful work closely examined observed parent–infant interactions among families to determine normal development (Ainsworth, Blehar *et al.* 1978; De Wolff and van Ijzendoorn 1997). Others have extended their study of the patterning of attachment behaviour to families where child maltreatment and parental mental health are major concerns (Crittenden 1985; Dozier, Stovall *et al.* 1999; Howe, Dooley *et al.* 2000). Identifying parental Insecure attachment style as a risk indicator for negative parenting style and neglect/abuse of offspring is of central interest in both research and Child and Family Services. Professor Pat Crittenden has done much to highlight the role of child abuse in distorted attachment patterns and repetitions of poor parenting across generations (Crittenden 1997), with other researchers looking at impacts of adoption and fostering on abused children and their adjustment to new families (Dozier 2003; Steele, Hodges *et al.* 2003).

Earlier chapters have shown how Insecure attachment style in adults is at a confluence of risk factors, involving stressful circumstances, problem partner relationships, lack of support, low self-esteem as well as early life maltreatment. These factors can all contribute to negative impact on the children in the family. Models of parenting that incorporate all these factors have been outlined by Professor Jay Belsky and colleagues, and are gradually becoming incorporated into a unified attachment model which encompasses social factors and past history, but is in need of additional empirical evidence (Belsky and Vondra 1989).

The transmission of attachment insecurity across generations in normative samples is argued to be through maternal insensitivity, intrusiveness or detached interaction and poor emotion-regulation when in contact with the child (De Wolff and van Ijzendoorn 1997). The starting point for testing this is to examine the concurrent association of maternal attachment style and her infant offspring's pattern of attachment behaviour. The degree of similarity between the two is taken to reflect transmission. Thus it is argued that a Secure mother will have a Secure child, and similar transmission is argued for varieties of insecurity of style. Most studies have used the AAI to examine attachment style in mothers, and then compared this for concordance with infants scored on the video-taped SST. Thus the interaction within the mother-child dyads plays out the expression of the internalised Secure, Anxious-ambivalent, Avoidant or Disorganised working models of attachment in both participants (Main, Kaplan *et al.* 1985). High concordances (65%–72%) have generally been found in the two generations, and these taken to indicate transmission of style from mother to infant (Main, Kaplan *et al.* 1985; Main and Cassidy 1988; Steele, Steele *et al.* 1996; van Ijzendoorn and Bakersmans-Kranenburg 1996).

Such concordances have also been shown prospectively when assessing attachment style using the AAI during pregnancy and in the infant at three months with the SST (Fonagy, Steele *et al.* 1991; Steele, Steele *et al.* 1996) and then 12–18 months of age (Steele, Steele *et al.* 1996). A 75% concordance was found and it was argued that Secure (autonomous) parental representations were more likely to be associated with Secure attachment behaviour in the child. This study goes further than the others in suggesting the presence of the attachment style in the mothers at the prior point creates a mechanism for predicting transmission to the infant after birth, rather than merely reflecting an interaction in parallel. The ASI has similarly been studied in pregnant women in the TCS-PND project (Bifulco, Figueirido *et al.* 2004) and the study extended to look at the mothers antenatal attachment style in relation to interaction with the baby at six months of age. This was assessed using a five-minute video-taped interaction around play from the Global Rating Scales (Murray, Fiori-Cowley *et al.* 1996). Mothers' global sensitivity ratings were related to lower social class, poorer support from partner pre-birth and poor infant communication (Gunning, Conroy *et al.* 2004). Anxious ASI styles (Enmeshed or Fearful) were significantly correlated in the mother–baby interaction with absence of global sensitivity (0.26, p<0.01) and Avoidant (Angry-dismissive or Withdrawn) styles correlated with remoteness (0.25, p<0.01). Subscales showed those with maternal Anxious attachment styles in pregnancy were more demanding in the interaction (0.38, p<0.001). Avoidant styles were significantly associated with silent (0.24, p<0.02) and non-energetic (0.23, p<0.03) interaction with a trend towards non-intrusive speech (0.20, p<0.06). None of the independent infant behaviours (such as attentiveness to mother, being actively engaged, positive vocalisation, being inert, distressed or fretful) were, however, correlated with the mothers' antenatal attachment style. Thus mothers' ASI attachment category during pregnancy can take predicted forms of interaction with her child at six months and maybe a precursor of her developing parenting style (Bifulco, Gunning *et al.* 2006).

Even in early adulthood, associations have been shown between parent and offspring attachment styles, but these are sensitive to gender (Mikulincer and Florian 1999). In a study of Israeli university students and their parents from intact families and using self-report measures, correlations were found for mothers and daughters and fathers and sons. For mother and daughters significant concordances were found for Secure, Avoidant and Anxious-ambivalent styles. For fathers, the concordance was with sons' Avoidant or Anxious-ambivalent styles, but not for Secure (op cit). Thus attachment style in both parents is clearly important as the child develops.

6.1 Partner, couples and family systems

It has been argued that previous attachment research has been limited in several respects (Kobak and Mandelbaum 2003). First, it is focused more on the child's experience rather than the parents' motivation for maintaining the relationship. Second, it gives only limited acknowledgement that caring for children occurs in the context of a parent's relationship with other adults where 'caregiver alliance' is a crucial aspect of childcare and family dynamics. Finally, parents' own attachment relationships can determine whether or not a secure base exists for the children. Kobak and Mandelbaum (op cit) describe how three relational systems: the parent–child relationship, the caregiving alliance and the adult attachment relationship can enhance or impede caring for children and need to be incorporated into attachment approaches to the study and treatment of families. Thus, feelings of anxiety or anger generated by the parent may be misdirected at the child or alternatively absorb the parent's attention thus detracting from parenting, and may include failure to encapsulate stress generated from adult relationships thus creating additional burdens for the child. Clearly the wider family need to be considered in determining intergenerational transmission of risk in attachment approaches.

In order to understand how attachment style in partners might influence parenting and the 'caregiver alliance', it is first necessary to look at the impact of such styles on each other. Attachment style assessed in couple relationships shows that most people prefer Secure partners (Chappel and Davis 1998) and these can buffer the effects of insecurity (Cohn, Silver *et al.* 1992). By encouraging openness and mutual expression, the Insecure partner can modify maladaptive behaviours associated with insecurity. However, sometimes the impact is not beneficial and a couple with at least one Insecure partner can also erode the sense of security in both its members (Rothbard and Shaver 1994; Feeney 2003). Thus even Secure individuals can become anxious about loss and rejection in the face of emotionally distant partners (Feeney 2003). Findings for mixed couples (one Secure and one Insecure) are therefore inconsistent, sometimes highlighting the Insecure (Senchak 1992) and sometimes the Secure (Feeney 1995), particularly when lower in conflict (Cohn, Silver *et al.* 1992). Destructive 'pursuer-distancer' cycles can emerge when couples struggle to regulate proximity and control the emotional tension of the relationship.

In partnerships, both men and women with Anxious attachment style report feeling more distress and hostility during problem-centred discussions, while Avoidant men are rated as engaging in lower quality interactions (Simpson, Rholes *et al.* 1992). Avoidant partners are argued to project their own unwanted self-traits on to their spouse and then use this to criticise and reject the spouse while boosting their own self-image (Mikulincer, Horesh *et al.* 1999). Individuals with Anxious styles tend to project their 'actual self' onto others and view themselves as overly similar to others. This allows them to feel closer and more similar to others and is an imagined basis for sharing each other's pain. Avoidant attachment style is associated with ineffective support seeking and Anxious styles with poor caregiving (Collins and Feeney 2000). Wives of Secure husbands are shown to be less rejecting and more supportive during problem-solving tasks and husbands of Secure wives listen more effectively in confiding tasks (Kobak and Hazan 1991). Relationship repair is seen to be easier in cases where at least one spouse is Secure (Feeney 2003). Relationship quality is predicted best by men's low Avoidance and women's low Anxious styles (Kirkpatrick and Hazan 1994).

Volling and colleagues looked at attachment patterns in relation to partner relationships, parenting and wellbeing in 62 married couples with a one-year-old child (Volling, Notaro *et al.* 1998). Self-report measures of attachment style were used and the SST for infant insecurity of attachment. Findings showed:

- In half of the couples, both members had Secure styles and in only 7% of couples did both members have Insecure styles.
- In the remainder where the partners had different styles, the most common pattern for a third was Secure-Avoidant combination.

- Where both members reported Secure attachment style, the marital relationships and support networks were better and fewer symptoms reported.
- Among the mixed attachment style groups, those where the wife had Secure attachment style and husband Avoidant style fared better in terms of their relationships, than where the wife had an Insecure style.
- Whilst relationships were found between Secure style and feelings of competent parenting, no relationship was found with parent's Insecure attachment style and infants Secure or Insecure style, either for individual parents or for couple attachment style combinations.

Thus whilst relationship and wellbeing outcomes were supported by attachment combinations in partners, this approach to intergenerational transmission did not yield positive results. However, only self-report measures of attachment style were used (with their focus on relating to others) possibly not a comprehensive enough tool for assessing parenting related aspects of attachment style.

The relationship with a partner is known to be critical to the effectiveness of parenting in the family (Cummings and Davies 2002; Cowan and Cowan 2005). Whilst a supportive partner can be a key resilience factor, for example in improving a mother's parenting capacity, the reverse is also true with problem partner behaviour and negative interaction between the couple, adding to risk of poor parenting and maltreatment of children (Forehand, Wierson *et al.* 1991; Kaczynski, Lindahl *et al.* 2006). Parenting quality is known to have multiple causes of which the partner relationship is one important element. In addition, stress, lack of other support, psychological state and a developmental history of abuse are all known to exert an influence (Belsky and Vondra 1989; Rodriguez and Green 1997). Attachment style as described in this book is related to all these factors and is thus a significant candidate for driving poor parenting.

In earlier chapters, the key role of partner relationships in a woman's attachment style has been described including problem partner behaviour involving violence. Partner behaviour can contribute simultaneously to Insecure attachment styles in the parent and poor parenting of children and their witnessing of domestic violence. Therefore women who find themselves in domestic violence situations, with partners with psychiatric disorder, antisocial behaviour, criminal behaviour or substance abuse, have a higher likelihood of having both an Insecure attachment style and being a poor parent (Johnson, Cohen *et al.* 2001; Kaczynski, Lindahl *et al.* 2006). Such women are likely to have their own attachment problems and deficiencies of parenting. Together these can be an explosive combination for the children in the household.

Family systems approaches have added to the parent–child focus in intergenerational transmission studies, by examining the contribution of both parents' attachment style, as well as the effects of the relationship between parents on children's development (Cowan and Cowan 2005). Studies by the Cowans' and their colleagues have specifically explored the quality of the parents' relationship as partners, the attachment characteristics of each, and problem behaviour in their preschool age children (Cowan, Cohn *et al.* 1996). In a sample of 27 couples and their first-born child, the AAI was administered to both mothers and fathers, together with assessments of marital quality, parenting style and child problem behaviour of both internalising (introversion, distress tension and depression) and externalising (antisocial behaviour, hostility, negative engagement, hyperactivity) types. Instead of deriving categorical attachment styles, continuous variables representing coherence, perceiving mother and father in childhood as loving, and anger towards parent figures were utilised.

Path analytic models showed different outcomes for mothers' and fathers' behaviour and for type of child disorder outcome. Mothers' attachment characteristics, quality of marital relationship and parenting style provided the best fit for explaining internalising behaviour in the child. For fathers, attachment characteristics followed a similar model but for externalising behaviour in the child. For mothers, the quality of marriage was found to be independent of attachment-related characteristics but adult attachment status with positive marital functioning was found to act as a buffer, protecting the child against the negative impact of Insecure attachment in one or both parents. The authors argue that the assumed intergenerational transmission through observable interaction with the child, and individuals' internal working models of attachment, need to be supplemented by the couple relationship and a more overtly family approach (Cowan and Cowan 2005).

This review shows that mother–infant interactions, parenting behaviour and partner relationships are all interwoven in family relationships and these can confer risks for all family members, but crucially for the children involved. Different findings emerge for different measures used, in different age groups of offspring with some variation by gender and when fathers are brought into the picture. The findings of the London studies will look at mothers' attachment style with the ASI, their reports of fathers' problem behaviours and then the independently interviewed young adult offspring. The outcome examined is the young people's experience of neglect or abuse from their mother, and their emotional disorder outcome. This will revisit findings from the last chapter, but taking both mother and offspring data and perspectives into account. The mothers' retrospective reports of her parenting behaviour when the child was growing up, is used to link the elements in the model.

6.2 Two London intergenerational studies

Intergenerational transmission of risk in the community has been investigated over two decades of study of London women and their offspring. An earlier study undertaken in the 1980s investigated representative London mothers and then followed up their young adult offspring to look for intergenerational transmission of risk (Andrews, Brown *et al.* 1990). Since the manner of selecting the dyads was identical and measures the same, the data was combined with the data reported in this book on the high-risk mother–offspring pairs. Unfortunately the first representative phase of the study did not use attachment style measures. Other measures used were the same, including self-esteem, support and the CECA for childhood experience and clinical interview measures of 12-month disorder in both generations. This will be summarised as background context for the high-risk part of the study to be reported.

6.2.1 Representative and high-risk groups combined

The combined samples yielded 276 mother–offspring dyads The mothers' ongoing adult vulnerability factors involved negative interaction with partner or child, lack of close confidant and low self-esteem (Bifulco, Moran *et al.* 2002) . In addition, the mother's childhood experience of neglect or physical or sexual abuse was also assessed. For the offspring an index of severe neglect, physical abuse or sexual abuse from any perpetrator was used, as well as any case level disorder in the year of interview. The path model developed from the analysis undertaken is shown in Figure 6.1 with combined data from both samples and from mother and offspring independent interviews. The significant associations (shown by continuous lines in the model) are:

- Mothers own childhood neglect or abuse relate to her adult vulnerability or depression.
- Mothers' vulnerability and depression are associated with neglect/abuse of her offspring.
- Offspring neglect/abuse related to offspring clinical disorder. An additional link was found between mothers' vulnerability and offspring disorder.
- Importantly, there is no direct link from mothers' early adversity and her offspring's neglect/abuse, nor of her early adversity and offspring disorder (see Figure 6.1, dotted lines).

This shows that the specific pathways identified imply intergenerational transmission of risk, with mother's vulnerability playing a critical role in the neglect/abuse of her children. Such vulnerability can be a magnet for a number of family, partner, individual and other risks for the child. So this model, whilst indicating transmission through the mother, does not necessarily imply this is as a result of her parenting. Transmission could also be through her attracting other risks to the family, such as through unsuitable partners. This model will be further explored with greater specificity and including attachment style, on the high-risk part of the London sample.

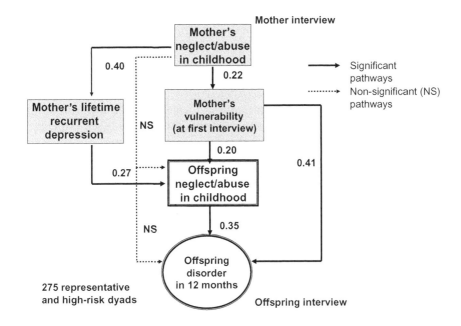

Figure 6.1 Mother's lifetime experience and disorder in offspring

Fathers were not interviewed as part of the study which is a weakness in developing the beginnings of a family model. However, this was impractical since a third were absent from households, and previous partners who may have parented the children were no longer involved. Instead the mother's account of her partner's behaviour was utilised, and by implication supported by offspring accounts. This is therefore, at best, a partial model and would need replicating but at least provides some exploration of pathways of risk transmission. On the basis of the links shown between mothers' vulnerability and offspring neglect and abuse, a more detailed investigation was undertaken with the 146 high-risk dyads (samples 3 and 4) in relation to mother's attachment style and neglect and abuse described by her young adult offspring.

6.2.2 Attachment style and intergenerational study

Previous analyses have already described psychological disorder in both mother and offspring samples, as well as the association of partner relationships and childhood experiences to attachment style for each. In order to examine transmission of risk from mother to offspring the lifetime measure of stress and of previous partner relationships (derived from the ALPHI) as described in earlier chapters was used, together with the

Parental Role Interview (PRI) measure of parenting which is now described further. Both were applied in the mother interview to measure the mother's earlier life experience as well as her parenting capacity while her children were growing up.

Two specific indicators of difficulties with partner were utilised. The first, 'severe and chronic marital/partner difficulty', was a binary index of 'marked' or 'moderate' peak difficulty associated with the partner relationship and present in two or more previous adult phases. Such difficulties included conflict in the relationship, physical violence from partner, partner infidelities, threatened separations or partner work difficulties. The second related index was 'problem partner behaviour'. Characteristics of the cohabiting partners were assessed in terms of treated psychiatric disorder, violent behaviour, apprehended criminal behaviour and antisocial behaviour described earlier and present in any current or prior cohabiting partnership lasting at least six months.

The PRI (Bifulco, Moran *et al.* 2009) is a measure that includes the assessment of chronic and severe difficulties in the motherhood role, positive and negative interaction as well as competence and incompetence in the parenting role. Competence/incompetence in the motherhood role involved asking mothers about their coping with the demands of motherhood around care, control and parenting of their children. Whilst the measure is currently used for ongoing relationships with children, this was applied retrospectively to the children as they were growing up, although supplemented by interactions with children assessed at first contact with the women. This reflected all the children in the mothers' care and not only the paired ones in the study.

Around half (52%) of the subgroup of 146 mothers had Insecure attachment styles at marked or moderate levels, with similar proportions (59%) having severe and chronic marital problems in their adult lives, and 47% having past or current partners with problem behaviours. Parenting findings included:

- Estimated incompetent parenting (interviewer rating) of the mother was rated in 41% of cases with a lower rate of 30% of women reported feeling incompetent (subjective rating). The two scales were highly correlated (0.42, p<0.001).
- Mothers' Insecure attachment style was significantly associated with her estimated incompetent parenting (0.26, p<0.01). The association was somewhat higher than for her reported felt incompetence (0.17, p<0.05).
- Partner's problem behaviour was associated with the mothers estimated parenting incompetence (0.25, p<0.01).
- There was no association of chronic marital/partner difficulty and parenting or attachment style.
- Logistic regression analysis showed that partner's problem behaviour, and mothers' Insecure attachment style provided the best model for predicting mothers' estimated incompetent parenting.

- Chronic marital problems or mothers chronic or recurrent depression did not add to the model of mothers' incompetent parenting.

Some further specification by attachment style was possible although numbers were too small to differentiate Dual/disorganised styles. It can be seen in Figure 6.2 that Enmeshed style and Angry-dismissive style had the highest rates of estimated incompetent parenting. When feelings of incompetence in parenting were examined all were rated lower than interviewer estimated and only Angry-dismissive style had a raised rate.

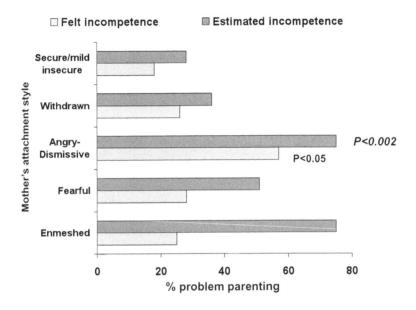

Figure 6.2 Mother's Insecure attachment style and parenting

When more fine-grained analysis was undertaken in relation to mother's individual attachment subscales, correlations showed that mothers' estimated incompetent parenting was significantly related to her:

- poor ability to relate to others (0.33, $p<0.0001$);
- mistrust (0.30, $p<0.0001$);
- constraints on closeness (0.24, $p<0.004$);
- fear of rejection (0.17, $p<0.04$); and
- anger (this showed only a trend, .14, $p<0.07$).

Mothers were also asked about how anxious they felt in their parental role when their children were growing up. High levels were reported by those with Dual/disorganised attachment style (60%) as well as those Enmeshed/Fearful (56%) and those Angry-dismissive (50%). This was double the rate expressed by those Withdrawn (23%) and those Secure (28%) (p<0.05).

In the offspring, the CECA measure of poor mothering in terms of maternal neglect, antipathy or physical abuse was used as an independent outcome of her incompetent parenting. This showed:

- 45% of the mothers who were estimated to be incompetent as parents were reported by their offspring as being neglectful or abusive, compared with 14% of the mothers estimated by the interviewer as competent in the parenting role (p<0.0001).
- There was, however, no significant association of mother's feelings of incompetence in parenting and child ratings – the figures were 30% and 26%, respectively.

Maternal neglect/abuse: In logistic regression analysis, mothers' estimated incompetent parenting, and severe and chronic partnership difficulty provided the best model for offspring-reported neglect/abuse. Partner behaviour problems fell just short of adding to the model and mothers' Insecure attachment style or her history of depression did not contribute.

Emotional disorder in offspring: Further analysis examined the various risk factors in relation to emotional disorder in the offspring. Only offspring report of maternal neglect/abuse was directly and significantly associated with emotional disorder in the young people. Mother's estimated incompetence in parenting fell just short of a significant contribution. Mother's Insecure attachment style, her lifetime depression, her chronic marital difficulties or partner problem behaviour did not add to the model predicting disorder in offspring.

6.2.3 An attachment model of intergenerational transmission:

A path analysis was undertaken to examine the associations between the mothers' characteristics, their report of their partners' behaviour and the offspring maternal neglect/abuse and disorder (see Figure 6.3). It can be seen that mothers' attachment style and partners' behaviour problems were associated with mother's estimated incompetence in parenting, but did not show a direct contribution to her neglect/abuse of her children. There was an independent contribution of marital adversity and mothers' estimated incompetence on offspring report of maternal neglect, antipathy or physical abuse. Only offspring neglect/abuse from mother was directly related to emotional disorder in the young people.

Thus an intergenerational model confirms the linkage of mother's Insecure style to her parenting, and from that to the offspring's report of

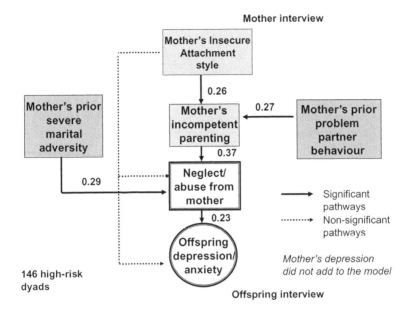

Figure 6.3 Attachment model of intergenerational transmission

her neglect, antipathy or physical abuse. However, partners play a critical role, and in this model mothers' lifetime recurrent depression did not add to the model. This model will now be illustrated in some paired case examples.

6.3 Case examples – mother and offspring

Two paired case examples are presented from the intergenerational study. The first pair is Alma with Angry-dismissive style who is mother to Felicity, whose Fearful style was described in earlier chapters. This is followed by Wendy who initially had Withdrawn style, but later changed to Angry-dismissive and is paired with daughter Donna who has a Dual/disorganised style. Donna has also been described earlier.

6.3.1 Alma's Angry-dismissive attachment style and parenting

Alma is described in earlier chapters, her Angry-dismissive style outlined and her severe abuse, particularly psychological abuse, from her stepfather in childhood is detailed. Alma was divorced from her first husband and living with her second husband and three young sons aged 2, 4 and 6. Her older children Paul (22) and Felicity (19), both offspring from the previous marriage, no longer lived at home. Her current partner was not very supportive. He had long-term physical disabilities, ill-health and had not worked for a number of years which had led to financial difficulties. At the time of interview there was negative interaction in their relationship. In terms of the risk indices, Alma was rated as having prior partner problem behaviour and chronic marital difficulties (with first partner). As described in earlier chapters Alma's Angry-dismissive attachment style included mistrust, overly high autonomy and high anger. She needed to feel in control and felt everyone relied on her, but she in turn could not rely on anyone. This prevented her from asking for help but also made it difficult for others to get close due to the anger and denigration of others she expressed.

Alma's disorder has been described earlier – she had had two episodes of depression in her life, once when her father died and again when her daughter Felicity ran away from home. She had had chronic GAD since the children were young but did not have NES.

Parenting: Alma was rated as having interviewer-estimated incompetence in parenting but she did not see herself as an incompetent parent. When asked about her difficulties with her children she was able to list them all: '*I've had problems with my older children – my eldest daughter Felicity has run away from home in the past, and she has problems with eating that I'm worried about. She did well at school, but worries about her appearance too much in my opinion. She never let me take her to a specialist. Then my older son, he's been involved in drug-taking and petty crime and has a police record.*'

She describes herself as a good parent: '*I always gave them enough time and affection. I always made sure that they got identical things so that they wouldn't fight. You can really work at it and hope that by sitting reading with them, teaching them things at home, they have that little bit extra . . . it gives them a better chance at life. I always want to give them a bright wide outlook on everything and to be quite frank with them . . . both my two teenage children know everything about my first marriage and how it went wrong and why it went wrong.*' Her views on fair parenting involve giving the children identical items, rather than focusing on individual likes or dislikes and she has inappropriately confided in her children about her first marriage and its problems.

When asked about discipline and control, she said: '*I'm a fair mother, I might be too strict, but I'd say that I work at trying to be a good parent. We have to do our best. I think I've strived for the kids and tried to give them a good quality of life. I can be too lax and my husband will step in and discipline them. They were good and well-behaved when young, but as teenagers they have gone completely off the rails. I tried to keep a tight rein on them when they got to secondary school – I didn't allow them out, didn't let them wear the latest fashions. But they still turned out badly. I blame the company they got into. There's no more that me and my husband could have done for them. We've slaved for them.*' When asked if she was ever too sharp and irritable with them she said: '*Oh yes, I think we all get our bad days, and I can scream like the rest of us. I do scream at them and I do get very angry if they have been out late. I bawl them out, and my daughter reduces herself to tears because she can't cope with being screamed at. Then she will say sorry. With my son it's not quite so good. When I see him, a couple of times a week, I'll scream at him. We have rows, but nothing we can't handle. When we have a row, it will be over the same day.'* When asked about her patience with the children she said: *'They have got a lot of respect for me. They tend to give in if they see me tearful. I throw a guilt trap on them. They feel obliged to say "I'm sorry". I have been irritable – sometimes I can say things that can cut them to the bone. My two teenagers are a handful at the best of times. My mum thinks of reasons why the kids behave badly... not the real reason that they are spoilt and they get too much of their own way.'*

When asked if she ever found herself unable to cope with motherhood she said: *'Well yes, my daughter's eating problems do get to me – I do think that it's her genetic inheritance though – my sister's had the same problem you know. My sister was worse though – she's even had psychiatric treatment for years. But I don't think my daughter has anything to complain about in her upbringing. If she hadn't run away she wouldn't have got into trouble. It's her own fault really. I don't see what else I could have done.'*

Comment: Alma does identify problems her children have had, but is unable to link any to her own behaviour. She describes herself as a highly committed mother who made sacrifices. However, her extreme insensitivity can be observed from her own account (for example making her daughter cry), her rigidity about rules and punishments and her blaming attitude towards her children. This, together with high negative interaction with them (she openly describes screaming at them), was taken to denote high estimated incompetence in parenting. Thus the atmosphere in which the children were raised was one of hostility and lack of affection and their mother's need to dominate the family group. This is consistent with the Angry-dismissive style and the need for control and blaming of others when things go wrong.

6.3.2 Daughter Felicity's Fearful attachment style:

Felicity is Alma's daughter and she was described in Chapter 3 where her symptoms of depression and deliberate self-harm were outlined together with her Fearful attachment style. She had just stopped cohabiting with her drug-addict boyfriend, and was working to improve her career prospects. In this she has been helped by her friend's father who is a close confidant. She did not have any children. She had suffered several psychological disorders. From the age of 13 she made three suicide attempts and reported major depression from 13 to 16, for which she was referred to the family doctor for treatment and later to a hospital for counselling. She then developed bulimia age 16 which was chronic.

Support and attachment style: Felicity had no support from her boyfriend Kevin and her only close confidant was her friend's father who was supportive. She described not being close to her mother: '*I feel I can't really talk to her, everything is too much of a mess. She depresses me. Sometimes I feel let down by her.*' She viewed her mother as too critical and unsympathetic and they also argue a lot. '*I want to get away from my past, but when I'm with her it all comes back, If I challenge her about the past she starts crying and says she was always a good mother and that now it's my turn to give – like money – it's weird.*' She was brought up by her stepfather to whom she was not close. She did not see much of her birthfather while she was growing up. When she occasionally bumped into him, he was usually drunk.

Felicity's attachment attitudes involved mistrust and constraints on closeness: '*I try to cope on my own, but sometimes I will ask for help. I feel uncomfortable being close to Kevin because he can change his mind so easily. I trust my friends to a certain extent, but I won't let them be close. A lot of the time I can't talk about my feelings of depression. I hold things back from everybody, I'm quite evasive.*'

She also had fear of rejection: '*I can't trust because I have been let down so often. I have been let down by my Mum, by my brother, my partner and my friend. I'm afraid of getting close in case get hurt. I'm really wary about men. I'm weird – I feel horrible if someone whistles at me. If someone says I'm pretty, it's threatening. Sometimes I can't go near my boyfriend – I can't face him. He gets to me – I can't see why he wants to be with me. I want to be by myself.*'

Childhood experience: Felicity was separated from her birthfather as a baby (see Chapter 4 for Alma's description of the domestic violence prior to him leaving). She reported experiencing a high level of antipathy, neglect, physical abuse and psychological abuse from her mother. She described the antipathy: '*She didn't pay that much attention to me. She was never one to hug me and tell me everything will be alright. I felt like she didn't like me in a way, but then she also loved me because I was part of her – her daughter – but she didn't like me as a person in general. Yes, she always criticised me, she humiliated me. She distressed me, she used to confuse the life out of me – I never knew what she was doing from one minute to the next*'. Her mother would disorientate her. She would say: '*don't you think that is really bad? If I agreed then she would tell me I was wrong and stupid.*'

She was also neglected: '*I took care of myself a lot – everything from 13, cleaning, cooking, washing my own clothes. Mum just told me to get on with it.*' Her mother didn't spend time with her, Felicity would just sit quietly in front of the TV and mother was often out. '*She wasn't there that much, my brother and I would get home from school and she would be in the pub opposite – she would make us dinner – then go out. I never saw her that much. She didn't pay that much attention to me. She didn't really give me the support and help I needed, I could not talk to her. She wasn't there for a lot of things she should have been. She would say "just get on with it, don't question, don't be stupid". She was not sympathetic.*'

Felicity was hit regularly by both parents, with mother assisting when stepfather beat her and her brother: '*I only had to look at them the wrong way and I'd get punched. Got hit if mum said we had done anything wrong – anything. As far back as I remember I can remember being hit. Twenty or 30 times I was really bruised a lot, from the age of 10. I could not go swimming a lot because of the bruises. But from age 13 I got hit a lot more. I was tied up and beaten with a cane because my brother had accidentally set light to something – Mum tied us up and beat us for hours – that was when I was 7. My feet and hands and tops of legs and arms were to my waist with curtain wire. A lot of the beatings were from my stepfather, he once punched me in the head. One time my brother painted graffiti on his computer – when they found out, Mum held us down and stepdad came upstairs – I was hiding in my room and hadn't even done anything – we both got beaten really badly. I knew what was coming, I could hear my brother screaming. I still have nightmares now – where I feel out of control – feel that people don't care. They both used belts or sticks, and I got punched in the face, punched in the head. I would be hit with a cane or stepfather's belt. Mum hit me with a mallet once – the prints were all over me. It was easily weekly, sometimes every day. I think they were careful not to bruise where it would show. I remember I had to have a few days off when they beat us severely – mum would keep us off school – summer holidays were a nightmare.*'

There were extreme forms of psychological abuse. For example, her mother Alma would buy a present for Felicity at Christmas, let her see it and then promptly take it away and say she could not have it. She took away her favourite dog, with no warning, no explanation and had it put down. She would make Felicity eat spicy foods like hot chillies: '*She used to do things like that with chillies – she used to put them in my mouth and they burned severely – I remember crying and screaming and she held the top of my head and my jaw so I could not spit it out.*'

Eventually the situation got so bad that Felicity ran away from home at age 14. When she was eventually found by the police, she insisted on going into local authority care and refused to go back home. While living on the streets she was raped by an ex-boyfriend and although she took police action he was acquitted at court. She also had a termination around this time.

Comment: Much of Felicity's later disorder – her depression and self-harm behaviour can be understood in relation to her very adverse childhood experience. Added to this were trauma experiences when she ran away from home. This has ruined her self-esteem, made her very mistrustful of others and increased her fear of rejection and being hurt. Her account of neglect and abuse from her mother while at variance with Alma's account, but the domineering, blaming and insensitive elements do emerge in both reports.

Comment – Alma and Felicity: Alma's poor insight to her shortcomings as a parent fits with her attribution of blame, including the children themselves, rather than take responsibility herself. Her account shows that she views herself as a good mother, but she gives enough examples to show her incompetence in this role. Her attachment style shows her poor ability to relate and access support, combined with mistrust, high self-reliance and anger towards others. The anger that characterises her adult relationships spills over into her relationship with her children. From her daughter's account she was hostile, critical, neglectful and physically abusive as a parent. The anger and denigration present in her attachment style are consistent with the hostile treatment of her children and her attribution of blame towards them rather than herself. However, Alma was a woman who had many difficulties in her own life. She had a neglectful and abusive childhood (see Chapter 5) was married at 16 to a man who was alcoholic and violent, and on leaving him found herself alone with two young children in a new city. Her second marriage was less fraught but also contributed to the poor parenting of the children. As a parent Alma lacked support, not only from partner but from others, including her very hostile mother. Her initiation into parenthood as a 17-year-old came when she had little experience of her own to bring to the role. During her adult life she has experienced periods of depression and anxiety. Her vulnerability, together with her husband's behaviour, has been transmitted with crushing effects, to her daughter through their poor parenting behaviour. And yet Alma could be seen in some ways as a survivor of her own abusive past. Her self-esteem is good, her functioning in many areas is adequate (for example, she has a good relationship with a friend and with siblings; she manages the household; she has kept her family more or less intact). The biggest casualty from her past, in addition to her choices of partner, is her deficiency as a parent.

6.3.3 Wendy's Withdrawn attachment style, changed to Angry dismissive style and her parenting

Wendy is a Turkish–Cypriot woman who was 35 years old at first interview. She is married to Lenny who is African–Caribbean and they have four children of whom Donna is the oldest (Leah, Claire and Richie are still at home). Lenny does not work and Wendy has a part-time job. Finances are thus difficult. Wendy lived in Cyprus with her Turkish–Cypriot parents for the first three years of her life before coming to London where she grew up. Whilst close to her partner at first interview, it was evident that the relationship had been problematic in the past and problems re-emerged by the follow-up interview three years later. Wendy had no other support. She was rated as having Withdrawn attachment style at first contact, but Angry-dismissive at follow-up.

Support and attachment style: At first contact, Wendy felt close to her husband and did confide in him. '*I usually tell him things. It takes time for me to open up, and even then I don't talk about feelings easily. But I can go to Lenny* *and he does always help me with things I am worried about. We talk a lot about the housing situation as well as our money problems. We are always trying to find ways of sorting things out. He is a good listener and he will offer advice when he can.'* She had contact with one of her two sisters but was not close and she had broken off contact with her oldest sister. She has one friend, Lorraine, but did not feel she could confide and had not told her about her problems. She was rated as having 'some' ability to make and maintain relationships and thus moderately Insecure.

She expressed mistrust of people: *'I'm very suspicious of people I don't really know – I think because of past experiences where people took advantage of my good nature and I've been let down. I do question people's motives, a lot of them are just out for themselves.'* She also had a moderately high level of constraints on getting close: about asking for help she said *'it depends on the problem'.* When asked about confiding her problems she said *'sometimes, yes. Sometimes I open my mouth when I shouldn't. I could kick myself after I've done it and wished I hadn't told them'.* Other people find her reserved and hard to get to know. Wendy was highly self-reliant and described herself as a bit of a loner. She also liked to spend time on her own. Privacy was important to her, as was having control over her life. *'I get frustrated when things don't go the way I plan them'.* Her desire for company was low: *'it's not important to have people around, I like being on my own'.* She didn't need to see people often, did not find it easy to initiate friendships and she had no social life. Despite a recent fall-out with her older sister, which she was irritated about, she did not express other sources of anger.

At first interview Wendy's profile fitted a moderately Withdrawn attachment profile, but her mistrust was atypical of this style. At follow-up interview 3 years later, her attachment style had changed to Angry-dismissive because of increased anger. This followed her husband having had an affair. He was no longer considered a confidant and she felt a high level of resentment towards him. *'Our marriage shouldn't have happened. I don't deserve to be treated like that.'* She also started rowing with the children and becoming resentful about things that had happened in the past. She also got angry with people at work, but found it hard to express it at times. Thus her earlier detachment had been activated by angry and mistrustful feelings.

Disorder: Wendy had recurrent depression in her life. The first episode was aged 18 following the birth of her baby and problems in her marriage. Her next episode was aged 34 when she experienced GAD followed by depression aged 35. This was again in relation to both partner events and problems with her children. She then had another episode of depression at follow-up following her partner's affair. This is untypical for someone with Withdrawn style, but common among those with Angry-dismissive style.

Self-esteem: She was rated as having NES at first contact, but this was a threshold example: She felt positive about her attributes and roles, but lacked self-acceptance: '*I don't feel I'm very good as a person, not as good as others.*' However, at follow-up her self-acceptance had improved.

Childhood: The main problem in Wendy's childhood was the relationship with her mother which was high on antipathy and physical abuse. Wendy's mother showed her no affection and spent very little time with her. '*I can never remember my mother showing any real affection to me. I've always felt that there's some kind of barrier between us. She was not affectionate. Never kissed and cuddled me. She never spent time with me . . . My mother said awful things to me. She often said she wished I was dead. She was very hard to please. We argued all the time when I was a teenager. After I started getting interested in boys that's when all the real bad problems started. We argued over my mother's attempts to arrange a marriage for me. At one point she wouldn't talk to me for months when I was 14.*' She also felt her mother was very controlling and that she interfered in her life: '*She wanted to know far too much about my life and secrets.*' There was no neglect, but discipline was very strict and authoritarian.

Wendy was also hit by her mother. '*She hit my sister Sara and I got involved and got hit as well. We both had bruises. I remember plenty of times getting beatings. My mum used to beat the girls, my dad used to hit the boys. I've been hit by my mother with belts, with shoes – with anything that would come to hand.*' Wendy was, however, closer to her father. '*My dad was more affectionate towards me than my mum. I was much closer to him. He would kiss and cuddle me. My dad was very easy-going. My mum always used to say I was my dad's favourite.*'

Partner relationship: Wendy had only ever been in one partnership which was from the age of 14. She met Lenny at a time when she was already depressed. She became pregnant by him a year later and was pressurised by her mother in having a termination, which she bitterly resented. When she was 16 she left home to marry Lenny. She also felt pressured into the marriage because her mother would not allow them to live together otherwise. Even on their wedding night her mother wanted them to sleep separately. Wendy had difficulties with her husband. He had been in trouble with the police and they had marital adversity, particularly involving his extra-marital affairs and marital conflict including his violence. Early on in the relationship they separated because of Lenny's infidelity: '*It was a nightmare, he's had quite a long relationship with this other woman for over five years. After my daughter was born, a year later I found out that the girl he'd been with was also pregnant. But he agreed early on in the relationship that no matter what happened he would always be there for my children.*' There was conflict and violence in the relationship: '*He's hit me on and off in all the years we've been together.*' As a couple they did not have a social life and she could never depend on him financially.

Parenting: While Wendy felt competent in her parenting, she was an anxious parent, helpless at times, admitting to hitting the children and tending to confide in her daughter when her marital problems became too much. She was rated as having interviewer-estimated incompetence in parenting. She had always worried about the children: *'I always got anxious when the girls go out. I worry about their safety. But I don't lie awake once I know where they are. If Leah was back late I would be looking out of the window and there have been times I have been out searching for her. I think I coped better as a mother when they were younger. I regret I have been like my mum, smacking them.'* She described the discord in the home when they were young: *'Lenny raises his voice to them all except Claire. He especially does not get on with our son Richie. There is a lot of screaming in the house. A lot of arguing with the kids as well. Lenny really hit me hard across my face once in front of the kids. Donna would have been about 10 years old. Most of the time she could come to me if upset. I think I managed to keep the children in check but I wasn't fanatical about discipline. Their father was more strict. We got on alright me and Donna. But we did argue. I've always tried to praise her for smallest things. I was proud of her art work. She did try to please me. She became really secretive as a teenager, and was very irritable. I found her difficult to like from age 13. I really beat her at times. I regret it. She used to lie to me a lot. I confided in her because she took an interest in my problems. She knew the things that were going on, but I wouldn't have told her details of my marriage.'*

'I blamed my partner for the problems she has had. I told him he should sort his life out. He was strict. And they all got on his nerves at times. But he was a good father. He would cook for them and bathe them and was interested in their school work and friends. He was physically abusive and would hit Donna. I think he once hit Donna really hard around the head when she was 15. He really lost it a couple of times. It was like he was fighting an adult, really hitting her. I was there at the time. But I couldn't do anything.' Wendy also hit Donna: *'I hit her from when she was about four until she was in her late teens. Usually several slaps around the face, couple of times around the legs, maybe weekly. It was the only way I could get through to her. I really bashed her a couple of times and lost control. Once when she was four I hit her so hard across the back of the head that she fell into the dressing table corner. I don't think she ever told anyone.'*

Comment: Problems with Wendy's parenting had several influences. First her partner was violent and having affairs outside the marriage which caused her a lot of stress. This made her depressed at different times when the children were growing up. Her partner was also physically abusive to her daughter Donna and she felt unable to protect her. The other influence, historically, may be from her own childhood where her mother showed marked levels of antipathy to her and would physically abuse her. She commented on the fact that she has repeated this. So she had no childhood role model of how to be a mother. The other issue is her Avoidant attachment style. Whilst this was rated as Withdrawn the first time she was interviewed, it then changed to Angry-dismissive at follow-up following another severe life event with her partner. As a Withdrawn mother this would be consistent with a remote and passive parent lacking in affection. However, Wendy sounds much more hostile and volatile suggesting that her earlier style may have been Angry-dismissive. From Donna's point of view there would have been difficulties with both parents although she and her mother became close later and her mother helps her a lot with her children.

6.3.4 Daughter Donna's Dual/disorganised style

Wendy's daughter Donna , a 24-year-old woman living with her two-year-old daughter is described in Chapter 4 in relation to her Dual Angry-dismissive and Fearful style and her history of substance abuse, depression and self-harm. She was separated from her partner who was extremely volatile and violent when they were together. She took out an injunction against her partner seeing their daughter and stayed with her mother Wendy for a few months. She felt that she should leave her partner but also said that the chances of her doing so were quite slim. She went around to her mothers three or four times a week for help with her own daughter, but otherwise was isolated.

Support and attachment style: In terms of support, Donna had lost contact with a lot of her friends through lack of trust. She had also fallen out with her sisters and had no close relationships. Her partner relationship was low in support with high conflict. She named her mother as her only VCO and although initially saying that she could confide everything, her confiding proved to be low – there were many things she would not tell her, for example about her relationship with her partner and his violence, because she knew that her mum would tell her to leave him. She showed some typically Angry-dismissive characteristics such as mistrust as well as anger in her close relationships, including violent outbursts to her partner. She also exhibited Fearful characteristics including fear of rejection being worried about disclosing in case others let her down *'best friends always turn out to be enemies – I would not tell my friends anything because they cannot keep a secret. I just feel you can't trust anyone. Only my mum'.*

Childhood experience: Donna was brought up throughout her childhood by both birthparents along with her three younger siblings. She had antipathy from her father and was physically abused by him on a daily basis, as he would hit them all with a belt, slipper or with his hands, all of which would leave marks and bruises. Her mother would also hit them but not as hard. Donna felt that her mother actually favoured her over her siblings as she would be given more pocket money. But she also felt that her father would hit her more than the others because she was the eldest. Her father would threaten to throw them down the stairs and that he would leave them if they did not behave themselves. The relationship with her mother was not hostile until Donna was 15 when her mother packed her things and told her it was time to go. There was constant tension in the house.

About her father she says: '*He was never satisfied with anything. Dad would say he would throw us down the stairs, then would say 'I was only joking'. He would say he wished he'd never had us, and he'd pack his bags. If he had punched me, I would have bloody punched him back – it is scary when you are young and when his friends came into the house he was as nice as anything. I hated him. There were loads of times he would send us to bed without food but my mum always fed us'.* Her mother would give her more things and would say that Donna was her favourite. She would give her money to go and buy things for herself. Father would give her sister Claire things and would tell her not tell Donna.

There was no neglect, both parents would look after them in terms of their material needs – their father would cook the meals and take them to school since he was unemployed during their whole childhood. Her parents would argue and when her father was angry he would throw bottles and other things around the room. She didn't recall him being physically violent to her mother. However, from around age 11 Donna's mother started to confide in her about the problems she was having with her husband which made Donna feel very uncomfortable. When she told Donna her problems Wendy would start crying. She also told her stories about her father as she felt that she was at the age that she needed to know: '*It made me feel sick, really sad and angry. She would also tell her how miserable she was. But what could I do?*'

Donna did not do very well at school and left school when she was 16 and was truanting for the last year. She was not happy at school, other children used to tease her about her mum being Turkish – called her a 'Turkish Delight' and would ask her if she ate kebabs and why her dad (who was Black) went out with a Turkish lady. Donna didn't tell her mother about the bullying because she felt she would be hurt by the comments. She did, however, develop a group of friends and did have one close friend. When she was aged 10 she was sexually abused by her mother's younger brother. She said that she remembers him taking her into his bedroom at her grandmother's house and sitting her on his knee. He touched her between her legs under her knickers and tried to kiss her. She thinks it may have happened more than once, but she never told anyone.

Donna left home when she was 16 after she met her first partner Nick. She had a lot of arguments with her mother before she left and one day decided to leave suddenly. She moved in with Nick at his mother's house. After a few months she moved into a hostel and found out that she was pregnant with Nick's baby. Both her mother and Nick wanted her to have a termination and so she did. She also discovered around this time that Nick had been sleeping around with a lot of other girls and she decided to finish the relationship. At this time he went to prison for aggravated burglary and attempted murder. She then started to go out with James whilst she was living in the hostel but continued to see Nick in prison. James did not know that Nick was still on the scene and this continued for several years into their relationship. James, is her current partner, and is violent.

Comment: In this case much of the harm done to Donna as a child was from her father, but her mother's helplessness, role reversal with her daughter and high antipathy during her teenage years contributed to Donna's burden. Her mother's chronic marital difficulties impacted on both her parenting and on harm to the children. The dynamics in the family seem to reflect mother and father favouring different children and giving them money, perhaps as a bribe instead of affection. The closeness to her mother has continued in adult life, but her mother's helplessness does not provide good enough support for Donna. Donna has in her own life repeated her mother's problem partner history. Whilst we do not know about her parenting of her child, her references to being hostile and violent do not bode well for the child's care.

Summary of intergenerational findings

- Prior investigation of a related representative mother–offspring dyad study showed mother's vulnerability and her recurrent depression contributed to offspring report of neglect and abuse in childhood. The mothers' own childhood had no direct impact either on the rate of neglect/abuse or on the young person's disorder. Attachment style was hypothesised as part of the maternal vulnerability and thus explored in the high-risk paired 147 mother–young adult dyads studied.
- Mothers' parenting was assessed using the PRI which questioned about difficulties in the parenting role retrospectively, involving quality of interaction with children, feelings of competence and interviewer-estimated competence and incompetence as a mother.
- Insecure attachment style in the mother at interview was significantly correlated with her prior estimated incompetence in parenting. This was also related to her prior partner problem behaviour (violence, antisocial, criminality).
- Mothers' incompetence in parenting was in turn associated with offsprings' independent interview accounts of neglect, antipathy or physical abuse from mother. A further contribution was from mothers' chronic marital difficulties. Only neglect/abuse from mother predicted offspring emotional disorder.
- Mother's estimated incompetence in parenting was a better predictor of offspring neglect/abuse than reported incompetence which tended to be reported less often.

- There was no direct association between mothers' Insecure attachment style and offspring neglect or abuse, or disorder.
- Mothers with Angry-dismissive and Enmeshed style showed highest rates of interviewer-estimated incompetent parenting.
- When mothers were asked about how anxious they felt as parents, highest rates were by those with Enmeshed, Fearful but also Angry-dismissive styles.
- Those with Withdrawn style had no increased rate of poor parenting behaviour.

6.4 Discussion

The research literature on transmission of risk to children through parents' attachment behaviour emphasises the modes of transmission through the parents insensitive, hostile or remote interactions. To this should be added parents' helpless behaviour. These collectively indicate a lack of attunement in being able to interpret the child's needs, inability to nurture the child, poor coping in the parental role as well as hostility if the child was competing with the parents own needs. It is clear from the analysis reported here, that attachment style assessed from problems in making close adult relationships also extends to interactions with children suggesting that internal working models are indeed involved. Partners, however, also play a large part, both in directly maltreating children, but also in terms of impeding the mothers' parenting through their problem behaviour or through marital difficulties.

The intergenerational study reported supports an attachment model, but also includes family systems and social factors, in which the mothers' reported prior relationship with her partner in terms of severe and chronic difficulty and his problem behaviour are associated with *her* neglect, antipathy or physical abuse of her children. Although mothers' Insecure attachment style contributed to understanding variance in her estimated incompetent parenting, it is important to note it had no direct link to maltreatment of her offspring, nor to disorder in offspring. Only neglect or abuse predicted emotional disorder in the offspring with mothers' own history of disorder not adding to the model prediction. These results have many parallels to those reported by Cowan and colleagues (1996), when looking at parents' relationship and attachment in relation to their young children's disorder. They similarly found no direct link between parents' attachment categories and the child's problem behaviour, but as in this data set, found an association between mother's parenting and offspring internalising or emotional disorder. The London study showed father's had a greater role in offspring behavioural disorder, but no information on father's attachment style was available.

Although mother's Insecure attachment style is significantly correlated with her estimated incompetent parenting, this generalisation does not hold for all those with Insecure attachment style. Only just over half of the mothers categorised as having Insecure attachment were rated as incompetent parents, showing that Insecure attachment style in mothers is not a sufficient indicator alone of parenting risk. Furthermore, similar proportions (around a quarter) of mothers with Insecure attachment or Secure attachment style were described as neglectful or abusive by offspring. While it can be shown that a number of other risk factors play a part in poor parenting from the mother, it can also be argued that the presence of positive factors (the father's relationship with the child; the quality of the couple relationship) may act as a buffer against mother's Insecure working model protecting against mothers' incompetent parenting and child maltreatment. This would be consistent with findings from Cowan and colleagues' showing that positive marital functioning is a buffer in parenting behaviour (Cowan, Cohn *et al.* 1996) and will be explored in the next chapter.

The distinction between reported and interviewer-estimated incompetence in the motherhood roles is a potentially important one. There are pitfalls in purely self-reported assessments of parenting given biases in self- and other-perception of those with Insecure styles consistent with the distorted internal working models. Taking self-reported experience at face value may thus distort the reporting of actual behaviour and characteristics of relationships and roles. Interviews which differentiate factual information from the person's perceptions are critical and need to be considered in relation to service-based assessment and parenting programmes. Understanding the lack of insight into parenting behaviour in some cases may aid the process of correcting incompetent parenting. It should also be noted that in this analysis it was only possible to assess parenting effectively through the more oblique means of asking about 'competence' in the role, rather than through a more investigative approach focused on the mothers neglect or abuse of her children. Such questioning has been shown in the same programme of research to have poor agreement with the child's account and likely to yield a major underestimate of maltreatment (Fisher, Bunn *et al.* 2011). This may hold an important message for services in how to question parents suspected of maltreatment.

Insecure attachment style has been shown to be primed and fuelled by stressful experience both in partner relationships, but also more broadly. The level of personal agency in marital and motherhood difficulties of those with Insecure styles is not known. However, the extremes of partner behaviour described go far above the negative interaction which may be contributed to by insensitive, or unattuned responses in partner relationships on the part of the woman. It could be argued that the selection of an inappropriate partner may be influenced by a young woman's Insecure attachment style with an element of 'assortative mating' occurring, whereby vulnerable or dysfunctional people are attracted to each other which increases risk to children (Quinton, Rutter *et al.* 1985). However, it should be noted how young many of these women were (e.g. age 14 or 15) when these violent partnerships were embarked on. This is too immature an age for a considered choice of marital partner and is perhaps more suggestive of lack of parental guidance. Alternatively, partners can have a beneficial effect and provide buffering against effects of stress and thus correct parenting style (Quinton, Rutter *et al.* 1985). Factors affecting such resilience will be examined in the next chapter.

7 Resilience

7.0 Introduction

In previous chapters, a range of risk factors associated with Insecure attachment style have been outlined. Here factors which might act as protective or resilience factors are considered. The aim of this chapter is to examine aspects of adult attachment style and associated experience which can protect against the experience of clinical disorder. This is central to understanding why many individuals survive early childhood adversity to function well in adulthood. It can also help point to effective intervention approaches.

Resilience is a somewhat complex notion, but is seen here as normal development taking place under difficult conditions (Rutter 1990). In this we will look to positive experience which may buffer against adversity experienced in childhood, and locate resilience in the individual and their prior interaction with the family and social environment. Resilience outcomes studied have included the absence of disorder, the presence of health and wellbeing or social competence (Garmezy 1985). A range of potential protective or resilience factors have been identified in the research literature including factors in the home environment (e.g. competent parenting, closeness to a parent) in the school or leisure arena (e.g. good support, good educational experience, religious participation) as well as in the individual (e.g. high IQ, good coping skills, autonomy, empathy and sense of humour) (Masten, Garmezy *et al.* 1988; Rutter 1990; Luthar 1991; Fonagy, Steele *et al.* 1994). The presence of such factors help explain why all individuals do not succumb to adversity, by identifying positive factors which may mitigate against developmental damage. There are also likely to be biological factors which act to enhance resilience. Gene variants have been identified which reduce the usual resilience most individuals experience (Caspi 2002; Moffitt, Caspi *et al.* 2005) or provide differential susceptibility to harsh environments to increase vulnerability or resilience (Belsky and Pluess 2009). However, the focus in this chapter will be on psychological and social factors.

Resilience will be tested in three ways. First, social competence in the form of Secure style will be examined and the good relationships and self-esteem with which it is associated. We have already discussed how those with Secure style have lower rates of disorder outcomes, and where this occurs despite neglectful or abusive childhood experience, this would qualify as a resilient outcome. Similarly those with mild levels of Insecure style have been shown to have lower disorder rates and in this way mimic those 'clearly' Secure. Second, another candidate for resilience is Withdrawn style. Whilst this could not be described as high social competence given its detached characteristics and tendency to isolation, it does carry a lower risk valence for clinical disorder and does exhibit competencies in coping as well as operating as a 'stress-avoidance' strategy. These styles will all be examined in relation to childhood adversity and positive experience to see whether they help buffer against clinical disorder. Third, positive change in attachment style in adults, from Insecure to Secure, will be investigated to further help to establish how increased resilience can be attained even in adult life.

7.1 Achieving Security despite adversity

Most people in the population are Secure in their attachment style as adults, and Secure attachment style tends to remain stable across periods of time (Hazan, Hutt *et al.* 1991). This, together with the fact that most children receive 'good enough' parenting, means that development of Secure attachment style is normative. Family contexts are varied and most have considerable positive input into the child's life. In addition to that provided by parents, or other people in the family, other sources are those outside the family, through friendships or positive school experience. When these co-occur with maltreatment in the family they can have a protective effect on development. The developmental task of attachment is to learn to form stable relationships, with expectations of trust and care, and to inform positive internal working models which generalise such expectations to other future relationships. We need to investigate how much positive experience, and from what sources, is needed in the face of ongoing neglect or abuse to enable such positive development to occur.

In the course of the interviews conducted during the London studies there were many examples of positive experience running alongside accounts of neglect and abuse. For example in Deirdre's childhood – despite high antipathy from mother and physical abuse from her father, she had a grandmother in the house to whom she was very close, and who provided care for her and her siblings. In Emma's childhood whilst her mother was prone to violent mood swings, it was her father who provided the day-to-day care and structure for the children and kept the family together. Even in the case of Alma's traumatic psychological and physical abuse at the hands of her stepfather, she did well at school and a sympathetic teacher believed her story, offered support and contacted social services. All of these experiences *could* have provided resilience, and may indeed be responsible for these women living relatively normal family lives in the community, not marginalised by extreme psychological disorder or social exclusion. But these positives did not ultimately protect them from recurrent emotional disorder in their lives. Previous research indeed confirms that being close to one parent, having a support figure and high educational attainment in childhood can all act to protect against depression for those with neglect or abuse (Bifulco and Moran, 1998). The way in which such experience impacts on adult attachment style needs to be further investigated.

7.2 Positive changes in adult attachment style

Attachment researchers consider the attachment system to be active throughout the lifespan and thus open to change (Collins and Read 1990) (Bowlby 1980; Mikulincer and Nachshon 1991). This is because adult internal working models, central to the attachment system, are modified by relationships with peers, partners and close others at different life stages (Collins and Read 1994). There has been substantial effort to investigate the stability of attachment style from childhood in order to show lifetime continuity. Less focus has been placed on circumstances under which it might change at later stages, despite the clear message in attachment theory that attachment style adapts with life change (Bowlby 1988). Recent research has shown that approximately 30% of adults report change in their attachment style over time (Baldwyn and Fehr 1995) (Hazan and Shaver 1987; Scharfe and Bartholomew 1994; Davila, Bradbury *et al.* 1997) (Hazan, Hutt *et al.* 1991; Keelan, Dion *et al.* 1998; Shaver and Brennan 1992; Ruvolo, Fabin *et al.* 2001); with accumulating evidence that such change is related to life events or new relationship experiences (Kirkpatrick 1994).

Few research studies have specifically investigated whether attachment style changes occur in a positive or negative direction (i.e. towards security or insecurity of style), nor have they studied changes in the instability of *specific* attachment style subtypes. Investigating the process by which people change their attachment style in a positive direction (i.e. towards a more Secure or adaptive orientation) has significant implications both for attachment theory and therapeutic intervention. The challenge for attachment researchers is to identify the personal, interpersonal or contextual factors that predict meaningful change in attachment styles over time (Davila, Karney *et al.* 1999; Cozzarelli 2003). A contextual approach views the change of attachment styles as occurring with important transitional life events associated with acquiring individual relationship status such as marriage, parenthood, beginning college education or first employment. Such roles are enhanced when acquiring new intimacy or support. Of course change can be negative and have a deleterious effect on attachment behaviour. Thus losing key relationships or roles through divorce, break-up of friendships, separation from child or loss of employment, can lead to deterioration in security status or change in style. All such changes need negotiating and potentially have implications for changes in levels of autonomy, mistrust, fear or anger in relationships. A four-year longitudinal study showed people with Secure attachment style who suffered from partnership break-ups were found more likely to become Insecure in their attachment style over time (Kirkpatrick and Davis 1994). A reciprocal relationship is argued to exist between adult attachment style and romantic relationship status, with changes in the quality of the relationship to be particularly important for attachment style expression. Both cross-sectional and longitudinal studies have shown that partners recently married became more secure in the relationship with each other and less anxious over time (Hammond and Fletcher 1991; Davila, Karney *et al.* 1999) (Fraley, Davis *et al.* 1998; Klohnen and Bera 1998; Crowell, Treboux *et al.* 2002). Other life changes such as adjustment to college life can result in a move to greater insecurity associated with problem coping styles and increased levels of distress. Changes to greater security are associated with positive change and lower distress (Lopez and Gormley 2002). More frequent fluctuations in attachment style may in themselves be a manifestation of insecurity (Davila, Karney *et al.* 1999).

Changes in adult relationships are clearly central to attachment style status. Failures in support from close relationships at the time of a crisis, are particularly associated with an increased disorder risk (Brown, Andrews *et al.* 1986), which might reflect the blocking of the proximity seeking function of the attachment system. Research has shown that women who become Secure over time show greater improvements in their perception of support and greater decreases in social conflict compared to women who remain stable or change to greater insecurity (Cozzarelli, Karafa *et al.* 2003). Thus individual's feelings about relationships are primed through different types of attachment experiences (Baldwin, Keelan *et al.* 1996).

Stability of attachment style as measured by the ASI was examined in the European TCS-PND project, in the perinatal period to see if there was change after the birth of the baby. This is important information for practitioners working in the perinatal field to be able to predict risk from mothers' attachment style during pregnancy. The ASI was retested with 96 low-risk mothers during pregnancy and then again six months after the birth (Bifulco, Figueirido *et al.* 2004). Attachment style proved to be relatively stable with 85% of women retaining the same scoring of either clearly Secure or some type of midly, moderately or markedly Insecure style at both interviews. This is despite the fact that the birth of the baby could be said to represent an attachment event which requires some accommodation, albeit a positive event for most of these women. When mildly Insecure was combined with Secure, then the stability was 77%, with greater movement towards security postnatally. Correlations between antenatal and postnatal ASI subscale ratings (e.g. mistrust, fear of rejection) were all significant and ranged from 0.57 to 0.63 (p<0.0001). Therefore, substantial stability was found in the perinatal period, with changes that did occur showing a move to greater security suggesting a grounding or anchoring effect of the birth and new family member.

7.3 'Earned' security

The attachment researchers working with the AAI have developed the concept of 'Earned Security' to explain how individuals reporting adverse childhood relationships with parents can provide coherent adult accounts categorised as Secure (Hesse 2008). It is argued: '*Coherent collaborative speakers could be judged secure-autonomous despite the coders estimates that during childhood parents did not show loving behaviour, and such transcripts were informally identified as 'earned-secure*' (Hesse 2008, p.586). Such status was much more common in adults than adolescents using the AAI, suggestive of a longer-term period of acquiring the necessary buffering experiences. Both those 'continuously Secure' (ie with good childhood experience and reported coherence) and those 'earned Secure' (with negative childhood experience and reported coherence), were less likely to have substance abuse than those Insecure (Caspers, Yucius *et al.* 2006). But those 'earned-secure' scored higher on depression scales (Dozier, Stovall-McClough *et al.* 2008). The latter were more likely to have spent time in psychotherapy than either 'continuously-secure' or insecure, suggestive of intervention impact (Jacobvitz 2008). As parents, those earned-secure were equally warm to infant offspring and provided equal levels of structure as those continuously-secure (Pearson, Cohn *et al.* 1994) and maternal sensitivity to offspring held up even under stressful conditions (Phelps, Belsky *et al.* 1998). In terms of marital relationships, earned-secure wives showed similar quality of marital interaction as those continuous-secure (Paley, Cox *et al.* 1999). The same findings were not supported however for adolescents or young adults (Roisman, Padron *et al.* 2002).

The 'earned-secure' label implies that individuals who started life insecure have worked towards gaining security through personal effort and professional intervention, in adulthood. However, this is not the only route to security and the possibility of acquiring security earlier in life in spite of neglect/abuse, perhaps through parallel positive experience, but without formal intervention, needs to be acknowledged. This can only be studied through careful measurement of childhood context involving both negative and positive experiences, including that in the school and peer group. Resilience may lie in various configurations of experience given the individual sensitivity to difficult parental relationships, the timing, severity and chronicity of negative experience and the co-existence of positive factors. Only through the careful mapping of details of childhood experience can the development of security be established.

This chapter will explore resilience in the London sample in terms of three possible models: (a) positive childhood experience which mitigates against adversity to produce Secure styles (positive buffering); (b) Withdrawn styles as potential drivers for stress-reduction through harm-avoidance (of roles and relationships); and (c) change in adult attachment style in positive directions due to positive relationship change (acquired-security).

7.4 Research findings in the London studies

7.4.1 Confirming Secure style as resilient against disorder

The first step was to examine in midlife women whether having a Secure or mildly Insecure adult style at interview was related to lower rates of disorder in those with childhood neglect and abuse, suggestive of its role as a resilience factor. Relevant rates were described in Chapter 5, where in the full midlife sample, amongst those with neglect/abuse in childhood 59% had highly Insecure attachment style, 21% mildly Insecure style and 20% Secure style. This shows that as many as 41% could be considered resilient. Chronic or recurrent depression over the lifespan was then examined as an outcome for those with different degrees of attachment style insecurity, in those with and without neglect/abuse. Figure 7.1 shows the findings graphically. It can be seen that for those with *no* neglect or abuse in childhood the dose effect is evident – with a downward stepwise rate of lifetime disorder – at 50%, 31%, 21% and 12% according to reducing level of insecurity (shown in the right hand column). For those with childhood neglect or abuse, however, the relationship appears less 'dose-like'. Those with highly Insecure styles have similar rates (58% and 54%) as do those with mildly Insecure or Secure styles (38% vs 37%). This suggests a resilience effect of the latter. However, findings only showed a trend in significance. Similar findings occurred when 12-month depression before interview was examined.

7.4.2 Positive childhood correlates of Secure style

The next question concerned identifying childhood experiences associated with the Secure style. This was examined in the sub-sample of 198 midlife women (sample 1B and C) where detailed childhood experience was collected, including that positive. Findings showed Secure attachment style was associated with early childhood experiences of:

- affection from either parent (0.37, p<0.001);
- companionship from either parent (0.23, p<0.001);
- parental concern (0.17, p<0.05);
- support in childhood (0.21, p<0.001);

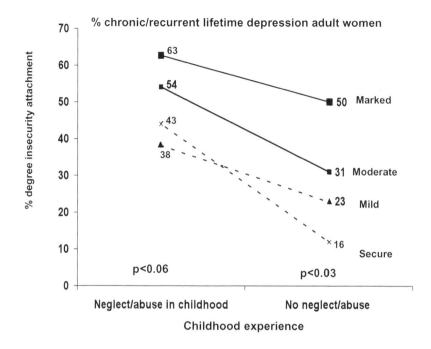

Figure 7.1 Degree of attachment insecurity, childhood neglect and abuse and depression

- child's social involvement (0.41, p<0.001);
- child's competence in either academic or non-academic subjects (0.25, p<0.001); and
- parental interest in child's education (0.28, p<0.001).

These positive experiences were then examined in relation to Secure style among those with neglect/abuse in childhood to test resilience. An association between Security and adverse childhood experiences were found:

- **Closeness to a parent** comprised an index of either high affection or companionship from either parent. Significant associations of such closeness with Secure style was found among those with neglect/abuse (0.20, p<0.03) indicating resilience. For those without neglect or abuse this was not significant (0.17).
- **Social involvement** of the family correlated with adult Secure style among those with neglect/abuse (0.33, p<0.0001) as well as among those without (0.36, p<0.0001), indicating resilience.

In both instances the correlations were *higher* if mildly Insecure style was combined with Secure.

This suggests that being close to a parent and having a high level of social involvement in childhood can create conditions for later Secure adult attachment style even where neglect or abuse is present. Both provide opportunities for acquiring the developmental tasks of attachment around trust and having positive views of others.

The next section will focus on positive experiences during adolescence as promoting resilience, utilising the Offspring sample. This sample has the advantage of a shorter recall period for childhood and mid-adolescence, and more details of school and peer-group experiences measured. Further details can be found in published papers (Bifulco 2008; Schimmenti and Bifulco 2008).

7.4.3 Positive adolescent experiences and Secure attachment in the Offspring sample

Positive experiences in peer group and school experience at age 15–16 were examined together with prior neglect and abuse from parents as potential contributors to Secure attachment style and thus markers of resilience.

Positive characteristics of peer group: This included having a confidant, being accepted in a group of friends, having positive interactions in the group, being popular and where the group activities were social (not criminal or antisocial).

Positive school characteristics: This involved reports of the school as a pleasant environment, as a place where the child felt accepted by peers and teachers, was able to study the subjects they enjoyed and being able to keep up with the workload. In addition, 'school attainment' assessed how well the young person performed in school-leaving exams to enable access to further education. Finally 'felt competence as student' reflected the degree to which the young person felt they were a capable, hardworking and good students, proud of their educational achievements.

Whilst the offspring sample involved high-risk young people as described in earlier chapters, in fact positive experience was also common, with the majority (80%) having at least one of the positive experiences outlined above in mid-teenage years, and 43% of the young people having had *both* a supportive friend and good peer group and 40% experiencing all three positive school factors. Secure attachment style at interview was then examined in relation to these positive experiences. Clearly Secure attachment style was related to:

- support from friend (0.23, p<0.01);
- positive peer group (0.19, p<0.05); and
- positive school characteristics (0.19, p<0.001).

However, Secure attachment style was unrelated to:

- academic performance (0.09); and
- felt competence as a student (0.09).

When logistic regression was utilised to determine the best predictors of Secure attachment style, an index of positive peer group was the only significant predictor, positive school experience did not contribute. These experiences were then examined in combination with childhood neglect/abuse and clinical disorder to determine their resilience status.

7.4.4 Secure attachment style and resilience against depression

The relationship of Clearly Secure attachment style and disorder for those with and without childhood neglect/abuse is shown in Figure 7.2 in the Offspring sample. Here 12-month case disorder of any type is investigated. Secure attachment style was negatively related to 12-month disorder, with a 'dose' effect for highly Insecure, mildly Insecure and Secure. However, it can be seen that mildly Insecure style had relatively higher levels of disorder than in the adult sample.

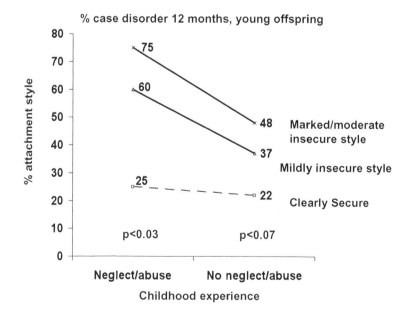

Figure 7.2 Neglect/abuse, Secure attachment style and disorder in 12 months in Offspring

The positive factors described earlier were then examined in relation to 12-month case disorder in the young people to see if they were significantly and negatively related.

- Only positive character of peer group and high academic attainment were significantly (and inversely) related to disorder.
- In binary logistic regression with the outcome of 12-month case disorder, Clearly Secure attachment provided the best model (negatively related to disorder) with peer group and academic attainment not contributing. Secure attachment also contributed when neglect/abuse was added to the model.

Thus it appears that whilst Secure style can be linked to early life and teenage positive experiences around care, peer group and education, it is a better predictor of absence of disorder.

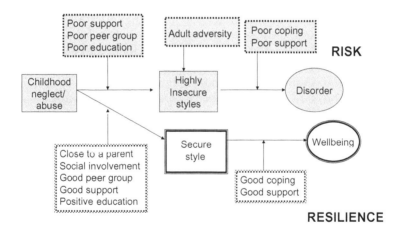

Resilience through positive childhood experience — buffers to neglect/abuse

Figure 7.3 Model of positive childhood experience and resilience

We will now outline two cases, one from the adult sample and one from the Offspring sample to illustrate these findings.

7.5 Case examples

7.5.1 Sheila's Secure style – her childhood school attainment and social involvement

Sheila is aged 29, living with her older sister Brenda and working as a journalist on a magazine. She comes from a working class background, her father was a lorry driver and mother worked part-time in a factory. Sheila did very well at school and when she left home she got a degree and later an MA. She has had relatively little change in her life; having completed her studies she has been at the same job and had the same boyfriend. Her living arrangements with her sister have also been stable. She does not have any financial difficulties. She has no history of clinical depression.

Support and attachment style: Sheila has had a boyfriend for seven years. They lived together for only six months, but then decided they preferred to live apart. The relationship had been 'up and down' but she was able to confide in him, he was sympathetic and responsive, and it was rated as good support. She also has good support from her sister Brenda who was named as her first VCO and also from her second VCO, a friend, Rita, who was a good support figure. Whilst in contact with her birth family, she was not very close to her brother and other sister and found her parents irritating, but tried to see them at least monthly. Her ability to make and maintain relationships was rated as 'moderately' high and therefore her attachment as Secure. This was confirmed by her lack of any negative attitudes around closeness or autonomy.

She was able to trust: '*I don't find it hard to trust people, but I won't trust people completely initially. I'll sort of suss them out first of all. But I don't put up barriers to actually trusting people.*' Whilst she had been let down in the past she didn't let it affect her attitude to others: '*No, I don't think so because I tend to look at the individual, and not assume anything.*' She did not find it hard to get close and could ask others for help when she needed to. She could make decisions alone, but after seeking the advice of others close to her. She did not have any conflict in relationships and did not get angry easily. She therefore had no negative attitudes related to attachment, had optimal levels of autonomy, showed neither anger nor fear in relating and was rated as clearly Secure.

Self-esteem: Her self esteem was good: '*I have intelligence, humour, ability to get on with people, fairness, awareness. I'm a good friend, trustworthy, and I'm just wonderful, that just about sums it up! [Laughs] My worst qualities are indecisiveness and worrying about things. I feel I haven't really established a career yet, I see that as a problem really. I don't think I'm any better than others, I think I'm a reasonable human being. I think I'm sympathetic. I think it depends on who the person is but I'll be sympathetic and also take responsibility for other people... I'd like to be more assertive.*' She felt proud of what she had achieved at work: '*Yes, the things that I've done that are really good I'm really proud of, yes.*'

Childhood: Sheila described her mother in childhood: '*When we were really young I remember her being affectionate, but as we got older, no, she wasn't. Before I went to school I remember spending a lot of time with her doing things together. And she'd always sit and watch* Watch with Mother *on the television with us. As we got older she opted out a bit more and let my dad get on with it. I think in preschool and primary school I probably was close to my mother. It may have changed when my younger sister was born.*' She then experienced antipathy from her mother. '*She was constantly criticising me. I could do nothing right in her eyes.*' Her mother would hit her from when she was four years old. '*She would slap me around the face at least once a week for something I had done wrong. I think she would just lose her temper and hit me. When I was a teenager she became more remote, more absorbed in her own problems.*' The parents took good care of the children in practical ways. They took a very keen interest in Sheila's schoolwork. She was favoured by her father due to her academic ability and outgoing personality: '*He was proud of my friends. I worked hard, and got a lot of positive feedback. They both had time for the necessary things.*' However, at one point when Sheila was about 13, her mother became very unhappy, possibly depressed, and there was role reversal whereby Sheila and Brenda shared the housework and looked after their younger sister because their mother wasn't coping. At this point her mother relied on Sheila for emotional support and would cry in front of her. Sheila felt a lot of concern and responsibility for her mother at this time.

Her parents' marriage was poor. '*It was a terrible relationship between my parents. They were always arguing, for weeks at a time. Mother would hit and throw things, it was always, constant. I don't remember a time when they were happy. I remember them hating each other. Dad would try and pacify her. Dad wouldn't criticise her, but she would be terrible to him. She would moan at him for days, or not talk to him. Arguments continued for weeks. She'd hit him and throw things at him. It was a very tense house, if things were good you always knew bad was coming.*' She and her sisters were close, however: '*I would say that my two sisters and I were close. My memory is of being close to Brenda and of being close to Tricia, being a bit distant from my brother and then my parents were just "there" but not close. We did spend time together as a family when we were a lot younger – we used to go on holidays. We would maybe go out for a day out, but obviously as we got older we didn't want to do that type of thing anymore. That's when we grew apart more.*'

Social life and education in childhood: '*I didn't belong to any clubs or Brownies, but I used to go to a group now and again, which was attached to the school I went to, which a lot of my friends went to. I also belonged to a swimming club. As a family we went to church regularly when young. I did have a lot of friends and I was invited to birthday parties. My parents didn't mind me mixing, but they didn't encourage it particularly. They would take me and my friends to places.*' Sheila had close friends at school and could confide in them. '*If had a problem I would have talked to Brenda or a friend at school.*' Her role model was her English teacher: '*I could always go to her with a problem. I probably would not have gone to my parents.*'

As well as achieving very good final end of school exam results (10 GCE O levels and four A levels), she was also good at sport and drama: *'I was good at everything. I was really good at sport.'* She also had confidence as a child: *'Yes, I thought I could do anything. I was capable but I don't remember feeling all that independent because I think I was sort of tied in with Brenda so I never remember feeling independent of her.'* She would plan the future: *'Yes. I wanted to be a lawyer and thought I would marry and have children.'* Her parents encouraged independence: *'It depended on what the problem was, but yes, they did like us to be independent. I can't remember them being that aware of our problems, so yes in that sense I think they sort of opted out I think.'* The children grew up looking out for themselves and each other.

Comment: Whilst Sheila did describe difficulties in her childhood with her parental conflict, and her antipathy from her mother and low level physical abuse, she appears to have been close to her parents in earlier childhood, and indeed was her father's favourite. This was because she did well at school and he took great pride in this. Her high level of educational attainment means she now has a rewarding job. She described being a sociable and competent teenager. She was always close to her older sister Brenda who was, and still is a confidant, and may have been her main attachment figure throughout. She has close support around her still. Therefore, her early life attachment to parents may have given her the basis for positive development, sustained by her older sister, and then developed a positive trajectory in terms of her school and social life success. This and her good sibling relationships and school and social competencies contributed to self-esteem which has been sustained. Added to these personal characteristics is an adult life which has been relatively free from major adversity and she has achieved stability in the main roles and relationships in her life. This underlines her resilience.

The following case study shows a young man with a mild level of Insecure style who seemed similarly resistant to disorder despite having childhood adversity.

7.5.2 Ethan's mildly Enmeshed style and high self-esteem

Ethan is a 25-year-old man who lives with his partner Carol, and their 18-month-old son in London. He is working as an area sales manager, but also pursuing an acting career. He has two close confiding and supportive relationships as well as closeness to his partner and his mother. He had a high level of self-esteem. His only sibling was a 22-year-old brother who still lived with their mother and who was seen weekly. His father lived in Scotland and he saw him only once a year. Ethan had no psychological disorders and functioned well in his family, work and social life.

Support and attachment style: Ethan had a range of good support figures, a close relationship with his mother and a strong confiding relationship with his partner with whom he had been living for six years. About his mother he said: '*She will always, always be there. If I needed warmth, support and love she will be there. Knowing she is there is important.*' They got on well together with occasional tension: '*She can annoy and upset me. She does not value herself enough. She enjoys moaning. She lets herself be used.*' However, they had never had any big argument or falling out. (Closeness rated 'marked', antipathy 'some'). He also named his mother as a support figure and could confide in her if he has a problem.

Ethan could confide in Carol. He could talk to her about everything that worried or upset him, and she was very supportive. Their interaction was good and they rarely argued. He felt he needed her to be there and would feel lost without her. The relationship was rated as 'very good' support.

He also had a friend and VCO, Adrian, seen twice a week. He confided in him about his work and acting, about financial difficulties, about his family and his partner. He would go into detail about issues. He got good support back: '*Very straight advice, which is good. Sometimes too straight! I can rely on him 90 per cent of time. Would miss him if he were to move away, but would keep in touch.*' While he was not very reliant on Adrian he did value his practical help. Their interactions were very good: '*We can have a laugh, but also straight conversations, we have the same sense of humour.*' This was rated as 'good-average support, no discord'. His second VCO, Martin, was seen every two weeks. With Martin he was less candid, he would not talk to him about problems with his mother, about money but could about work. The support received was '*good, very responsive – 70 per cent of time he listens. We are great friends. I would miss him if he moved away.*' Interaction was positive: '*We can laugh and have good times. We have the same belief system and we communicate well. Sometimes things are left unsaid. But there is no big tension.*' This relationship was rated 'insufficient support, no discord'.

With two close confiding relationships, Ethan was rated as 'moderately' high on ability to make and maintain relationships and therefore in the Secure range in his attachment style.

However, his overall attachment style proved to be 'mildly' Enmeshed because he had low autonomy in relationships as evidenced by high need for company and fear of separation. In general he considered himself very sociable, liked to have people around him as much as possible and didn't feel them to be a nuisance. '*I love meeting new people. It is generally important to have people around. When alone in the house I just get bored or feel a bit lonely, I suppose. What usually happens is I just realise no one is there and I go downstairs, pick up the phone and just talk to my mum. She'll say "why did you phone?" and I'll say, "I don't know, just for someone to talk to."*' He enjoyed meeting new people and found it easy to initiate new friendships: '*I like being sociable. I like having someone around to talk to. I don't like silence. If I'm at home on my own I've always got music on and I'm so bad I end up putting it on in every room on the same station. I'm into crowds.*' He was also anxious about separation, for example when his partner Carol was away or if she got back later than expected. *'Just for a while I feel something missing from me. I just get upset. I don't know if it's because I'm worried. But what usually comes out my mouth when she returns is "Look, why haven't you phoned to say you'll be back later when you have a go at me for doing it?"'* When his parents were away, he missed their company. He also finds it difficult to say goodbye: *'I usually feel that I haven't said goodbye properly. I'm sort of too scared that I've given the impression that I'm happy they've gone.'* Therefore, he was rated as mildly Insecure in his attachment style with Enmeshed characteristics.

Self-esteem: Ethan had high self-esteem. When asked to describe himself and his characteristics he was highly positive: *'I'm very energetic, very open, very direct. I'm an achiever. I think I'm nice to be around. I am friendly, reliable and trustworthy. I am very driven, very motivated and very positive!'* He thought he was attractive, intelligent and sympathetic. The only negative he could think of was that he was sometimes self-absorbed: *'If I've got something on my mind. Also, I can procrastinate sometimes.'* He was also very positive about his role performance. *'I am a good father.'* About his work he said: *'I'm good but improving. I'm very young. I've still got a lot to learn but I'm very good at dealing with people. Being dynamic and making decisions and achieving things. It's improving.'* He thought he was good at homemaking *('I can do the dishes')*, good at socialising *('Easy to get on with, I make a good friend')* and good at his hobbies (surfing was his passion: *'I'm standard, but still very decent at it'*). As a partner he described himself as *'Fabulous!'* and as a father, *'Great!'* He was very accepting of himself, would not want to change places with anyone, *'Still happy being me.'* He wouldn't really change anything about himself.

Childhood experience: Ethan's positive attachment style and self-image had developed in spite of difficult childhood experience. He was brought up by both parents until he was seven years old, then when his father left, his mother looked after him and his brother alone until he was 15 years old. Then he left her to go and live with his father and stepmother until age 17. His father was an excessive drinker who used to beat his mother and physically abuse the children. Ethan once witnessed his father trying to strangle his mother. His father was neglectful and took little interest in his care, schoolwork or friends. There was also antipathy from the father towards him and he was frightened of his father's unpredictable moods: *'I was tense and fearful of him. He was hard to please. I was frightened and would stay out of his way. He would beat us then apologise. You always did what he told you. He was strict. You didn't mess about. If he told you to do something you would do it.'*

In terms of physical abuse, he remembered an incident when his father had belted him around the head. He also knocked him off a chair once with a punch. *'Once he picked me up by the neck and punched me against the wall. I would regularly be slapped more than punched. It happened about twice a week.'* Once when he was little he brought some puppies home and his father threatened to throw them off the balcony. Ethan pleaded with him: '*At first he wouldn't listen but then relented and my mum took the puppies back to the shop. I have memories of him fighting with my mum. There would be physical violence. I would hear slaps and hits. I saw him slap her across the face – I think she had black eyes from him punching her. I remember seeing him once strangling her, his hands round her neck.*'

However, his mother was affectionate, loving and uncritical. His relationship with his mother was always close: '*We got on well. She looked after us, supported us. She allowed us to be who we wanted. She was affectionate, very loving and warm. There were times when I did shout at her, would sometimes swear at her and say I hated her – when I was in my teens. From the age of seven, I was the man in the house. I would help mother around the house, for example tidy the house and do the shopping. It didn't interfere with my social life. My mother didn't badmouth father – she was always fair about dad.*'

Once Ethan's father had left the household there was generally a much happier atmosphere at home. Although his mother remained affectionate her supervision and discipline with the two boys became lax. At around 10 years old, Ethan started to rebel, truanting from school, and shoplifted, amongst other conduct problems until he was aged 13. He went to live with his father because his mother couldn't cope. Although his father continued to drink, he stopped being violent. '*I wasn't fearful of him then. There was no hitting at all. He still drank but wasn't violent anymore.*' However, there was still criticism and antipathy from his stepmother who resented his presence: '*I didn't like her. We moved into her house. I kept out of her way and would creep around the house and stay in my bedroom. She would criticise me to dad. He felt he was 'piggy in the middle', acting as an intermediary.*'

School and peer group at age 16: Ethan was difficult at school – always in trouble, getting into fights or stealing. He disliked school. However, he was good at English, had a talent for spelling and was active at sports. He felt he was a good student but with poor teachers. '*School was a waste of time, the teachers weren't responsible for me and didn't nurture me. One of my teachers basically let me have a year off to go out. I pretty much failed in everything except English and craft and design.*' He had lots of friends at school who did not get into trouble and of whom his mother approved. He also had a close confiding friend when he was 16. At age 18 he left home in London to study drama in Scotland. After a one-year course he returned to London to continue his studies. He found it financially difficult since he was not entitled to a grant, but then he got an offer of help from an eccentric wealthy benefactor who funded his first year. He met Carol at drama school and they lived together whilst still studying.

Comment: Ethan's good adjustment and resilience is probably in part due to his close relationship with his mother throughout childhood. Although he experienced maltreatment from his father, his absences allowed him to develop further closeness to his mother. Whilst he has experienced some problems in school and with antisocial behaviour for a few years in adolescence, he has come through this without generalised mistrust or fear of rejection, and with an ability to make close friends and relationship. His career development also shows ability and motivation and has helped him find rewarding activity to complement his stable relationships. This exemplifies his psychological resilience which has in turn led to a stable social environment.

7.6 Withdrawn attachment style category as resilience factor

Previous chapters, have shown that Withdrawn attachment style, unlike the other Insecure styles, is related to lower rates of disorder, less childhood adversity, fewer severe life events, better coping strategies, less NES and less conflict in relationships. Its main Insecure characteristic is around absence of positive support. In Chapter 4 those with Withdrawn styles were shown to be the most likely to lack a close confidant, the second most likely to be single parents, but least likely to have partner separations. Their relationships were highest on 'indifference' rather than conflict. Withdrawn will therefore be examined in the adult sample as a potential resilience factor for those with childhood adversity, with particular emphasis on its correlation with lower adult adversity as a 'stress-avoidance' factor.

Those with Withdrawn style were shown to have similar rates of childhood adversity to those Secure. However Withdrawn style was not significantly associated with any of the positive childhood experiences. Therefore adult experience was examined to see if these individuals had somehow avoided more adversity. There was some support for this, those with Withdrawn style were less likely to be working class, had less total adversity in different domains in adult phases and during change points than those insecure (see Figure 7.4).

Lifetime depression was then examined in relation to Withdrawn and other highly Insecure attachment styles and childhood neglect and abuse and lifetime chronic or recurrent depression (Figure 7.5). It can be seen that those Withdrawn had the lowest rates.

Therefore it would seem that Withdrawn style may prove to be a resilient style because of its detached, avoidant characteristics which lead to reduced adversity and stress. Avoiding closeness, whilst reducing quality of life, nevertheless means a likelihood of experiencing fewer life events, for example those involving partners, family and close friends. Thus separations, divorces, loss of friendships and conflicts with close others are highly unlikely to occur. This style therefore uses a 'stress-reduction' approach to keeping equilibrium by reducing involvement with others.

Individuals with such style may have a biological predisposition suggestive of less sensitivity to the environment (Belsky and Pluess 2009). The differential susceptibility hypothesis described in the introduction states that individuals vary genetically in their developmental plasticity with more

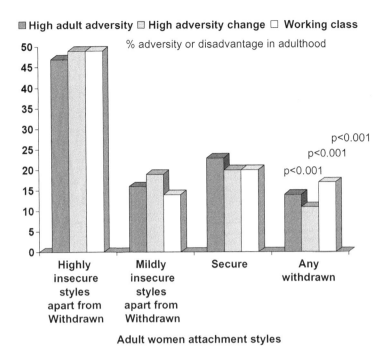

Figure 7.4 Adult adversity and Withdrawn styles

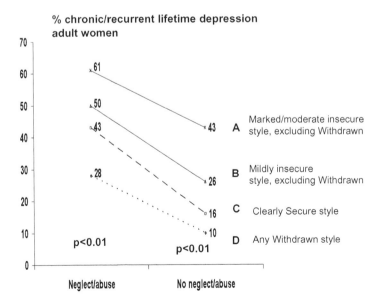

Figure 7.5 Type of highly Insecure attachment style, childhood neglect and abuse
and lifetime recurrent depression

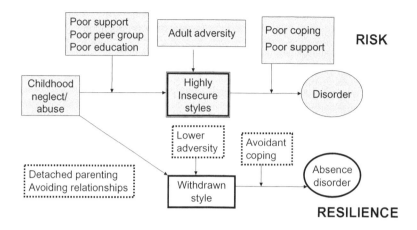

Withdrawn resilience — reducing adversity

Figure 7.6 Model of reduced adversity and resilience

plastic or malleable individuals more susceptible than others to environ-mental influences in a for-better-or-worse manner. Thus a proportion of individuals (those less malleable) may be less affected developmentally by adversity in childhood. Those with Withdrawn styles may constitute such a group.

The following example is of a woman in the adult sample with a moder-ately Withdrawn style, already described in Chapter 2.

7.6.1 Whitney's Moderately Withdrawn style and resilience

Whitney is a 45-year-old woman living with her 43-year-old husband Tony and their six-year-old son Simon (see Chapter 2). Whitney works as a nurse part-time, being available for her son after school. She trained as a nurse after leaving school and remained single and unattached until she married in her thirties, having her only son when she was 37. At interview she was experiencing some difficulties in her marriage. However, she had had no clinical disorder in her life

Support and attachment style: She did not receive any support from her husband Tony, but did receive support from her friend Sara, named as a confidant, but not as 'very close'. Her father had died a few years ago and Whitney had regular contact with her mother to whom she did not feel particularly close and who she found distant and unsupportive ('some' closeness; 'little/no' antipathy). With one support figure she was rated as moderately Insecure. She had constraints on closeness, and did not expect help from others: *'I think that a lot of people tend to gloss over your problems and you tend to simplify them when you tell them, and other people will just agree with anything you say, or else people have got the same problems and can't help.'* She also had high self-reliance: *'I've had to be. I need to make my own decisions and have control over what happens to me. It's too important to ask other people what they think.'* She was therefore rated as having moderately Withdrawn style.

Self-esteem: Her self-esteem was in the moderate range, scoring as neither negative nor positive. She was not particularly self-critical, nor self-praising, *'I'm probably average. I'm probably absolutely boring! [Laughs] I've travelled around a bit but I've never rebelled or done anything outrageous. I'm not outstanding. I'm not the 'life and soul of a party' type. I'm not intelligent, not at all. I don't know, I think I just get by and manage my life quite well. I can be efficient, but there is always room for improvement. Some days are better than others. I do give way to other people. I think I tend to put myself last. I think I am probably a bit too caring sometimes. I do say what I think, but I get into trouble for it. No, I have to be honest, if I think something is wrong I have to say it, yes, and I am proud of that. I'm not really attractive but ok – average. I never had too many dates. I'm not a model-type girl, I'm just not that type at all.'* She described herself as 'good' at her job, and 'average' as a mother. As a wife *'I'm probably just as hard to live with as he is.'*

Childhood experience: Whitney was brought up, together with her brother, by both parents in a stable childhood. But she found it difficult to get on with her father, who had high antipathy towards her: *'I think dad thought I was really stupid because I didn't do very well at school – but his view was "at least she is a girl – when she grows up she'll get married and as long as she can count the money in her purse she'll be okay". But of course I didn't get married till I was 36! I think I did disappoint them. But then even my brother who was their favourite disappointed them as well.'* Her father was a disciplinarian: *'He was terrible. He had a stick – he had a cane at one time and he used to hit me across the hands. Mum said it happened once when I was a baby. I must have caught a cold or something, and I just cried a little bit and he smacked me right across the leg and she thought he was really being mean, hitting a baby like that.'* Her parents were not neglectful and cared for her practical needs.

When she was aged 14 Whitney was sexually assaulted by two boys at school. They caught her in a classroom when the teacher was not around before the lesson began but when all of the students were present. The two boys (whom she had known throughout her school years) grabbed her and pulled her tie, blouse and bra off so she was half-naked in front of the class, to 'see what sort of tits she had'. No one intervened to help her. The headmaster was later told, as well as her father, and the boys were reprimanded and a note of the incident was made on their records but they were not sent home or suspended. *'My dad went mad. You can imagine it – he was up at the school seeing the headmaster. I suppose he was protective, he was fuming with rage.*

Why wasn't there a teacher there, why were we left alone? There was no support after-wards from other pupils – in fact rumours started circulating about me being promiscuous. It made my school life difficult.'

Therefore Whitney did have sufficient adversity in childhood to increase her risk of depression – both her high antipathy from father and moderate severity of sexual abuse. She would be scored in the neglect/abuse index even though she did not have the unstable childhood and multiple adversity present in some of the other cases described.

Adult experience: Whitney had little adversity in her adult life and low experience of adverse change. She was determined as a teenager to leave home and start a career. Since she was able to get a room in the nurse's hostel when she started training she was able to leave home and simply said to her father '*"I'm off." He never stopped me, which was a miracle, and my friends were already in there so it was easy to settle.'* Her early adulthood was stable while she was single and training as a nurse and there were no major difficulties experienced. She did not have many boyfriends and no cohabiting relationships until she met her current partner before marrying. Her problems only emerged in the last few years before interview. Therefore her lack of prior clinical disorder could well be attributed to an adult life where she had few interpersonal roles and was focused on a career as a single woman.

With her current difficulties she used a lot of normalising in her coping and a focus on positives. About her husband, who had a drink problem, she said: '*You see, sometimes he's really nice, because he'll help me do things. He will go out with Simon . . . he does go out with us for the day, to the park or picnics, whereas I know some guys wouldn't do any of that. There are two Tonys there. There is the one who is drunk, that couldn't care less about us – doesn't care about anybody, who needs a good kick up the backside, and there is the other Tony who is extremely nice and very kind and very thoughtful. A woman I spoke to was telling me about her friend's grown-up children, who are divorced, separated, gone off with other people, cracked up or whatever. Let's face it, it's a fact of life isn't it, especially today, that marriages don't last? My mum and dad will have been married 50 years next year but it's going to be a very rare thing for any one of our generation to be married that long. It's just incredible that people used to stay together like that.'* She seemed reconciled to the fact that their relationship could end.

Comment: Whitney had a great deal of forbearance about her situation, was accepting, used minimising or normalising strategies to reduce any anxiety or distress about her situation and tried to focus on some positive aspects. In this way she regulated her emotion, and this was consistent with her Withdrawn attachment style which involved high self-reliance and detachment from others. She preferred to rely on her own resources – she had a number of reasons why she didn't get close to others nor asked for help, intimating that this would be pointless. Not confiding fully in others and getting their reaction helped her to continue to minimise her difficulties and tell herself that the situation was acceptable. The benefit of this was that she had not experienced any clinical level of depression in her life, although she did describe some non-specific tension symptoms. Of course the disadvantage was that the situation could have deteriorated further until it was at a level which she could no longer manage. It was of interest to note that her mother had a very minimising approach to problems also, and was dismissive in her response when Whitney had asked for her help in the past. Whilst her mother's parenting in childhood was adequate, it was never very warm or close, and this together with her father's hostility and perhaps together with her sexual assault experience which was not well managed, had left her reliant on herself rather than others for support.

7.7 Attachment change

In order to look at possible improvement in attachment style over time, and thus increase in resilience, the attachment styles of adult women assessed twice were examined (154). Over the average three-year follow-up there was evidence of high stability of Secure attachment style with 73% of women remaining broadly Secure or Insecure at both time points. Other findings showed.

- Attachment style ratings showed significant correlations at follow-up with highest stability for Fearful style (0.44) as well as Clearly Secure style (0.43 p<0.001).
- Enmeshed and Angry-dismissive were somewhat less highly correlated at 0.22, (p<0.01).
- Withdrawn style was similarly correlated at both times at 0.24, (p<0.01).
- The behavioural scale of ability to make and maintain relationships had the highest correlation at both interviews of 0.51, (p<0.001).
- The attitudinal attachment scales most highly correlated at both interviews were Constraints on Closeness (0.47), Fear of Rejection (0.40), Fear of Separation (0.32) and Mistrust (0.29). (All p<0.001).
- The least correlated were Self-reliance (0.14), Anger (0.15) and Desire for Company (0.03) (not significant).

The characteristics of those rated Clearly Secure at follow-up was then examined in relation to status at first interview, to look for positive change in security. Findings showed:

- Most (67%) were also clearly Secure at the first interview.
- The other styles most likely to change to Clearly Secure were those Enmeshed (14%) and those Withdrawn (12%).
- Those styles least likely to become clearly Secure at follow-up were those Fearful at first interview (5%) and those Angry-dismissive of whom only 2% were rated clearly Secure at follow-up.

A more sensitive marker of change in attachment style was devised by taking incremental change of one point or more on the 13-point overall scale of type and intensity of style. In this scheme 53% of women showed small degrees of change, equally in a negative or positive direction. Other variables such as positive changes in support including a newly confiding VCO relationship, or improved partner support as well as changes in self-esteem and changes in employment were examined. Findings showed:

- Positive incremental changes in attachment style were associated with increased VCO support (33% vs 5% with no improved support, p<0.0001) and with improved partner support (33% vs 9% with no improved support, p<0.008), and being in a partnership at follow-up, but this did not reach significant levels.
- However, there was no difference in rate of adversity in different role domains in the intervening period for those with positive change.
- When positive attachment change was used as an outcome in logistic regression analysis, positive changes in support predicted positive attachment style change. This included increased quality of relationship with partner, having a new partner or new VCO or improved quality of VCO relationship.
- Changes in depression level had no impact on changes in attachment style.

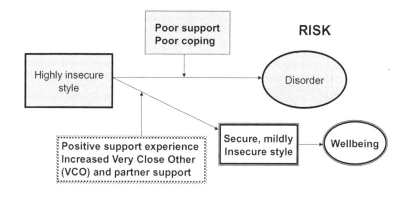

Figure 7.7 Model of attachment change through positive support

Finally, the matter of treatment in relation to clinical disorder was examined as a possible factor in positive attachment style change. In the midlife women followed-up, 30% described having some sort of treatment or intervention in their lives, 20% of which involved psychotherapy. Of these 19% had received treatment in the year before follow-up interview, with 10% receiving therapy. This was usually tied to clinical disorder rather than vulnerability, so is likely to be more common in those with higher disorder rates. In fact having either general treatment or psychotherapy was not linked to positive attachment style change: 21% with treatment vs 19% without had positive change, the figures for psychotherapy in the year being 14% vs 9%.

The following example is of a woman with a moderately Enmeshed style at first interview, who became clearly Secure at follow-up due to changes in her life. She was described together with her childhood experience in Chapter 5.

7.7.1 Eloise's Moderately Enmeshed style changes to Secure

Eloise was aged 43 years at first contact, divorced and had been living with her second partner of nine years and her two children: a son then aged 14 and a daughter aged 11. At first interview she and her partner were arguing constantly with threats of violence. She had already asked him to move out when first interviewed, but he only went to his flat upstairs. Eloise had poor support from her partner (inadequate support with discord), and she had two VCOS, but only one was also a confidant. Eloise was rated 'some' on ability to make and maintain relationships and had a moderately Insecure style. She had a high need for being with people and fear of separation: *'Being alone in the house – sometimes I get very scared – it sort of depends how I'm feeling – when I do get scared, I do get scared and I think you know, I have to make sure the windows are all locked and doublecheck things and it doesn't feel very nice.'* She worried when her partner was away: *'the thing that I'd feel anxious about was that he'd have a motorbike crash or something like that, that he'd get beaten up or have a crash or something. So I was anxious that something would happen to him.'* She found it difficult to make decisions alone and needed constant reassurance. She had a moderately high rating on anger – repeatedly referring to her resentment to her mother, as well as being angry at her partner. She exhibited Enmeshed style with anger expressed to her mother and her partner.

Changes in support: By follow-up interview three years later, Eloise had formally left her husband, moved house, started a new job and taken up spiritualism. She met her current partner Geoff at the Divorced and Separated Social Club and they began cohabiting within three weeks. Their relationship was good and Eloise hoped to marry him one day. She had also intentionally lost contact with her mother although she still sees a sister weekly. She felt breaking off with her mother would facilitate her 'psychic growth' although her children did retain contact with their grandmother. Her relationship with her son was now close – much improved from the previous negative interaction. However, her interaction with her daughter was less good and characterised by more irritability, and they spent little time together. She had also made new friends one of whom became a confidant. By follow-up she had lost contact with the previous VCOs Sue and Cathy but named new VCOS, one of whom Liz, a work colleague was a confidant. *'We've become close and talk quite a bit about things. I can tell her every-thing and she is always sympathetic, interested and concerned.'* She did, however, acknowledge it was an 'office relationship' so felt attachment was low. The relationship was rated 'good-average relationship, no discord'.

She describes confiding fully in her new partner: *'The moment I stepped into his arms I knew I was going to marry him. I can confide easily in him about anything. We discuss money, things to do with the children. He is sympathetic, listens and offers everybody advice.'* He can be critical however, mainly about finances. She describes him as mean with money, *'but it's his way of being helpful – but it has annoyed me in the past and we do talk about it. He's very loving and very compan-ionable. We sit and hold hands and watch television together. We get on very well. We just do everything together.'* (Rated good-average support, no discord).

Secure Attachment attitudes: When asked about her self-reliance she said she could cope on her own *'to a point yes'.* When asked if it was important to be independent: *'I never used to think so, but as I get older I can see that I quite like it in some ways. There are times when I would much rather be making a decision with someone else, but on the whole I don't have those problems. Its important for me to understand that I'm responsible.'* This was rated as in the moderate/average range, and an increase on her previous 'low' self-reliance where she needed other people to make decisions for her. This seems to have been due to her decisiveness in moving house and job and leaving her partner.

She described her need for company as *'in transition. I used to always have the radio and television on upstairs and downstairs. But now I don't mind being in and quiet and just pottering around the garden. Having someone close is still impor-tant and I would like to see friends more often. But I can be on my own more now.'* This was rated as in the moderate/average range, previously rated 'high' When describing her fear of separation she said: *'The only people I get anxious about are the children. With my daughter it is not as much anxiety as a constant threat – where is she? what's she doing? I hope she's all right and no-one is taking advantage of her. I have grown out of the panicky life and death worrying over my children. Geoff would probably say I am overprotective, but I don't think I am. I don't mind being in the house alone now'.* This was rated as 'some' fear of separation and a reduction in the previous 'moderate' level. Her anger had also reduced, mainly because she had broken off contact both with her previ-ous partner and her mother who had been the source of her hostility.

Another new element in her life was her 'psychic awakening', an experi-ence similar to a religious conversion. She began to feel over time that she had psychic experiences and joined an organisation where she was intro-duced to a psychic healer who put her through a trance session during which she said 'black negativity' rose out of her. She went on to train as a spiritual healer and worked helping other people. As a consequence of these experiences Eloise reported using different coping strategies. She was now able to downplay her problems by seeing them 'in the distance of eternity'. She appeared far more self-accepting and calm about things in general and her self-esteem had improved.

Thus effectively her life had changed fully and her attachment style at follow-up was rated as clearly Secure from the previously Enmeshed style.

Summary of resilience factors

Adult sample Secure style correlates

- Women categorised as Secure, but also mildly Insecure and Withdrawn showed significantly lower rates of lifetime depression than their counterparts with 'marked/moderate' levels of other attachment styles. These three categories were investigated as possible resilience factors.
- Secure adult style related in the adult women to childhood experiences of closeness to a parent, support, social involvement and competence at school. Social involvement and closeness to a parent related to Secure style even in the presence of childhood neglect or abuse suggestive of promoting resilience.
- Those with mild levels of Insecure style have lower lifetime depression than those with 'marked/moderate' levels of Insecure style and this holds among those who have experience neglect and abuse in childhood.
- Those with any level of Withdrawn style also have a reduced rate of depression even when experiencing neglect and abuse in childhood again suggestive of a resilience factor. They had lower experience of adult adversity. These individuals may have a genetic propensity to be less sensitive to their environment, and thus less harmed by it.

Offspring sample Secure style correlates

- Positive experiences in mid-teenage years around peers and school life were surprisingly common in this high-risk group of young people.
- Support and positive peer group and positive school experience aged 15–16, were significantly associated with Secure attachment style.
- Peer relationships were found to predict Secure attachment outcomes.
- In logistic regression analysis, Secure attachment style related to lower disorder outcome in the presence of neglect or abuse in childhood confirming its role as a resilience factor.

Attachment style positive change

- Attachment style (Secure vs Insecure) was stable across an average three-year follow-up period for three out of four adult women. Change occurred for 20%, equally in a positive (towards greater security) and negative (towards greater insecurity) direction.
- Clearly Secure or Fearful styles were the most stable over time.
- Of those Clearly Secure at follow-up, two-thirds had been Clearly Secure at first interview with similar rates of Enmeshed and Withdrawn (14% and 12%) but few rated as Fearful or Angry-dismissive at first interview contact.
- Incremental positive attachment style change was related to positive change in support with VCOs and partner.
- Change in attachment style was unrelated to depression at follow-up, changes in self-esteem or receiving treatment for clinical disorder.

7.8 Discussion

It is clear that a good proportion of individuals survive harsh family treatment if they have other positive experiences in childhood or during teenage years with parents or peers or at school, which helps them to function well as adults. The Secure and mildly Insecure styles show increased levels of positive experience in childhood and adolescence to buffer against negative experience. Those with Withdrawn styles offer a different version of resilience. They deactivated emotion and were distanced from others and the social world. The implications involve having less emotional entanglement and therefore less stress and adversity arising from other people, less negative interaction and conflict. Lacking confidants may reduce quality of life, but not having to confide about problems also means that any cognitive minimising of difficulties can go unchallenged. Of course such styles may be open to other disorders not measured in these studies, for example somatising disorder or physical illness.

It is suggested that individuals with Withdrawn styles may be less 'plastic' or malleable in their susceptibility to the environment (Belsky and Pluess 2009). That is, they are less sensitised to both negative and supportive environments with less adverse developmental sequelae (Belsky, Bakermans-Kranenburg *et al.* 2007). Those with other Insecure styles are likely to be more malleable and more sensitive to their environment than those Withdrawn and thus suffer more from inadequacies of care.

The samples quoted here were community-based and mainly selected on the basis of psychosocial risk factors in the adult women (e.g. childhood neglect/abuse or ongoing relationship problems or low self-esteem). In contrast to many research samples, they were not selected as a psychiatric sample, nor were they selected for clinical disorder or for service use. This allowed for an analysis of resilience to take place and a number of resilient individuals were found which might be missed in samples using clinical services. There was perhaps a surprising amount of positive experience recorded given the frequent adverse experiences also described. This held for both the adult and Offspring samples. A recent United Nations Children's Fund (UNICEF) report has shown how in rich developed world countries, the UK has the worst level of wellbeing for children and young people, together with the USA (UNICEF 2007). This analysis utilised average data taken in the early 2000s from nationally representative school samples and household data on income and living conditions. High ratings for negative perception of health, school life and personal wellbeing were found in UK series, based on the responses to single items such as 'I feel lonely' or 'how much I like school' or 'how good is my health'. Whilst the findings may indeed accurately reflect worse quality of life in UK youth, the narrow range of measurement may have failed to highlight co-existing positive attitudes and experiences, which paradoxically may indicate very good quality of life consistent with improved material conditions and greater availability of educational opportunities. This may be due to a polarisation where wellbeing is very high for some young people and very low for others with the average tending towards the lower end, but it may also reflect the complexity of modern life in metropolitan areas where good and bad experience are often juxtaposed. Thus it may be possible to simultaneously have good and bad experiences of school or home or health. The results found in the London studies reported here suggests such juxtaposition does exist and that full analysis of quality of life and wellbeing is a complex field of study where negative and positive experiences need to be separately assessed and not merged into average ratings in order to reflect the true patterning of contemporary life. Perhaps this would lead to a more optimistic view of how our children will fare in future life.

Family contexts are complex, with ecological and psychological factors providing layers of influences, any one of which could have positive, negative or mixed valence for disorder outcomes. Past research has been successful in identifying direct effects of negative risks for disorder outcomes and outlining negative trajectories from childhood to adult life, with adolescence frequently a critical juncture. Integrating protective or resilience factors into such schemes has been the object of much investigation, but these effects are often harder to study, given that many research samples are either representative series where risk factors are low or clinical samples where the negative outcome is predetermined by selection. High-risk community populations can therefore be highly advantageous in studying the overlap of risk and resilience factors with both disorder and well-being outcomes identifiable. This can help with identifying protective or positive factors in the natural environment, which can guide preventative interventions to enhance such elements in the community at large (Bonanno 2004).

Utilising contextual interview measures can help not only with exploratory study of risks and resilience, but also aid in the identification of such experiences when interventions are planned. The context of experience is usually critical in determining the meaning of the experience for individuals. Thus an abusive parent, whose impact is defused by a close friend or relative, or being in a violent household buffered by positive school experience, may result in a different interpretation of experience forestalling future negative generalisation. It can potentially avert the generalised beliefs that the world is hostile, that people cannot be trusted and that the self is unlovable. Such characteristics form the nexus of Insecure attachment style and related low self-esteem and are the schemata from which adult disorder emerges (Beck 1967). Being able to hold on to a secure internal working model, which is based on trust, optimism and self-acceptance can provide the basis for a more fulfilled and healthy transition from adolescent to adult life.

Being able to chart positive change in attachment style in adults is also important. As 'working models' it was always anticipated that the cognitive templates underlying attachment insecurity could change over time with positive experience. This of course provides the rationale for intervention, and the next chapters will look at attachment style in relation to interventions and clinical practice.

8 Attachment-based interventions and services

8.0 Introduction

This and the following two chapters will look at the relevance of attachment theory for psychological and social care practice with children, adolescents, parents and families. This will draw from child and family services in the UK, utilising attachment models to inform assessment and intervention. This will include reference to couple and family therapy, child psychological services, child protection and safeguarding services as well as adoption and fostering. It is not within the remit of this chapter to review all the various early interventions, parenting programmes and psychotherapeutic approaches available or applicable. Instead some of the more prominent ones and those representative of a general approach with an explicit attachment perspective will be outlined. However, there will be no details of their formal evaluations and tested efficacy. The aim is to outline and discuss the 'translation' of knowledge gained about attachment and its application to the treatment and intervention field. This will be extended with practice examples in the following chapters. A particular plea will be made for effective assessment acknowledging adolescent or adult attachment style as a crucial element.

Services for children and young people in the UK are focused not only on safeguarding or protecting those already affected by neglect and abuse and related family difficulties, but also on prevention and early intervention to tackle the multiple problems faced by children, young people, their parents and families prior to serious child protection concerns developing. A multi-agency approach is acknowledged as central to effective intervention or treatment for the complex range of psychosocial risks involved. This requires in-depth assessment of child and family circumstances and behaviours easily communicated across agencies to other practitioners involved. Alerting practitioners in the field of social work, psychological services and education to identify the early attachment-related markers for parent and child vulnerability and risk is discussed within the broader context of family dysfunction, childhood risks for psychopathology and treatment.

The approach to assessment and service provision in the UK tends to be largely ecological (Bronfenbrenner 1979) and emphasises the different levels of social impacts on the child as covered in the statutory Assessment Framework approach to case analysis (Department of Health (DoH) 2000). This specifies the importance of the parents' or main carers' parenting behaviour, the family context and the developmental impact on the child (Bentovim and Bingley Miller 2001). Attachment theory, or attachment indicators are not mentioned specifically. However, parental unavailability, neglect, abuse, conflict, and the family's poor functioning are identified as critical in effective assessment, to establish if abuse thresholds are reached and the child and family need treatment or intervention. There are, however, benefits in specifying attachment perspectives and assessment tools for the purposes of safeguarding and family support when identifying child neglect and abuse.

In spite of large-scale concern and legislation to eradicate childhood neglect and abuse (National Society for Prevention of Cruelty to Children (NSPCC) 2011), many children and adolescents are still subject to maltreatment with only a proportion reaching relevant services (Tunstill and Aldgate 2000). Those who do reach services and are removed from abusive parents suffer discontinuity in care, are often in repeated arrangements throughout childhood, with poor outcomes from residential and fostering placements for psychological disorder and schooling (Rushton 2004; Chamberlain, Price *et al.* 2006). Rates of disorder in childhood and adolescence attributed to maltreatment are high, and these continue into adulthood resulting in lifetime vulnerability and disadvantage. The aim of services in this area is to provide stable and caring alternative arrangements for children removed from their parents, together with psychological and educational service aid, to decrease risk and aid resilience for the children and young people concerned. For those labelled as 'children in need' who are provided with family support and remain with their biological families, the aim is to reduce risk and increase resilience in existing families with a focus on working with parents.

In the child protection field in the UK, there are highly developed methods for assessing children and their families and analysing such information (for review see Bentovim, Cox *et al.* 2009). The Assessment Framework, utilised by social workers and by other professionals as the Common Assessment Framework, covers a range of family characteristics to be assessed from family environment, parenting capacity and child developmental needs. The parenting aspects identified in the required framework include emotional warmth, stability, safety and care. Attachment to the parents or carers or disturbances in attachment patterns in children are not specifically identified in the model. Instead the child's emotional and behavioural development, identity and family and social relationships more generally are labelled (DoH 2000). There are a series of assessment tools social workers can use to aid with this assessment such as the Home Observation and Measurement of the Environment (HOME) inventory (Cox 2008), Family Pack of Questionnaires and Scales (DoH, Cox *et al.* 2000) and the Family Assessment (Bentovim and Bingley Miller 2001). The ASI has recently been added to this, and the Safeguarding Assessment Analysis Framework, SAAF (Bentovim, Cox *et al.* 2009) and the training is now rolled out for both adoption-fostering and for other childcare/protection services.

Whilst there is still emphasis on evidence-based models and methods for assessing and analysing cases, recent developments following the Munro Review are beginning to advocate more creative approaches to assessment, and those less technologically driven (Munro 2010). It is in this context that whilst examining different interventions related to Attachment approaches, we also consider the utility of the ASI for assessment.

8.1 Family support/children in need

The requirement for UK services to provide preventative family support emerges directly from the Children Act (1989) and is amplified in the updated law (2004). This entails recognising and building on protective factors to identify family strengths to avoid social exclusion, poverty and poor functioning. Family support applies to families with dependent children who are at risk of family breakdown through violence or neglect (May-Chahal 2003). The emphasis is on good parenting, and the aim of providing support is to prevent future difficulties for the children and, at the extreme, preventing the need for the children to be taken into care and accommodated by the authorities. The services included are those psychological, medical, social, educational and criminal justice, working closely together.

Definitions of family support may be family-, parent/carer- or child-centred and involve the creation or enhancement of locally based, accessible activities, facilities and networks for families in need. These include those which alleviate stress, increase self-esteem, promote parental/carer/family competence and behaviour and increase parental capacity to nurture and protect children (Hearn 1995). Family support may be provided by a variety of means – for example through financial security, provision of health, education and welfare services, assurance of safe streets, good environments and strong communities. It may also refer to services where social or emotional support is the main provision. Here the focus may be on a particular child or on the whole family, and be either broad or narrow in terms of the service being offered. A narrower focus more relevant to psychological services is often on parenting skills and, when children are seen to be at greater risk for emotional and behavioural disorder, therapeutic work is addressed with the individual child or with the family as a whole.

8.2 Working therapeutically

Since the publication of Belsky and Nezworki's (1988) *Clinical Applications of Attachment*, the last two decades have seen a considerable focus in the literature on the aims, claims and outcomes of attachment-based therapies. In step with the burgeoning research interest focused on risk and intervention outcomes of attachment insecurity, attachment-based clinical interventions have proliferated to address the relational disturbances and sometimes extreme behaviours seen to emanate from attachment failures.

Michael Rutter and colleagues' recognition that Attachment theory's attention to real-life experiences require attention to interpersonal rather than intra-personal defences raised awareness that attachment classification, whether Secure or Insecure, tended to be applied to the individual rather than to a specific relationship (Rutter and O'Connor 1999). Since then, the perspective has shifted in recognising that in birth families both adult and child co-exist with their own unique attachment style, the adult style being based on the individual's own experience of early care and later socio-emotional development and the child's style developed in reaction to the specific ongoing relational and parenting style available. In foster and adoptive populations the child's relational dynamic has usually been formulated within a previous potentially abusive or neglectful dyadic relationship and is imported into an independently formed attachment dynamic in a new family. This may then challenge the new carer's own Secure or Insecure attachment characteristics. The tensions implicit in such relational reactivity contribute to further risks for insecurity, behavioural disturbance and disorder.

In keeping with advances in identifying specific individual, familial, social and intergenerational risks for Insecure attachments, clinical applications have also become increasingly focused on interactional and contextual factors intergenerationally. Thus targeting the parent–child dyad and family context advocated in the 'vertical' treatment approach crossing generations is now widely advocated. Specifically, the association of maternal sensitivity , shown to be associated with the different patterns of organised attachment in the child (Ainsworth, Blehar *et al.* 1978) has focused therapeutic work on the enhancement of this quality of attachment. Enhancing parental sensitivity to the child through altering parents' internal working models, are components which distinguish attachment-based therapies rather than therapies in general.

The American Professional Society on the Abuse of Children (APSAC), led by established researchers and clinicians in the attachment field, recommends that first-line services for children and families showing relationship difficulties should be based on the core principles of attachment theory. Such theoretical basis of attachment as a therapeutic framework for clinical intervention does not provide a prescriptive approach to enhancing the parent–child relationship. Most programmes, however, identify the 'client' as being the parent–child dyad, with focus on the relationship between the two, and the mother or caregiver as a main point of access for intervention. Treatment is mostly aimed at modifying interactions and improving attachment security through effecting change in maternal/main caregiver behaviour and representational models. These latter are the mental structures of self and of self in relation to other, which are developed through early experiences with caregivers as internal working models. To create such change, many programmes include play-based approaches in which parents are coached to alter their usual patterns of behaviour, and to be sensitive to the child's initiations and actions. However, the various approaches also vary widely in terms of the target populations, key components of the treatment, client characteristics, the specific techniques and practice principles relied on.

Underpinning many dyadic interventions are:

- The therapeutic relationship as a secure base through which new ways of thinking and feeling about the self, others and relationships are facilitated.
- Modification of mother's/carer's internal working model of relationships and of the child.
- Developing increased maternal sensitivity, insight into, and attunement to, the child's emotional cues.
- An emphasis on mother's emotional understanding, mentalising of her own and the child's state of mind, and emotion-regulation.

Approaches may either rely on coaching behaviours, or on video footage to reveal and illustrate harmful interactions, or may explicitly make the mother conscious of blocked feelings and memories that continue to hamper attachment interactions. The caregiver's capacity for mentalising emphasises the crucial role that the caregiver's thoughts, feelings and behaviour towards the child play in the pattern and security of the child's attachment (Ainsworth, Blehar *et al.* 1978; Main and Hesse 1990). This is increasingly emphasised as critical to facilitating change in mother–child attachment relationships. The theoretical framework provided by attachment theory also strongly links the programmes available in targeting behaviours that help parents become a reliable resource for modulating stress and arousal in the child. At a neurobiological level this leads to normalising HPA axis function. The role of the parent or carer to be reliably in charge of the child's regulatory system is thought to underpin the effects of such interventions although this is rarely measured. Additionally, few programmes systematically gather data that informs clinicians about the adult carer's capacity to modulate their own stress levels during interactions with their partner or child, or indentify the different strategies used by the parent for regulating attachment distress whether through hyper-activation, deactivation or dissociation as categorised within different attachment styles.

Given that the parent or adult is the usual 'port of entry' for engaging with the parent–child dyad, the absence of routine attachment-based assessment as a pre-clinical measure of the parent's attachment related functioning is notable in children's services. Thus the perspective on attachment remains very much with the child's viewpoint, perhaps not fully encapsulating one or both parents' or carers' complex attachment patterns. Thus the individual parent's capacity for engaging with others to help buffer against external stressors often remains unknown, even when parents are deemed eligible for participation in the therapeutic process.

Pre-clinical assessment tools used by psychologists and therapists, while raising awareness of specific risk factors that may contribute to medium- and high-risk of disorder in the children or young people, have very brief questionnaire formats, and do not allow for assessment that more closely investigates the characteristics of the parent–child and family relationship. More specifically, attachment patterns that both adult and child have developed in response to their respective caregiving and more recent relational experiences are not routinely investigated (O'Connor and Byrne 2007). There is an overall absence of a more holistic approach that incorporates scales which can assess the parent and child's interpersonal context and relating and Insecure attachment style, used routinely by either psychologists or social workers. It is established that this is an area of risk which, in conjunction with provoking stressors, can cause the onset of disorders such as depression and other internalising and externalising disorders. Yet, no complementary assessment is made of the specific characteristics of the parent/carer–child relationship or of the specific characteristics of the child's and parent's attachment style. This would provide crucial measurement of the way in which the child or young person's behaviour, whether emotional or behavioural may reflect developmentally salient functions in terms of self-protection. As such, no assessment is made of the emotional climate in which the child or adolescent negotiates daily interpersonal relational transactions and whether these may be characterised by a need to protect against anger, emotional withdrawal, fearfulness or emotional dependence and engulfment. Furthermore, assessment of general stress factors, those arising from attitudinal factors that underpin difficulties in relating to family members or from social contexts can provide key information in relation to risks for disorder and coping but are not routinely covered. It is this gap the ASI seeks to address.

The development and mainstreaming of treatments tailored for attachment issues have limited implementation due to a sometimes scant evidence base for the efficacy of the programmes. Below is a summary of some prominent attachment-based intervention approaches. In this summary, no consideration will be given to behaviour modification approaches such as Re-birthing, Rage Reduction, Attachment or Holding Therapy or any other controversial therapy that have had harmful outcomes (Prior and Glaser 2006).

Figure 8.1 seeks to map the more well-known interventions in terms of the different risks associated with attachment insecurity, although many of course do tackle more than one attachment aspect. (See below for fuller descriptions of interventions.) On summary inspection, this shows how most are directed at problem parenting, some mixed with interpersonal stress (e.g. Circle of Security (CoS)) and partner and family relating (Attachment-focused Family Therapy (AFTT), Filial Therapy). One is specifically focused on disorder (Watch Wait and Wonder (WWW)), one with the biological underpinnings of attachment problems (Attachment and Bio-behavioural Catch-up (ABC)) and one focused on mentalising (Mentalising-Based Therapy (MBT)). Otherwise the approaches in couple and family therapy have absorbed attachment principles into their practice, but without articulating specifc new techniques in intervention and without rigorous evaluation.

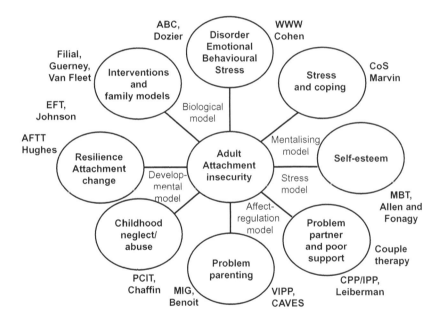

Figure 8.1 Focus of attachment-based interventions for children and families

A brief outline will be made first of couple and family therapy for adults, and then those interventions for adolescents and children, and finally those for parents and infants. In the next chapter, those interventions offered for children looked after by the state (in fostering, adoption and residential care) will be outlined. Whilst this is not intended as a comprehensive overview, readers are directed to more extensive reviews (Bakermans-Kranenburg, van Ijzendoorn *et al.* 2003; O'Connor and Zeanah 2003a; O'Connor and Zeanah 2003b).

8.3 Interventions for families

8.3.1 Couple Therapy

The application of attachment theory to adult relationships did not occur until the late 1980s and was considered a revolutionary event for couple therapy (Johnson and Lee 2000; Johnson 2003; Johnson and Whiffen 2003). The practice of couple therapy has obvious resonance with attachment approaches, particularly those using a social and relationship-based approach. Both couple therapy and attachment theory hold the following principles in common:

- Adult love relationships mirror past relationships with parents and actively re-create the negative elements of these relationships to resolve inner conflicts.
- Problems in relationships are due to developmental delays that cause partners to enmesh rather than differentiate.
- Partners lack skills, either communication or negotiation ones, with which to create good rational quid pro quo contracts with spouses.
- Enmeshment confuses caring and coercion.
- Quid pro quo contracts are generally found in distressed not happy couples (Johnson and Whiffen 2003).

Attachment perspectives on distressed adult relationships highlight the bond between the partners, and the need to define the relationship as a safe haven and a secure base to allay anxiety and fear. Proximity to an attachment figure serves the purpose of reducing fear and offers an antidote to feelings of helplessness and meaninglessness. Therefore, a key issue in distressed relationships is that partners need to be accessible and responsive to each others emotional cues in order to regulate each other's emotion. The spouse becomes the primary attachment figure for the majority of adults and as such the main source of security and comfort. The therapist not only needs to improve communication skills in the couple and increase insight into past and present relationships, but needs to address the need for comfort and promotion of safe emotional engagement and responsiveness as the fundamental basis of secure bond. The importance of soothing and supportive responses in defining close relationships is an important requirement for safe emotional engagement (Gottman and Levenson 2000).

It therefore follows that isolation, separation or disconnection from an attachment figure, or its threat, is inherently traumatising. Distressed partners who are emotionally disconnected tend to become immersed in fear and insecurity and tend to adopt the stances of fight, flight or freeze that characterise responses to traumatic stress. The more distressed and hopeless the relationship, the more automatic, rigid and self-reinforcing the emotional responses and the interactions between partners will be. From an attachment perspective the patterns of distress in couple relationships are quite finite and predictable and reflect the process of separation distress. Most often, one partner will pursue for emotional connection, but often in an angry, critical manner, while the other will placate or withdraw, to keep the peace or to protect him/her from criticism. Each partner's steps then call forth and maintain the other's in a reciprocally determining feedback loop. Critical complaining and defensive distance predict the continuing deterioration of a relationship. Occasionally couples will seek therapy when the pursuing spouse has given up and is beginning to withdraw as a prelude to detachment. Depression and anxiety naturally accompany relationship distress with its attendant loss of security and connection and debilitating sense of isolation, and such distress is likely to maintain these emotional problems. Attachment theory identifies specific associations between relationship distress and mental disorders, which most clients describe in terms of loss, aloneness and sense of helplessness (Johnson 2003).

Couple therapy is based on attachment as a theory of relatedness. It thus focuses on an evaluation of attachment needs and fears and the promotion of safe emotional engagement, comfort and support. It also involves a privileging of emotional responses and communication and direct addressing of attachment vulnerabilities and fears to foster emotional attunement and responsiveness. The creation of a respectful collaborative alliance in the therapy session can be a safe haven and secure base in which an explicit shaping of responsiveness and accessibility is made. Specifically detached partners will be re-engaged and blaming partners will be supported so that bonding events can occur and offer an antidote to negative cycles and insecurity. A focus on how the self is defined and redefined in emotional communication with attachment figures is also made. An explicit shaping of pivotal attachment responses that redefine a relationship is undertaken and an addressing of injuries that block relationship repair. Below are specific forms of attachment-related therapy (Kobak and Mandelbaum 2003).

8.3.2 Emotionally Focused Family Therapy

Emotionally Focused Family Therapy (EFFT)(Johnson and Lee 2000) is mainly focused on the adolescent in the family, and aims to modify the distressing cycles of interaction that amplify conflict and undermine secure connection between parents and the adolescent to improve responsiveness and the secure base. Therapy involves 10–12 sessions, mostly with the whole family to reprocess key attachment related emotions and revisions of patterns of interaction to approximate to those secure. EFFT in practice aims for the de-escalation of negative cycles such as 'attack-withdraw' that maintain attachment insecurity and block safe emotional engagement and responsiveness. The naming of these cycles and discussion of their impact helps the couples to see these cycles more objectively rather than labelling each other as the enemy. Critical pursuing partners can begin to ask for their needs to be met in ways that foster compassion and contact. Powerful 'bonding events' can then occur, that offer a new emotional experience of connection. The consolidation of gains, and the integration of the process of change into the couples' model of the relationship and each partner's sense of self can then occur. Core intervention techniques include: Reflecting on emotional experience, Validation, Evocative Responding, Heightening, Empathic conjecture or interpretation, Tracking, Reflecting or Replaying interactions, Reframing in the context of the cycle and attachment processes and Restructuring and shaping interactions. Such intervention has proved beneficial when compared to cognitive therapy in a study of young women with Fearful attachment styles and eating disorder (Johnson, Maddeaux *et al.* 1998)

8.3.3 Attachment Focused Family Therapy

Variants of general family therapy are Attachment Focused Family Therapy (AFFT) or Dyadic Developmental Psychotherapy (DDP) (Hughes 2009). This is an integrative method of psychotherapy that was developed in the 1990s for the treatment of children and youth who manifested serious psychological problems associated with complex trauma and serious failure to establish secure patterns of attachment. Most of the clients receiving this treatment were residing in foster homes, adoptive homes, and residential treatment centres. Over the past decade the therapy has maintained its attachment-focused, family-centred stance while continuing to refine its theoretical foundations and treatment interventions and to broaden its focus to include the treatment of all families (Hughes 2009). At the same time there have been two empirical studies that have begun to demonstrate the clinical efficacy of this treatment model (Becker-Weidman and Hughes 2008). Treatment is focused on helping children who have difficulty in responding to normative dyadic interactions by helping parents develop exchanges that contribute to felt safety for the child's neurological, emotional, cognitive and behavioural functioning. The model is congruent with attachment principles in promoting reciprocal non-coercive interactions that communicate acceptance, curiosity, playfulness and empathy.

8.3.4 Filial Therapy

Filial Therapy (Guerney 1964; van Fleet 2005) integrates attachment, developmental and psychodynamic theories in a strengths-based approach that combines family therapy with non-directive play therapy . The aim is to help parents develop increased attunement, strengthen attachments and prevent family disruption. It focuses on prevention and resolution of difficulties in family functioning rather than being child problem-focused. The basis of the approach is to address attachment difficulties and a wide range of behaviours associated with poorly managed family relationships as well as chronic and acute difficulties associated with traumatic experience. Drawing also on behavioural and social learning theory parents are taught basic child-centred play therapy principles and skills and then practise these skills under the close supervision of a trained therapist. Because Filial Therapy encourages working with both parents to effect change and promote secure parent–child relationships, it has a strong focus on parental attachment and behaviour, as well as on the whole family system and its dynamics so that the target child is not singled out. Its approach recognises the need for parents to be directly involved in building emotional bonds and thus become the stress moderators and behaviour managers. In acknowledging the parents as 'agents of change' it empowers them to become directly responsible for regulating the child's elevated HPA through the application of therapeutic parenting skills (empathy, reflective listening, structuring and limit setting). The skills are directed at providing real and emotional safety during perceived social and emotional threat and anger, fear or other distress enactments. The approach also targets behavioural and attitudinal parental reactions to the child's play and a key focus of the approach is the opportunity to process the child's thematic play as its is perceived and responded to through the parental attachment lens. Research outcomes demonstrate a reduction in child behaviour problems (Grskovic and Goetze 2008), decrease in parental stress (Kale and Landreth 1999), increased parental acceptance of the child (Bratton and Landreth 1995), increased parental empathy (Glover and Landreth 2000) and improved parent–child relationships (Grskovic and Goetze 2008).

8.3.5 Mentalising-Based Therapy

MBT approaches have been developed from attachment and psychodynamic concepts and, when applied to couples or families, also incorporate systemic practices and techniques (Allen and Fonagy 2006; Bateman and Fonagy 2012). It utilises varied formats working with individuals, couples and families, as well as with multi-family and multi-couple groups, through network meetings and supervision (Fearon, Target *et al.* 2006; Asen and Fonagy 2012). The emphasis is on techniques and pragmatic ways of using mentalisation-based ideas to develop practice as a complementary framework and 'add-on' to mainstream systemic approaches. It thus builds bridges between systemic and psychodynamic models of work. A main focus is on patients with Borderline Personality Disorder (BPD), where those with Disorganised attachment fail to develop mentalising capacity within the attachment relationship with parents. The object of treatment is that BPD patients increase mentalisation capacity to improve emotional regulation and interpersonal relationships. The major goals include better behavioural control, increased affect regulation, more intimate and gratifying relationships and the ability to pursue life goals. This is believed to be accomplished through increasing the capacity for mentalisation in order to stabilize the client's sense of self and to enhance stability in emotions and relationships with the enhancement of mentalising itself as focus of treatment. The focus is on the present state and how it remains influenced by events of the past.

MBT is developed for work with children and families in difficulty as a brief psychodynamic therapy, using attachment, relational and mentalising principles (Fearon, Target *et al.* 2006). The aim is to promote longer-term resilience in a family for example by promoting methods of coping in relation to supportiveness. It is manualised and lasts 6–12 sessions. It deals with issues of mentalisation defined as the capacity to interpret the behaviour of others and oneself in terms of underlying mental states – feelings, thoughts, beliefs and desires. This is taken to drive the way people behave towards others, as well as how they think of themselves in relation to others. This capacity is taken to be closely associated with Secure attachment style, and resilience. In common with psychodynamic treatment in general, MBT explicitly uses the therapeutic relationship to further develop mentalising within the whole family. The approach is described as having similarities with CBT, in that thought processes are mediators of experience and behaviour, but also with systemic family therapy in that the child's problem is a manifestation of poorly functioning family systems. In the course of the therapy the model is fully articulated to the family with directive and psycho-educational components included. During the therapy the family go through a process of understanding each other more clearly through observation and discussion. The impact of stress is identified and the difficulty of mentalising when stressed outlined. The association between mentalising, stress and behaviour is emphasised as leading to unsupportive family interactions.

8.4 Families in stressful and adverse circumstances

Some of the family-based approaches specifically target those families with adversity, those under stress and those where parental psychological disorder is present. Approaches are similar to those described above, as well as involving parental sensitivity (described below). Most focus on strengthening the attachment relationship between caregiver and child, in order to improve the child's self-regulating abilities and sense of efficacy and enhance the caregiver's sensitivity, for example Watch, Wait and Wander – WWW (Cohen, Muir *et al.* 1999). Others target disadvantaged and maltreating families including depressed mothers and those exposed to domestic violence such as Child Parent Psychotherapy (CPP) and its adaptation for infants (IPP) (Lieberman, Weston *et al.* 1991) in which an explicit attachment approach, combined with developmental, trauma, social learning, psychodynamic and cognitive behavioural frameworks are used in working with both parents and children.

The Circle of Security (CoS) (Marvin, Cooper *et al.* 2002) is a group-model intervention geared towards family support for children in need where there are parenting difficulties. In the USA it has been based on deprived Head Start (the equivalent to the UK Sure Start) families and uses an explicit attachment approach, teaching caregivers the fundamentals of attachment theory (for example parent acting as secure base for the child). In focussing on parenting behaviours and internal working models it provides caregivers with awareness and understanding of the non-conscious, problematic responses they sometimes have to their children's needs and thus increases parental sensitivity to children's cues.

Other interventions focus on parenting such as Manipulation of Sensitive Responsiveness (van den Boom 1995) provided for mothers from low socio-economic groups with irritable infants, and is based on Ainsworth's sensitive responsiveness components, namely perceiving a signal, interpreting it correctly, selecting an appropriate response and implementing the response effectively. Another approach, the Parent–Child Interaction Therapy (PCIT) (Chaffin, Silovsky *et al.* 2004) emphasises changing negative parent caregiver–child patterns and combines an attachment approach with developmental social learning theory. Parents learn skills when they interact in specific play with the child. It utilises a two-stage approach aimed at relationship enhancement and child-behaviour management.

Two other interventions use video techniques to show parents their behaviour when interacting with their infants. One of these is Video Feedback Intervention to Promote Positive Parenting (VIPP) (Juffer, Hoksbergen *et al.* 1997) and is aimed at promoting maternal sensitivity through the review of taped infant–parent interactions. The other, Clinician Assisted Video feedback Exposure Sessions (CAVES) is based on principles of mentalisation and emotion regulation and aims to help mothers traumatised by histories of abuse and violence, to think of their children in more adaptive, mental terms (Schechter and Willheim 2009). Most interventions are also largely focused on infants rather than older children. In recognising the important role of play in promoting healthy parent child relationships many use either infant-led play therapy as a way of expression for the child, but it is not clear to what extent maternal attachment issues are addressed. Partners/fathers are not explicitly referred to or included in these interventions. With the exception of a few programmes such as CoS or VIPP measures of attachment style in mothers do not seem to be used, nor of her relating in the wider family, as for example with partners.

8.4.1 Attachment and parenting sensitivity

Interventions which utilise adult attachment elements predominantly focus on maternal attachment style, parenting sensitivity and interaction with the baby or infant in dyadic therapeutic treatments. An extensive meta-review of evaluation of 88 interventions for early childhood attachment interventions has been conducted comparing the impacts on maternal sensitivity and child attachment style (Bakermans-Kranenburg, van Ijzendoorn *et al.* 2003). A number of these have already been described above, such as WWW, PPP, IPP and video approaches. There were, however, numerous others with varied types of intervention (e.g. those non-personal, conducted by either a lay person or professional) and interventions conducted in clinics or at home. The focus could include support, parenting sensitivity, representations of internal working models or these in combination. In terms of assessment methods, these included a range of child measures such as the HOME inventory or the SST, as well as Ainsworth sensitivity scales in addition to observational methods of the mother.

The effects sizes on average were higher for maternal sensitivity change (d=0.33) than child attachment style change (d=0.20) but both were significant (see Figure 8.2). In fact, those most effective for improving maternal sensitivity also improved child attachment security. Some results were surprising – briefer interventions were more effective, as were those by non-professionals, and those not involving contact (e.g. providing soft baby carriers to hold the baby close). Interventions worked whether single- or multiple-risk families were involved and those few which involved fathers were particularly successful, although had less positive effects on mothers also involved. Interventions focused on sensitivity rather than on support or on mother's representations were most effective. It was observed that attachment insecurity was harder to change and 'sleeper effects' were discussed whereby the attachment changes could occur at a later time. The focus was on positive parental behaviours including responsiveness, sensitivity or involvement, but these were restricted to observational methods of assessment. Findings showed that studies utilising SST showed less positive change.

8.4.2 Attachment and Bio-behavioural Catch-up (ABC)

Attachment models identify biological delays to development as important, these arising from poor parenting and problematic interactions between parent and child. ABC is one of the few interventions to assess biological processes to note the level of dysfunction due to attachment-related issues, and to identify catch-up as an effect of intervention (Dozier, Lindheim *et al.* 2005). This is undertaken through parent and foster parent training and with infants and toddlers. It is aimed specifically at infants who have experienced early adverse care and disruptions in care, with the programme providing specialist help for foster carers. It is designed to

Summary findings of meta-review
Bakermans-Kranenburg *et al.* 2003

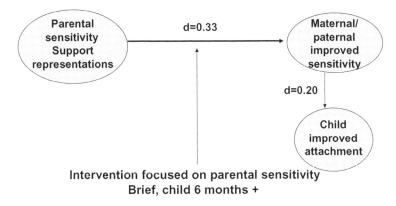

Intervention focused on parental sensitivity
Brief, child 6 months +

d=Average effect size, both significant.

Figure 8.2 Findings of meta-review infant intervention studies

strengthen the child's regulatory capacities, but with the intervention techniques focused on the adult as a resource for modulating stress and
arousal. ABC recognises the use of biological markers to look for change in
children. The effectiveness of regulating cortisol with children in foster
care showed diurnal cortisol patterns (as assessed by morning and bedtime
salivary cortisol measures) that were significantly different in the intervention and community comparison groups post-intervention providing
evidence for positive change (Dozier, Lindheim *et al.* 2005).

8.4.3 Multidimensional Therapeutic Foster Care (MTFC)

MFTC is a very widely used and studied intervention for fostercare, originally designed in the USA at the Oregon Social Learning Centre (Fisher
and Chamberlain 2000), and now used in the UK after an extensive trial
funded by the Department of Education (Scott, Spender *et al.* 2001). The
programme is aimed at working with foster carers to improve interaction
with the placed child and to improve behavioural difficulties in the child.
Whilst this is mainly a social learning and behavioural programme, in
recent years it has also examined attachment change as an outcome (Fisher
and Kim 2007). The aim is to give parents the skills to bring up their
children and cope with problem behaviour with target groups of children

with behavioural problems. Professional therapists are trained at the Oregon Centre and with weekly supervision undertake programmes for individual children that run for as long as necessary. From the 1970s, Patterson and colleagues at the Oregon Social Learning Centre studied the effect of different programmes on the families of antisocial boys in order to develop the MTFC. When evaluated, significant reductions in antisocial behaviour were recorded and the intervention is considered to be well-supported by research evidence. However, treatment effects were not very stable and longer follow-up uncovered mixed results. These were improved when programmes were extended for longer periods. Also, a fifth of families dropped out of the programme and another third refused to be contacted 12 months after completing the course.

One of the interesting evaluations of the preschool intervention has been the effects on cortisol regulation in the young abused children (Fisher, Stoolmiller *et al.* 2007). As described earlier, children who have been abused have atypical diurnal patterns of HPA axis activity shown as low early-morning cortisol activity that remains stable over the day. In a randomised, controlled study of maltreated children who were allocated to MFTC or usual foster care, the target intervention children exhibited cortisol activity (collected through saliva) comparable to the non-maltreated control group. This was unlike maltreated children in the regular foster care group who showed increasingly flattened morning-to-evening cortisol activity. However, no attachment measures were used in relation to this. In looking at attachment-related behaviours in preschoolers, the child's attachment was measured by means of foster carers diary at three-month intervals over a year (Fisher and Kim 2007). Children randomly assigned to the intervention showed significant increases in Secure behaviour and significant decreases in Avoidant behaviour. Both the target group and the usual foster care group showed improvement in Anxious-Resistant behaviour.

The intervention approaches with an attachment focus described are summarised below.

Summary of attachment interventions

- There are a number of existing interventions available for attachment-related difficulties in couples and intact families that are aimed at parenting. These focus on a range of attachment-related constructs (such as mentalising or parental sensitivity) and many use family-therapy approaches, often with a focus on families in adversity. The most common focus is parenting issues, particularly maternal sensitivity in relation to infants.

- Many of the interventions do not use an assessment of parent's attachment style at the beginning of treatment, and the style itself is rarely the main focus of the intervention.

- Most interventions which use attachment approaches are aimed at improving attachment between mother and baby around increasing sensitivity and parenting skills and most show positive impacts on maternal sensitivity and child attachment style. These impacts are also shown for fathers. However, most approaches do not include partners, nor do they explicitly look at the mother's support network in establishing her relating pattern outside the mother–child dyad.
- The age range for children involved is limited. Most interventions are geared mainly towards infants, preschool children or middle childhood. These do not seem to extend to teenagers.
- Some approaches are more psychodynamic, a number use dyadic therapeutic approaches, whilst others are psycho-educational. A number do attend to social issues such as domestic violence and social deprivation. A variety of methods are used – including video-feedback. There is no consistency of assessment for attachment style in mothers or children either pre-clinically, or to chart outcomes.

8.6 Discussion

Treatments tailored to attachment issues in the relationship between the mother and infant or child are available and many seem effective, particularly in increasing maternal (or paternal) sensitivity, with some effect in improving the child's attachment style. However, there is little focus on maternal attachment style, relationship with partner and support, for example in reducing barriers around Anxious-ambivalent and Avoidant styles. It also appears that most interventions do not usually extend to older childhood and teenage years. Thus a more systemic approach is rarely used and the range of tools used to assess parents is narrow. The approaches need further research in relation to comprehensive assessment tools used for children and young people around attachment. Such developments will help to provide more holistic and theoretically sound approaches to treating young people and their families with disorders and parenting difficulties.

Whilst a number of attachment-based interventions for children and families have been presented here, there has been a specific focus on family-based approaches. The advantages of family-based approaches are that since both parents and child are involved in the intervention there is more chance of change that can be maintained in the family system with improvements to communication and resolution of conflict to aid the family unit become more stress-resistant. The approach seems particularly well-attuned to social approaches to attachment. The approach incorporates the therapist's attention to the regulation, processing and integrating of the key emotional responses within the couple and parent–child relationship (Johnson 2003). In turn, emotion and emotional expression is a key link between the self and wider systems and an organiser of the interactional cycles. Attachment focuses on how the self is defined in the context of recurring interpersonal interactions. Models of self and other concern the loveability of self and the trustworthiness of others, and guide interactions with others. These models tend to be stable because they are continually confirmed in interactions with significant others. The therapist can actively use new positive interactions to challenge negative views of self and other and promote the construction of more positive sense of self.

The principle function of emotion is communication of the current motivational state of the individual (Johnson 2003). The therapist can help partners regulate reactive emotions that fuel negative cycles such as attack/defend and access and articulate marginalised emotions that can be used to move partners into new forms of emotional engagement. The need for secure emotional connection with key others is considered to be hard-wired by evolution and there are a few finite ways of dealing with the loss of such a connection. In terms of utilising attachment style, there are engagement styles/strategies which can be made explicit and correspond: first, is hyper-activating the attachment system and so becoming preoccupied with the relationship, monitoring it constantly and becoming coercive and aggressive. Second, attempting to deactivate the attachment system by 'numbing out' and 'shutting down' to care less and protect the self. Third, trying both of these in sequence (Kobak and Handelbaum 2003). This is used by trauma survivors who both desperately need and seek and desperately fear and avoid closeness.

Effective assessment of different family members, to highlight attachment in the family as well as elucidate communication patterns, conflict, and support needs is central to both assessing need and evaluating effectiveness of treatment. To date, measures such as the ASI have only been piloted in Filial Therapy, but the potential fit of the interview is likely to be good in the other therapies outlined. These relationship aspects are likely to mirror the underlying affect-regulation, mentalisation, self-perception and parenting behaviours underlying them.

It can thus be seen that couple and family therapy approaches to treatment fit well with social approaches to attachment style, extending this to all the family members involved. This in turn requires complex patterning of the permutations of hyper-activating/preoccupied styles with the deactivating/shutting down styles and the effects that these can have on the partners involved and on their parenting. This will be developed further in later chapters. The next chapter will illustrate the use of the ASI in identifying adult and adolescent attachment styles in child and family services.

9   Attachment Style Interview use in child and family services

9.0 Introduction

The last chapter looked at a range of interventions currently available which in adult attachment is part of the focus of work with families to improve parenting and child–parent interactions and to reduce disorder in both generations. This chapter will focus on the relevance of the ASI as an assessment tool in practice contexts with case material to illustrate its use in case analysis.

Of the 9.5 million children and young people in the UK, 400,000 are labelled 'in need' and 60,000 are Looked After Children (by the State). When placed with foster or adoptive families, such childrens' needs are complex, with ecological and psychological factors providing layers of influences, any one of which could have positive, negative or mixed risks for development and disorder outcomes. Research identifying risk trajectories from childhood to adult life can help identify protective factors in the natural environment to guide preventative interventions in the community at large (Bonanno 2004).

The relevance of attachment theory for adoption and fostering has long been recognised and 'translating' its concepts into practice when placing children with new families has progressed in recent years (Howe 2001). Much of the concern over suitable placement has been about the potential parenting capacity of the new carers and the psychological 'match' between carer characteristics and those of the child to be placed. This has perhaps had greater emphasis than the parallel concern over the carers' own attachment needs in relation to adult support in aiding resilience. These needs are identified in the practice guidance for adoption and fostering (Department for Education and Skills (DfES) 2006) which identifies the characteristics required of prospective carers in terms of both stable supportive relationships and parenting capacity. The former is needed to provide a consistent caring context for the child being placed, as well as to sustain the carers when facing the stress often induced by the demands of their new role. The guidance specifically outlines the need to assess 'ability to make and sustain close relationships', the 'capacity for emotional openness', the 'quality, stability and permanence' of the partner relationship and 'support networks for carers' (DfES 2006).

Attachment theory and practice has fitted well into children's services around the adoption and fostering context in finding replacement caregivers to ensure improved child development and wellbeing. Monitoring of Insecure attachment style both in children to be placed and with their adoptive or foster carers has been undertaken in research studies and has found that where the carers have Secure attachment style the children are more likely to develop greater security of attachment (Dozier, Stovall *et al.* 2001; Hodges, Steele *et al.* 2003). These studies have typically used the AAI to assess parental attachment style and the SST or Story Stems for infants and preschool children. However, all these measures are somewhat restricted in usual social work practice given their requirement for expert use and complex administration. More mainstreamed methods are needed to replicate such assessment and monitoring in everyday adoption-fostering processes.

Carers are required to build Secure attachments. The capacity to do so is evidenced through confiding relationships and can be assessed through exploring the existence of supportive relationships and the capacity to share difficulties and accept help. Thus, the role of support is likely to be critical to parenting capacity in determining the success and stability of future adoption or fostering placements. Assessments are therefore needed to measure the quality of support, and carers' ability to access it, in addition to their parenting competence. The problems surrounding the disruption of adoption placements and the need for additional post-placement support are well-established (Rushton 2003). The higher rate of placement breakdown in foster arrangements, particularly for children older at placement, are beginning to be equalled by those placed for adoption in recent years (Fergusson, Lynskey *et al.* 1995; Triseliotis 2002). Placement instability is related both to child and carer characteristics (Quinton, Rushton *et al.* 1998) but few studies have looked at fostering or adoption placement specifically from the point of view of carers' coping capacity and need for support. Earlier discussions in this book of stress models (Brown, Bifulco *et al.* 1990) indicate how vulnerability factors (identified as poor marital and other support, conflict with children or low self-esteem) interact with provoking agents (involving severe life events and difficulties, particularly in close relationships) to produce clinical depression. The likelihood of this occurring to carers post placement seems extremely high. Of particular relevance is the finding that stressful events linked to areas of high commitment are associated with a 40% rate of adult depression, those linked with a prior difficulty a 33% rate and those with both characteristics a massive 73% rate of disorder. This compares with rates of 8% depression resulting from other severe life events (Brown, Bifulco *et al.* 1987). This finding is relevant to the adoption and fostering situation given the high commitment to the caring role required and the difficulties that children bring to the placement, as well as the likelihood of severe life events occurring post placement that put carers at a particularly high risk of depression.

Investigator-based interviews such as the ASI and PRI collect narrative accounts of contextual material to investigate interpersonal relating and parenting. They offer narrative elements which can be used both qualitatively to elicit context and meaning of experience as well as quantitatively using benchmarked thresholds to ensure reliability of categorisation with the possibility of generating data across services for evaluative purposes. Utilising such contextual interview measures can help with the initial assessments of risks and resilience in carers and aid in identifying any areas where extra support or intervention is needed.

Thus accurate assessments of support networks and quality of relationships, however, are not only relevant for suitability of placement but are also important for anticipating the likely support requirements post placement of those accepted as adoptive parents. Figure 9.1 illustrates the impact a placed child can put on the carers and family to effectively generate a 'reverse transmission' of risk up the generations to effect carer's functioning. When support networks, individual relationships or support-seeking capacity look fragile, these elements can be strengthened through additional services, such as direct social work, support groups or befriending. Supportive contexts are relatively fluid and are thus amenable to erosion in deteriorating contexts as well as enhancement through use of appropriate intervention (Harris, Brown *et al.* 1999). Being forewarned about possible change promotes better provision and increases the utilisation of service-based support when difficulties arise. This requires the use of standardised interview tools for the reliable assessment of partner and other support and 'emotional openness' in accessing support such as that provided by the ASI.

9.1 Attachment Style Interview assessment in prospective adoption or foster parents

Experience shows that in using the ASI in practice settings, clients easily recognise the attachment profiles as applied to their own characteristics. This is because the styles are transparently based on information they provide directly. Thus someone who describes being fearful of rejection will usually recognise this in relation to Fearful category. If not then the practitioner can quote back statements made in order to illustrate the final style deduced from the interview. Summary sheets for helping explain the styles to clients are made available usually in short vignette format emphasising a strengths and weaknesses approach. Assessing a prospective adoptive carer as moderately or markedly Insecure clearly carries risks associated with the many factors identified in previous chapters. It is likely to be associated with poorer partner and support relationships along with attitudes which are Anxious or Avoidant and will make subsequent contact with services diffi-

'Reverse' transmission of risk, placed child to new carer

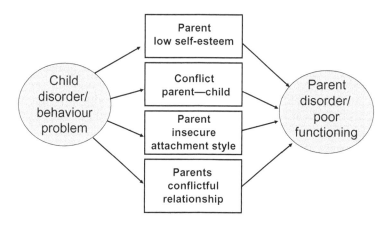

Figure 9.1 Transmission of risk from placed child to new carer

cult, relationships more likely to disrupt and parenting of children more problematic. The paired attachment styles of partners also needs to be taken into account and individual interviews undertaken. The ASI is never used as a collaborative couple measure, but only with each member individually to ascertain each ones perception and personally held attitudes. Having both parents with a highly Insecure style clearly increases risk for the child. The precise impacts of different style combinations are not known, but there is added impact to the mental health of each of the couple (Condé, Figueirido *et al.* 2011). The style shown to have less risk is that of Withdrawn. Anecdotally from assessments done in services, this seems more common in men. It carries with it the issue of a poorer range of support (often the wife is the only confidant) and attitudes of high independence and barriers to closeness. In itself it is not a disruptive style and is associated with less adversity but the lack of emotional expression may provide a somewhat distant environment for a needy child, and this needs to be considered alongside all the other characteristics assessed. However, if the main carer is Secure and the partner moderately Withdrawn, this may prove a suitable context for adoption or fostering and is often considered acceptable.

As described earlier, 'mild' levels of Insecure attachment style exert no additional psychosocial risk, hold some resilience and may prove to aid psychological matching of carer with child. For example, while Enmeshed style involves high dependence on others, at the 'mild' levels, where good support has been achieved, positive characteristics of sociability, warmth and frequent contact with family and friends are common. Such parents are likely to enjoy nurturing babies and young children who show high dependence and need for contact. Similarly, while those with Fearful style at high levels have an expectation of rejection, at 'mild' levels such styles involve sensitivity and awareness of other people's feelings. Such parents may welcome a timid or sensitive child who needs careful handling. Those with Angry-dismissive styles who have excessive mistrust at high insecurity levels, at mild levels are likely to show assertiveness and authority. Such parents may be effective for children who need boundaries, clear rules of discipline and effective champions in demanding resources and support from services. Those with Withdrawn styles, while overly self-reliant and isolated at extreme levels, can show high independence and practicality unimpeded by emotion. Such parents may provide appropriate parenting for children who are themselves detached and phased by expressions of emotions. Any of these mildly Insecure styles may prove to be strengths in certain adoption and fostering situations and their basis for matching to child attachment characteristics requires further investigation. The implications are the same for adoption, fostering or kinship care where children with complex needs are being cared for; without sufficient support and with attitudes which deter closeness and support-seeking, any carer will have reduced resilience to stress. In order to match parents and children, it may be necessary to also assess children's attachment style. However, there are few assessments for children, so this becomes difficult in practice contexts. Whilst a child ASI is under development, and an intensive Child Attachment Interview (CAI) is used for assessing children's attachments (Target, Fonagy *et al.* 2003), there is little currently suitable for practice.

Based on the principles discussed in earlier chapters in relation to attachment-related family therapy, and utilising findings from the research presented in this book, a schematic model can be developed to indicate the systemic flow of different negative elements emerging from Insecure style in both the relationship between parents as well as in their parenting of their child and the effects on the child. This is shown in Figure 9.2. Variations of this scheme will be used to illustrate different combinations of attachment style and parenting behaviour developed in this and the following chapter.

The following examples are disguised practice cases where the ASI has been used to assess parents in a range of contexts. Each raises a different issue around parental attachment, parenting competence and potential risk to the child.

9.2.1 Adopting Daisy – parents' anxious styles

The ASI was used as a preclinical assessment tool with prospective adoptive carers Erin and Frank to aid understanding of their support contexts, quality of marital and other close relationships as well as attachment attitudes of 10-year-old Daisy.[1]

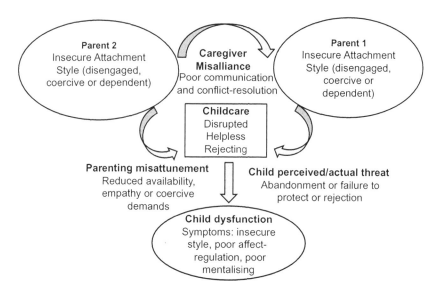

Figure 9.2 Developing a family-attachment model

Background: Referral information for Daisy included her history of severe neglect in a context of domestic violence. Attachment difficulties were indicated by her behavioural and emotional withdrawal, her inability to show affection and age-inappropriate demanding and challenging behaviour. A referral for Filial Therapy was made to support the parents in helping Daisy come to terms with her traumatic early life experience, to increase their understanding of the impact of the prior neglect and domestic violence on Daisy's early development and to develop empathy and a stronger attachment to their adoptive daughter.

Daisy had already been placed with Erin (aged 35) and Frank (aged 37), with a plan for adoption. However, the relationship with Daisy was strained and characterised by tension and disappointment. The carers saw Daisy as a self-reliant child with little interest in the care she received or affection for them. She was emotionally unpredictable, with moods inexplicably swinging between happy and thunderous, and they felt she was hard to get close to. Frank and Erin were disappointed that Daisy did not appear to need them as much as they would have liked.

An indication that Erin and Frank's own attachment needs, and the lens through which they viewed Daisy, may have obscured their perception of her attachment cues was suggested in referral information. This emphasised that Daisy's growing relationship with her carers was not developing quickly enough to satisfy their needs for attachment as indicated by her dependency. Whilst Daisy was beginning to be openly affectionate and on observation seemed to relate to both with warmth and caring, Erin and Frank felt that the degree of emotional closeness and neediness they desired was lacking. For the therapist, the opportunity for gathering information about the support and attachment characteristics of both carers in addition to behavioural question-naires and symptom based pre-intervention measures was felt to be critical to full understanding of the family and the success of the intervention.

Mother Erin's support: Erin reported a very close relationship with Frank in which there was high confiding and emotional support. She talked openly about her feelings about Daisy, and could also tell him about other things of an emotional nature. Whilst this was considered a close confiding relationship it was noted that she had a high level of felt attachment indi-cated high emotional dependency on her husband. She said: *'I could not manage without him. I would feel lost, lonely and unloved if Frank was no longer there.'* Her relationship with her VCO, a friend known for many years, was also a confiding and supportive relationship, but in Erin's view: *'She's quite independent and that makes me irritable with her. She does not ask for help enough. She doesn't want to bother you but does not realise that you'd be happy to do it for her, she's one of those people.'* Despite having other friends, no other confiding VCO relationship was described. Erin was rated moderately high on her ability to access support and make and maintain relationships and there-fore in the secure range of attachment styles.

Erin's mildly Enmeshed attachment attitudes: In exploring attitudes towards closeness and autonomy, Erin reported a high need for company and a high fear of separation that had been even more intense in the past. *'I used to hate being on my own but now I quite relish my time alone as long as it's not too long. Too long is more than a day. I really get worried after a day and if no one calls me I feel really lonely and start ringing round my friends to make sure they haven't forgotten about me.'* When describing brief separations from Frank, she said: *'We have been apart and I was quite depressed being away from Frank, but I never stopped him from going. Yes, I was anxious on my own and wished that Frank hadn't gone. If he wasn't there I would miss the feeling of being needed and loved. I call him all the time if he is away.'* A high rating for fear of separation was made for anxiety about separations. With these two anxious attachment characteristics this indicated Enmeshment in her style.

Whilst having two close, supportive relationships meant that Erin was considered potentially secure in terms of support, her dependent need in relationships meant that a 'mildly Enmeshed' rating was made. This provided insight into the high expectations of closeness placed on Daisy who struggled with her own avoidant attachment and anticipation that closeness with others could lead to being rejected, neglected and hurt.

Father Frank's support: Frank relied exclusively on Erin for emotional support. He was able to give examples of confiding in her about his health concerns related to his recent diagnosis of heart problems. They talked it all through in detail: *'down to my tablets, my diet, that sort of thing'* and he had also talked with Erin about his feelings of being let down by his family recently. They discussed issues around Daisy at length. Frank found that Erin gave him support and showed concern when he confided. It was considered a confiding and supportive relationship.

However, when asked about confiding in the two close friends he named as VCOs, whilst he said he *'probably could confide'* he was unable to describe a recent occasion when he had done so and rarely met with his close others on a one-to-one basis. *'I have never had to tell either of them my most personal feelings but I could if I had to. If we had problems with money or the family, maybe I would, but it hasn't really come up. And they know about the difficulties with my health. If I felt the need to confide in either of them I am sure I could.'* Yet he had never discussed his feelings about adopting Daisy. *'I've had no issues to talk about recently but my health issues are no secret. We meet up together as couples, there's never been the need for a one-to-one really.'* So despite naming two close others, there was insufficient confiding in either about emotionally charged topics to rate as high support. With only Erin as an emotionally supportive partner and confidant, Frank was rated as having only 'some' ability to make and maintain relationships and categorised as 'moderately' Insecure.

Frank's moderately Fearful attachment attitudes. Frank's attitudes showed his high mistrust and fearfulness of others: *'I don't trust outsiders. Yeah, I am suspicious of people. And yes, I do question their motives because as I've said I've seen and heard so many things in my life . . . I need to get to know someone really well before I can trust them or even confide in them. I wouldn't trust anybody until I got to know them. People are out for themselves, definitely. That's the way people are . . . I'm always wary of everybody.'* He also expressed fear of rejection: *'Oh yes, I've regretted being open with others. I've confided in others and they've gone and let me down. I need to know that I can trust someone. You become wary and you make that conscious decision that you're not going to confide in that person and trust that person because they are untrustworthy. Yes, I have been badly hurt, rejected and let down by my ex-wife and that possibly has impacted the way I now am with others. I also felt hurt by my family, my brothers and sisters over that.'* With high fear of rejection, Frank was rated as having moderately Fearful attachment style.

Comment: Erin and Frank both expressed a high need for emotional warmth but also heightened sensitivity to rejection and to separation. They also had high expectations of the relationship they would have with Daisy and had felt some disappointment about her apparent self-reliance. Although Daisy was gradually showing her wish for closer attachment, Frank's high mistrust and fear of rejection made him wary and suspicious of her affectionate overtures and Erin quickly felt abandoned if Daisy showed any sign of withdrawal. Daisy's lack of expressed emotional neediness towards her adopters and the cautious pace with which the relationship developed, further contributed to their perception of her self-sufficiency as rejecting and of her occasional shows of affection as being untrustworthy. The tension between the adults' needs and expectation and Daisy's self-protective independence threatened the adoption process.

ASI assessment revealed that Frank and Erin shared an emotionally dependent relationship from which all others, with the exception of Erin's one confidant were excluded. Daisy was also excluded. Erin's high need for love and high fear of separation was met by Frank whose high fear of rejection enforced a sense of completeness with Erin. For him all other emotional support was viewed as untrustworthy and unnecessary. For Daisy, feelings of being excluded and unwanted by her carers reinforced her existing strategy of isolation and emotional detachment. This was at times coupled with an over-compliance to try and win her parents love, the duality reinforcing her carer's lack of trust in her emotional responses and their feelings of not being needed or valued.

Assessment of the carers' attachment style contributed to enhanced understanding by the therapist of how Daisy's self-reliance and withdrawal activated their combined attitudes of mistrust, fear of rejection, high need for others and fear of separation. Information derived from the ASI contributed to the processing of each of the sessions with an added understanding that Erin's own need to be loved by Frank and Frank's exclusive trust in Erin made it difficult for Daisy to see a place for herself within this closed alliance. The therapeutic work revolved particularly around Frank's trust issues which had inhibited his other support-access as well as Erin's over-dependence on him which again made them a unit with little need for anyone outside. They became aware of Daisy's attachment needs, and how these were expressed in ways unfamiliar to them and how they had unknowingly rejected her. Since Erin's style was fundamentally in the Secure range, this helped her to grasp the issue quickly and help Frank to also see the situation more clearly. Subsequent work as well as in making them more sensitive to Daisy's tentative attachment advances, also focused on Frank's ability to relate to others outside of the marriage. The key elements in this case are outlined in Figure 9.3.

9.3 Attachment and child safeguarding services

9.3.1 Fern's anxious and David's Dual/disorganised attachment styles – a child protection issue

A referral to child protection services was made due to evidence of neglect of baby Elsa aged 18 months, in the care of her mother Fern (aged 25) and father David (aged 35) and with an older child Sophie aged six also in their care. The concerns were in relation to probable neglect around unhygienic living conditions, David's anxiety disorder and cannabis use and Fern's mild learning disability and prior post-natal depression. The primary

Both parents' Anxious styles

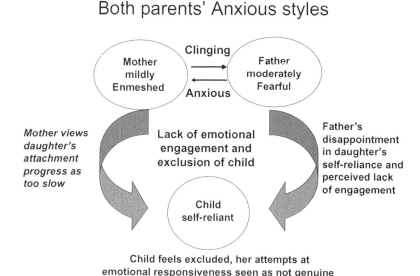

Figure 9.3 Parents' anxious styles

concerns were in relation to neglect of the baby, as well as the emotional impact on both the baby and on Sophie of David's unpredictable behaviour. Fern agreed to a mother and baby foster placement whilst further assessments were undertaken. David remained in the home on his own.

The ASI's undertaken with both mother and father were only part of a larger overall assessment, but provided valuable information that helped with overall decisions on whether the care of the baby should be left to this couple. Both parents had an Insecure attachment style: Fern was moderately Fearful (although also showed some Enmeshment in her relationship with David) whilst David was rated Dual/disorganised – combining markedly Fearful and Enmeshed style with anger. Thus both were potentially poor functioning and high risk as parents, but particular aspects of their attachment style needed to be considered in order to predict how they might function as parents in the next year or two.

Mother Fern's inadequate support: When asked about her relationships, it was evident that Fern confided in no one, although she named David, her mother and sister as close support figures. She was very dependent in her relationship with David, and idealised the relationship: *'I can talk to him. He is there when I need him. He comes to see me, because I don't even want to say it (that they are separated)... it makes me upset that I can't even be with him. I love him loads. He is my best friend really.'* However there was little actual confiding.

When probed about what she could confide, she said: *'I will confide whenever I feel like it . . . but very rarely. It is just when I am upset or need to talk to someone. I have just told him bits and pieces because I didn't want to say too much about my business, I only give the brief detail. Because I know he is very good at giving advice, but he can't take it'.* Their interaction is poor with a lot of arguments: *'Anything can make us both irritable.'* Arguing led to a split nearly two years ago, but they made up again: *'Every time we have fallen out, we are friends again. We have never massively argued. Only one big break-up. We haven't been together since we split up a year and a half ago. Well maybe longer. But I was living with him and we were sleeping together and that was it. It was like being friends but with extras.'* From this account it became evident that Fern was somehow unable to differentiate when she was together with David and when they were apart. So despite currently being separated she still saw them as a couple.

Although in close contact with her mother she did not confide in her: *'Very rarely, but I do when I can. Because I feel really weird talking about things I have done, because I think she is going to be ashamed. I don't know why, because I know I should be talking to her more than I should be talking to David. There are all sorts of things I could talk to my mum about but it isn't very private stuff. Say I was upset, I would just say, "yeah, I'm fine". I just put on a brave face.'* She was also unable to confide or get support from her sister: *'Because she is my sister, I don't think she is supposed to know my problems. It is hard sometimes, I don't know why. I wouldn't talk to her about most of my problems.'* Therefore despite fairly frequent contact with her family, she did not communicate her problems and therefore did not get any meaningful support. She was rated as 'little/none' on ability to relate to others and therefore markedly Insecure.

Fern's markedly Fearful style: Fern reported mistrust, barriers to closeness and fear of being rejected. Much of her mistrust was in relation to services which she felt had let her down. She found it hard to get close to people: *'Yeah, because of my school life. Women are more difficult to get close to because they are all bitches.'* If someone wanted to be her friend, she says: *'I would find it uncomfortable but I would try to be their friend. But it is something I am not used to.'* She couldn't ask for help in general and didn't like to ask her social worker: *'I don't feel comfortable around my social worker. She said she is not against me but I don't believe her at all.'* Fern felt she had been let down by services and this would stop her trusting or getting close to almost anyone. Fern was therefore rated as markedly Fearful in her style.

Father David's inadequate support: David's recent stressors concerned the sudden death of his grandfather who brought him up, money problems, separating from Fern and social services' concerns about the care of their daughter Elsa. David did not confide much in Fern: *'Sometimes I do, yes. I did tell her that I had a fight history in my relationships blah, blah, blah, and she understood all that, so she knew what I was like in that way. And other bits and pieces that* *she had to know, and then there are bits and pieces that I don't tell anybody. Well it's just like a sore subject, like my granddad and that. I've mentioned bits and pieces about how he died and that blah, blah, blah, but I won't go into detail.'* David couldn't report any recent incident of confiding. *'It needs to be the right moment. It is hard yes, but I've always kept myself to myself really. Last year I wasn't paying attention to bits and pieces, and having arguments for no reason, bad moods and things like that.'* He acknowledged that he did argue with Fern a lot, but did not consider it 'serious'.

David named his brother as his VCO: *'I confide in him the most.. Pretty easy, yes, whenever I need to, and about anything. Everything I worry about, blah, blah, blah. Everything. He basically knows me inside out really. The only thing we don't talk about is granddad, everything else we talk about yes.'* However, he does not talk about his relationship with Fern: *'Not so much. People I'm in love with no, I wouldn't no. I don't even talk to myself about such things, I just don't think about. I won't talk about love stuff or things like that really.'* He had not seen or spoken to his brother in the last six months and therefore this was taken as low-level confiding in actuality. He was therefore considered to have no ongoing close support and was rated as 'little/none' on ability to relate to others and therefore markedly Insecure in his attachment style.

David's Dual/disorganised style (markedly Fearful and Enmeshed): David found it hard to get close: *'Yes, to men, or women. No idea why.'* He can't ask others for help: *'No. I don't like it. I tend not to ask for help from family for money, although I know they would help me if they could. You know, unless I'm really on my knees, then I would have no choice, but if I've got £5 for the electricity and I need £4 to top it up, I won't go and ask and borrow a fiver to top it up, I won't do that. Or if I've got no food, I won't go down and ask them for food. I won't do that either, no.'*

He expressed fear of being rejected: *'I've got a couple of friends, I know them really well, but things that they have done to me, not personally or physically, mean they are just not trustworthy.'* He has been let down and this has made him wary of getting close. *'Yes ... I just get nervous. Like a relationship never lasts over four years, it's never gone that far I don't think. It just seems to get to the point like between the third and fourth year, and I just shut down, I have to end it. There's no reason for it. I can be fine during the relationship, it can be rocky but it just gets to the period where I shut down.'*

David's report of self-reliance was contradictory: About coping he said: *'Yes and no. I can cope with certain things but when it comes to travelling, I don't like it. Large crowds and things like that, I don't like feeling like I'm being backed into a corner.'* Neither can he make decisions easily. About feeling in control he said: *'I like to know what I'm doing, you know. I can look after myself. Even if I was in a relationship, I would always do what I had to do first.'* David became anxious when people close were away. *'I'm anxious in general ... I do get worried. If Fern is travelling back to where she's got to go, that will bother me until she texts me saying 'I'm alright' because you know she has Sophie with her as well. There is always that sort of general worry, like "oh my*

God she's had a crash". He found it difficult to say goodbye and would worry if Fern was back late: *'Depending on how late she was. If she was like three hours late I would get a bit worried you know, what's happening? I'm getting more and more worried.'*

When asked about anger and whether he had arguments he said: *'Sometimes, with anybody really. It depends on the subject. It could be anything that would start it, like if someone was picking on someone. I'd like to have a go (and answer back). It's not like a full-blown argument. I don't know how to explain it but it's not so much heated. It's a friendly geared discussion you know like there's no "I'm going to batter you", nothing like that, it's just verbal. It just like sarcasm yah, yahs, but heated you know.'* However, he had been observed by neighbours shouting at his daughter. When asked about it, he said: *'Yes, but not up at her face and grr, grr grr... you know. But we could be sitting right here, and Sophie would be in the corner and I would be saying "shut up" and things like that.'* It was an incident of extreme verbal abuse to both his daughter and Fern that led to the foster placement. Fern attested to their frequent arguments, and David acknowledged a history of domestic violence. He had also been aggressive to social workers who were dealing with Elsa's safeguarding.

Comment: Given that the couple had already separated as a result of social work intervention, the decision had to be made whether Fern could continue to look after Elsa and Sophie alone, and whether Elsa could be protected from David's potential dangerous impact. In considering what is required of good parenting, for example in terms of a close harmonious relationship, other support from outside to help with stress management and coping, ability to seek help with realistic awareness of who would provide reliable support, reasonable levels of autonomy and control over anger or fear – it can be seen that none of those apply. Whereas it was felt that Fern, with support, might be able to provide better parenting, David's presence was seen as dangerous. David had little insight in to his inability to relate – he was both anxious and aggressive towards others. He had no insight into his own anger, which he downplayed. When faced with the possibility of his children being taken away he coped by getting angry and violent. So a critical factor became Fern's inability to separate from David and her high emotional reliance on him. Although living apart because of the issue of David's danger to the children, in her mind they were still together and she would allow him whatever contact he wanted. An in-depth assessment contributed to the decision that David was ruled out as able to parent Elsa on his own. Fern proved unable to progress in the foster placement and was not willing to engage in any form of therapeutic input. The care plan was therefore for adoption of Elsa and Sophie. See Figure 9.4 for Summary.

Parents mixed styles — anticipating child risk

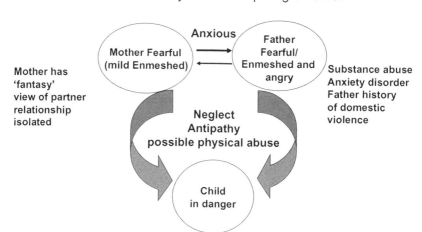

Figure 9.4 Parents' Insecure style and likelihood of future risk to child

9.3.2 Confirming custody arrangements – Father's markedly Withdrawn style

Warren is aged 53 and has four children living with him, the older two are mid- to late-teens (aged 18, 16) the younger ones six and nine. His ex-partner Astrid had mental health problems and was physically abusive to the youngest (six-year-old daughter). Problems with the children included nine-year-old son Craig who had been treated for attention deficit hyper-activity disorder (ADHD) and possible emotional disorder and Matt aged 16 who truanted from school.

ASI assessment of the mother indicated that she had a markedly Angry-dismissive style, with very poor parenting competence, and was highly hostile and physically abusive to the children. There was no recommenda-tion for her to look after the children, despite attending psychotherapy and parenting classes. The question was whether the father could continue to look after the younger two children, as well as the older teenagers, given his very Avoidant (Withdrawn) attachment style and some practical difficulties with parenting.

Father Warren's support: Warren had no support whatsoever and was very isolated. Whilst in the relationship with Astrid, who was very controlling, he did not make any friends and his family all lived at some distance. Since separating from his wife he had not made any new friends, although he had some friendly interactions with other parents at school.

Warren's markedly Withdrawn style: Warren had high self-reliance, and low need for adult company. He did not miss having others around, although he would miss the children if they were not there. He was not mistrustful, although he regretted the difficult time with his ex-wife and her treatment of the children. However, he was not bitter or angry towards her. Neither was he anxious or fearful about having been let down by her. He presented as very contained and self-sufficient with regard to his adult relationships. He did, however, describe great closeness to the children: '*The children are my life – if I lost my kids I'd have nothing left. We are all as one. I'm all they have.*'

Warren's parenting capacity: When asked about parenting using the PRI, Warren described spending all his time with the children, with whom he had good interaction: '*I am with the children 24/7. We do activities together like going to the beach or fishing. We cuddle up together and Matt reads to them, or they play on Wii or laptop. We always have a good time. When Craig and Matt go on the computer they have a smile on their faces. The kids will play football together or go scrumping for apples.*' He and the children go shopping together. '*When we are together it is like an explosion – everyone talking and wanting things. We talk and share things*'. There was little negativity, arguments were usually over the children using the PlayStation and he had to step in to handle bickering between children. He said, '*I'm patient, never raise a hand to them. They have never been slapped by me.*'

Warren felt he looked after them well: '*I would do anything for them. They are good kids, polite, don't swear.*' He gave them time and affection. He knew when to expect them in and didn't let younger ones off the estate. The older ones would ring him if due back late. He considered himself as good as other parents. '*I can keep them in check.*' In terms of care, the older teenage children helped him with cooking but there was not much variation in their diet. Warren would always ring the school if one of the younger children was sick , and took them to the doctor when needed. He let them socialise and Craig had friends over to stay. The social worker assessed there was moderate competence in parenting, summarising in the report that he: '*looks after the children single-handedly and, has high commitment to their welfare*'.

Warren was aware of some negative aspects of his parenting: '*I don't send them to bed when I should. I do worry that I can't read to the children and I feel overwhelmed at times about school issues and don't always visit the school.*' The social worker judged there was a level of incompetence, however, this was attributable in part to poor environmental conditions and partly to his inexperience. For example, whilst the children were well fed, their diet was unvaried; if the children truanted Warren would not take any action. He had not sought help for his son's ADHD. There were also too few opportunities for stimulation of the children and, as a family, they didn't spend enough time with friends or other adults. Also, hygiene in their living conditions was inadequate. Therefore, Warren's overall parenting was considered to be mixed with signs of both competence and incompetence.

Outcome: A decision was made for Warren to keep the children but with a high level of social work and other support. Thus although his attachment style was highly Insecure, Withdrawn style was not considered a threat to the children in terms of hostility or helplessness, and there was no anger to indicate abusive behaviour and no fear to indicate helpless parenting. His isolation was the main vulnerability factor and services arranged for the children to be more socially involved and further efforts were made to integrate Warren into the local community. His interaction with the social workers was good and he was prepared to improve his parenting where required. His affection for his children was genuine and they were clearly closely attached to him. So this example shows how the ASI and the PRI can be used to help support parents in continuing to care for their children. In the next section, children looked after in residential care will be examined in relation to attachment issues. See Figure 9.5 for summary.

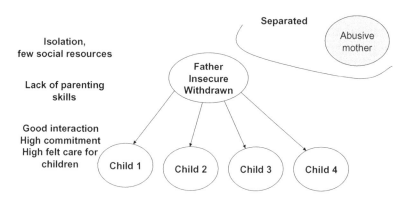

Figure 9.5 Father Withdrawn – parenting behaviour

9.4 Attachment and residential care

The policy preference in the UK is for children separated from their parents for child protection issues to be placed in foster care (sometimes with family or friends) or adopted. There are nevertheless young people in residential care, due to breakdown of other types of placement. This constitutes around 12% of the 60,900 children and young people Looked After in England in 2009 (Department for Children, Schools and Families

(DCSF) 2009). We know that children looked after by the State in any arrangement have poor outcomes, compared with the normal population of intact families, with half of these children having emotional and behavioural problems at clinical levels. However, the highest rates for poor outcome are for those in residential care which, at least in part, reflects their higher levels of dysfunction prior to being placed there (Ford, Vostanis *et al.* 2007). Longitudinal studies have found that, as adults, these individuals are more likely to become involved in criminal activity (Farrington 1990), to be referred to forensic psychiatric services (DCSF 2007) and high-security hospitals (Scott 2004). They have worse educational outcomes (National Care Advisory Service (NCAS) 2008), are more likely to be homeless and to become teenage parents (DfES and DoH 2004). Those placed in residential care in the UK are usually adolescents with complex needs who have often exhausted or disrupted other types of arrangements, with residential care increasingly seen as a last resort, so residential care is not the primary cause of the problem (Colton and Hellinckx 1994). With the Every Child Matters initiative (DfES 2004), there was a need to consider how residential care can become an appropriate and positive placement option for young people with difficult early-life experiences, for whom foster arrangements have failed and who usually present with complex mental health needs. An attachment approach can give added insight into these young people's difficulties in forming relationships and thus help create the required stable and caring residential environments required to develop resilience.

In line with attachment principles, in recent years there has been a move towards smaller residential care homes (Colton and Hellinckx 1994). The smaller units seem to better imitate the dynamics of a 'family' and shed the negative 'institutional' connotations of larger homes (Cameron and Maginn 2008). An emphasis is placed on attachment-related aspects such as security through stability of arrangement and bonding with the carers who in turn develop greater attunement in their care (Howe, Brandon *et al.* 1999). Therapeutic interventions in residential care have been shown to be effective (Dozier 2003; Zegers, Scheuengel *et al.* 2006). Attachment approaches are increasingly used to supplant the unstable family models experienced and build resilience (Moore, Moretti *et al.* 1997; Hawkins-Rodgers 2007). Interventions in residential care have included the therapeutic community approach, where planned therapeutic help as well as education is provided on site in the home (Stevens and Furnivall 2008). These involve a number of different theoretical approaches including CBT (Stevens 2004) but few are identified as attachment orientated.

There are a handful of studies of attachment style in young people in residential care in the UK and continental Europe. Many of these studies use the AAI to assess attachment style with nearly all young people in both German (Schleiffer and Muller, 2004) and Dutch (Zegers *et al.*, 2006) residential care homes were found to be Insecure (94%). There was some gender differentiation with more girls showing Anxious/Preoccupied styles and more boys Avoidant/Dismissive. As many as 46% exhibited complex (multiple) attachment styles or were scored as 'Cannot Classify' and therefore in terms of the classifcations in this book were rated Disorganised. Both genders showed antisocial or aggressive behaviours with girls also having emotional disorder. Similar results have been found in the UK (Wallis and Steele 2001) with 92% Insecure with the majority (62%) 'Unresolved/Cannot Classify' and 23% Avoidant/Dismissing. The findings thus indicate that Insecure attachment style is rife in residential care settings with varieties of Disorganised, and Avoidant/dismissive styles the most common category. We wanted to test the adolescent ASI in such settings to see if the same rates of Insecure style were found using a support-based approach. We also planned to use the ASI to inform practitioners working with the young people about their profiles to aid with more tailored interventions based on these assessments. In the process of doing so we found a need to provide workshops and training for residential care workers around attachment principles and categories to help them in their work of understanding the young people in their care.

9.4.1 The Attachment Style Interview in residential care

The ASI is being used in residential care practice by St Christopher's Fellowship (SCF) in relation to a structured, social learning and attachment-based intervention with adolescents. The manualised intervention is influenced by the Oregon model, but reapplied to residential care settings, where the residential care worker and not the parent provides the daily care record ratings. It also includes attachment principles based on providing a secure base through stability of placement, small homes and developing positive relationships with care workers. The scheme was developed in-house based on social learning models of behaviour modification using praise and reward through points systems for pro-social behaviour and sanctions (point deduction) for antisocial behaviour to encourage socialisation in the young people. In attachment terms, deficits in the young person's social support and close relationships and their barriers to trust and closeness are modified through the relationship with the care workers, with efforts around monitored home contact and development of positive peer relationships. The adolescent ASI is used to provide an enhanced assessment of the young people on entry to the programme to help work out the areas of need for the social learning intervention. At first the ASI university partners undertook the assessments, but subsequent trainings and workshops have been run for the care staff with ASI assessment training for selected staff across a range of homes. The programme has been disseminated to relevant agencies locally and nationally.

The first 28 young people assessed using the ASI are reported on here, most were boys (78%) with the mean age of 14 (range 11 to 17). In terms of relationships, a fifth of the young people had no contact at all with their mother and over a third had no contact with their father. For those with contact, when asked about the quality of contact with mothers a third reported no closeness and nearly half reported high antipathy to mother. For fathers, half reported no closeness and 43% high antipathy to father. When more general support was examined, only a quarter were able to name any Very Close relationship. For six respondents this included friends, one named a mother and one named a professional. However, only one of these was objectively assessed as supportive. On the basis of the absence of close support, most of the young people (71%) were rated as having 'little/no' ability to make and maintain relationships and therefore markedly Insecure with 29% rated as having 'some' ability to relate and therefore moderately Insecure. None were rated as having good relating ability required for a Secure or mildly Insecure rating.

The most commonly rated style was Dual/disorganised style (46%) usually combining Angry-dismissive and Fearful styles, but with one Enmeshed and Angry-dismissive style combination. There were also three young people with combined Anxious styles (Fearful and Enmeshed). When single Insecure styles were examined, most young people were shown to have Angry-dismissive (32%) with only two markedly Withdrawn. Four young people had Fearful styles (14%), with none having a solely Enmeshed style. These rates are similar to those reported in other residential care samples (Zegers *et al.* 2006). In community samples, only 9% are rated as Dual/disorganised, and only 39% Insecure among teenagers in UK schools using the ASI (see Figure 9.5) (Oskis, Loveday *et al.* 2011).

This serves to underline the high levels of vulnerability of the young people since none of them had close support from parents, other family members or friends, and all had difficulties in relating to others, particularly around mistrust, anger and fear of rejection. It also provides a guide for the carer in understanding the young person's behaviour in light of how they themselves report on it. For example, often a parallel presentation of Fearful style in young people who were predominantly Angry-dismissive had not been noticed by care staff at times, but explained the inconsistency and unpredictability in relating.

To date only a small number of follow-up interviews have been undertaken prior to the young person leaving care in this intervention. This proved a difficult task because it is common for placements to disrupt with little warning, for a variety of reasons which can be triggered by the young person or by services. This means that setting up the necessary assessment at a standard length of time after initial assessment, prior to leaving is difficult. However, of six completed to date, all have showed some positive albeit not radical change. Thus there was movement from 'marked' to 'moderate' levels of insecurity and from dual to single styles. There was increased ability to relate through improved confiding, leading to greater attachment to carers and encouragement to make new friends. There were

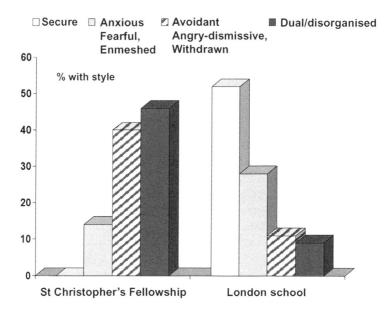

Oskis *et al.* 2011

Figure 9.6 ASI attachment styles in residential care and comparison school
teenagers

reductions in negative attitudes such as mistrust and reductions in anger
due to anger-management elements in the intervention. This is illustrated
in the case of Darren, described below.

9.4.2 Darren in residential care, his Dual/disorganised style

Background: Darren was 14 when he arrived at the residential care home.
He had been removed from his family by social services one year earlier
because of experiences of antipathy, neglect and physical and psychological abuse by members of his family. His mother had died after a long illness
when he was 10, the point at which the neglect and abuse started. Darren
had three prior placements during that year (two foster care arrangements
and one prior residential home). These broke down in part as a result of
his problem behaviour, characterised by impulsivity and aggression. Darren
was diagnosed with hyperkinetic disorder at age 13. At the time of interview, he was excluded from school due to aggressive behaviour, and was
considered to be behind his peers educationally. Darren presented as a
very talkative, excitable and likable young man who engaged well with the
ASI interview although he got distracted on occasion. At times he became

agitated and turned his back on the interviewer but answered all questions quite fully.

Support and family relationships: Darren was asked about his current relationship to his family. He was not close to his father, and he reported high antipathy towards him: *'I am not close to my father, I never see him. I used to have maximum respect for him. I don't now though. He took the piss out of me; I hate him and my brother for that.'* He was angry with his brother and had no contact with his siblings or stepsiblings, apart from one sister to whom he felt close and saw regularly: *'I am close to my sister who lives with my Nan. I get on ok with my sister. I am an ok brother to my sister but not to my brother. I would get angry with my dad and brother the way they treated me.'* When asked about sources of support, Darren reported that he was close to his Nan and sister but that these weren't confiding relationships. *'I don't confide in anyone. I can tell my Nan some things not everything though. I don't really talk to my Nan that much. I don't tell people things because they are private.'* He was therefore rated as having 'little/no' ability to make and maintain relationships and therefore markedly Insecure style.

Darren's markedly Angry-dismissive and Fearful Attachment attitudes: When Darren was questioned about his attachment attitudes he was found to display both Angry-dismissive and Fearful attitudes. He reported high mistrust and constraints on closeness: *'Yes, I find it hard to trust people. I think mostly people are out for themselves. I think people are against me in every way. I sometimes question people's motives. It's just the way I think. I sometimes trust people I know; I don't trust people I don't know, it depends on their attitudes. People have let me down, my dad my brothers and my friends. I want people to know how much my dad let me down.'* He also demonstrated high constraints on forming close relationships: for example even when talking about his sister and Nan he said: *'I wouldn't say I'm that close to them, I'm not close to anyone. I don't love anyone. I don't confide in anyone. I don't really care about having anyone to confide in. I would maybe like one person but I don't really care'.* When asked whether he found it easy to ask people for help, he said he couldn't. When asked whether he could go to others for advice if he had a problem, he responded: *'Yes I could ask somebody here for help.'*

Darren had extensive anger in relationships: *'I argue a lot with people. I would get angry at school. I would fight with people at school about normal stuff but we would make up. I sometimes argue with my Nan over police and stuff and living with her. I would get angry with my dad and brother the way they treated me. I would shout and swear.'* Darren had to be moved to the current residential home from a previous residential placement due to his constant fights and assaults on other young people and staff. He was excluded from school because of his disruptive and aggressive behaviour. Darren was still angry towards his father and brother. These attitudes are all associated with Angry-dismissiveness which was taken to be Darren's primary style of relating.

However, Darren also reported some fearful attitudes towards others. For example he was able to report clearly on his fear of rejection: *'I have been let down in the past. By my dad, my brother and my friends'.* When asked if he felt that he couldn't trust others in case they let him down he said *'Yes'.* When asked whether that was based on his experience, he said *'Yes. I sometimes back off. I just recently I've found myself backing off. I am not close to anyone. I don't mind somebody telling me things. I don't have feelings.'* Darren was able to articulate his high need for company. Whilst he had no friends and had no one with a high degree of contact, he said that it was important to him to have a lot of people around. Being alone bothered him. *'I like having people around me all the time, I get lonely. I get lonely on my own.'* As a common feature of Dual/disorganised style, Darren had contradictory statements on his self-reliance: on the one hand he indicated dependency – he stated that he didn't cope well with his problems on his own and needed a lot of reassurance, he reported that it wasn't important to be independent. *'I cope better with other people's help. I can make decisions on my own but I need others help.'* On the other hand, he had a high need for autonomy: *'Yes it is important to feel that I have control over my life. If things don't go the way I want them I get angry. I need to have some control.'* These characteristics also border on Enmeshed style, and it was considered that Darren may have a triple style with both Anxious elements of Fearful and Enmeshed.

Follow-up interview: At follow-up nine months later Darren showed improvement. Whilst still rated as Dual/disorganised style, he was rated as 'moderately' rather than 'markedly' Insecure. His relating style improved and he was beginning to be able to confide and relate to the care staff: *'Yes…I can talk to most of them, there are one or two persons that I can tell lots of stuff to. This is better here than other places I've been to. You can express your feelings, that is the best thing about here. The bad things about leaving here are the relationships that you've got, people you trust, the contact. Basically the people that you like most, the good times you have. I have talked to them while I've been here, or they would come to me, ask how I was feeling.'* His anger had reduced – it became less explosive: *'I would say I can still be an angry person…It is just me…but I don't know actually. I think I nag people now more than lose my temper.'* The staff observed him becoming calmer.

He became focused on school work and wanted to improve his education. He learned to swim and play tennis. Importantly he was persuaded to take his medication for his ADHD which also had a calming effect. Previously he had been too mistrustful to take it, considering it would do him harm. Figure 9.7 illustrates the reduction in the attachment subscales which relate to the overall style.

This example shows evidence of incremental change in this young person, but by no means does this lead to a Secure outcome over the nine months of the intervention. It was unlikely that a boy like Darren, with Dual/disorganised attachment, and no intensive psychological treatment

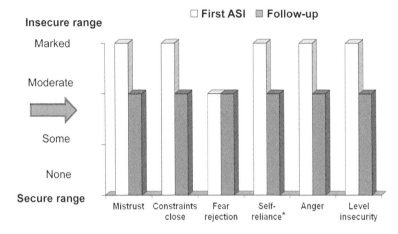

Figure 9.7 Darren's change in ASI scores

would become Secure in this time scale. The ASI shows a direction of change, and one which with a longer time period may have produced more dramatic results. However, a key finding from this pilot project was that the staff involved became far more attuned to attachment issues, welcomed additional training around attachment and found the intensive assessments helped them to understand the young people's behaviour better.

Summary

- The chapter outlines the need for accurate assessment of individual attachment styles in parents and carers responsible for children with high levels of need. Cases were provided to look at patterning of styles and parenting.
- A case was provided of an adoption placement where the carers with Anxious individual attachment styles had an inability to see the attachment cues provided by their child placed, which they experienced as rejecting.
- A case was also provided from child Safeguarding services to show how the parental relationship provided dangers for the children in the care of a Fearful mother who had an idealised relationship with the Dual/disorganised father. Another showed that a Withdrawn father while having some difficulties looking after his children after his abusive wife left, was learning to interact well and gradually provide better care.

- Attachment-related characteristics of intervention in residential care included the need for stable arrangements, for smaller care homes, and for staff to be trained in recognising attachment issues when forming relationships with the children in their care. It also included careful monitoring of contact with the abusive parents.
- Very high rates of Insecure style were found in children in residential care, in particular a high level of Dual/disorganised style typically involving Angry-dismissive and Fearful elements. This reflects early life trauma but also very problematic relating styles. The ASI was able to document modest change over time.
- Using the adolescent ASI has proved a useful tool for identifying both the characteristics of the young person on entry to the care home, as well as for charting change over time. It is now being piloted as an assessment undertaken by the care workers themselves in-house.

9.5 Discussion

At the outset of this chapter we emphasised the need for interview tools able to assess emotional openness in accessing support and stressed the need for more widespread use of an Attachment framework approach to achieve better understanding of the short- and longer-term developmental impact of parental style, behaviour and discordant environments on the child. The strength of such an assessment is that environmental and psychological risks for corrosive parenting contexts and developmental deviation in offspring are identified simultaneously. Holistic assessment of attachment style and its real behavioural consequences also highlights interpersonal contexts and specific parent–child interactions linked to anxiety and withdrawal disorders or to aggressive acting out behaviours and conduct disorders.

The ASI can aid in identifying risk and protective factors in adults who care for children entrusted to them through foster or adoptive arrangements. The case material demonstrates the elements of socially based Insecure styles relevant for specific interpretations and interventions to improve parenting and to prevent further familial abuse. In this way assessment is primed for early detection of risk and can fulfil the aims of both prevention and intervention in identifying safeguarding needs while also throwing into relief the specific psychological barriers to support and attachment formation in families. Adopted and fostered children who have had difficult and painful histories with birth parents and who have experienced abuse and neglect within caregiving relationships are at risk of developing severe emotional and behavioural difficulties as well as psychiatric disorder. These children require parenting that can not only help them rewrite their negative relationship templates but can also help reduce their risks for the development of disorder as adults. Parents who care for such children are required to respond to the angry aggressive, emotionally withdrawn or disordered strategies that the child brings without being encumbered by their own attachment anxiety, angry or detached avoidance. Children who have experienced painful histories tend to gravitate to the more secure parent in the family. This is likely to heighten attachment-related vulnerability in the less secure parent and challenge the parent's own fearful, hostile, withdrawn or dependent attachment style. As parents and carers embark on parenting children with challenging attachment behaviours, intense support is required to cope with crises and diffuse situations. More directly, poor parental functioning and disorder can be averted if the parental attachment vulnerabilities are identified and made available for supportive intervention.

In the arena of family support services accurate assessment of environmental risks, in terms of support networks, quality of relationships and support-seeking capacity, are critical for anticipating the likely requirements of those families for whom these aspects look fragile. Through early identification, potential risks to the optimal development of children can be mitigated by the provision of services such as direct social work, support groups or befriending each of which can be pivotal in preventing further family management difficulties and reduce risks for poor child outcomes. Profiling individual attachment characteristics that denote psychological risk in birth families and vulnerability in carers and adoptive parents, can focus direct work with both behavioural and attitudinal variables of each distinctive Attachment Style. This can also inform support needs and choice of treatment to address the psychological factors that contribute to psychosocial vulnerability, depression and psychopathology in adults. Also to identify the poor social and interpersonal contexts that are linked to anxious inhibited (internalising) and antisocial aggressive acting out (externalising) symptoms in children and young persons.

Thus the particular value of ASI assessment in child protection, intervention and adoption and fostering services is the ability to identify parental risk in the lack of support as well as in the intensity of parental negative attitudes. Conversely, strengths can be identified in the presence of supportive networks and mildness of style that may indicate resilience and an ability to overcome, and help children and young people overcome the experience of adversity.

The next chapter will look more closely at attachment dynamics in families presenting for therapy.

Note

1 Unlike the parents'/carers' names, those selected for children are random and do not reflect their attachment style.

10 Attachment style and family dynamics

10.0 Introduction

This chapter will look more closely at the family dynamics present in families who have approached services where the ASI has been used as an assessment tool with the parents/carers. The focus is on capturing the patterning of attachment style of the parents and its impact on the child and family functioning. The efficacy of any treatment will not be examined in detail.

Attachment theory and research provide a framework for understanding the way in which child, adolescent and adult disorders may reflect aspects of family functioning, relational failures and the process by which symptoms might have developed. The relational impact on the child's developmental organisation is revealed in the child's internalising (minimising-avoidance), externalising (amplifying anxious-ambivalence) or lack of such organisation as seen in the child's non-strategic freeze or disorientation. This indicates the way in which the child–parent relationship, whether due to lack of care or abuse, has contributed to the child's strategy to regulate emotions, maintain self-awareness, and feel in control within dyadic relationships. Insight into the child's disturbed attachment dynamic, further emphasises the need for enhanced assessment of the emotional climate in which these daily transactions take place and their link to difficulties with neurological and self-regulatory processes that lead to internalising (fearful, sad) or externalising (aggressive, disruptive, delinquency) or disordered (mixed) psychological difficulties.

One of the early tenets of Bowlby's theory was the influence of the experience of early rejection on later interpersonal functioning. The impact of parenting quality, whether characterised by hostility and anger, fearfulness or excessive dependency and helplessness is, regardless of intentionality, likely to be experienced by the child as different types of rejection. Each of these parenting characteristics forms the basis for the formation of generalised expectations that others will be punitive, rejecting, unreliable or neglectful of emotional and relational need. This becomes the basis for the development of behaviours inclined either towards attachment Avoidance and social withdrawal or attachment Anxiety and social preoccupation.

Negative care experiences impact the child's attachment security and development of strategies for coping with relational stress. Most significant among the consequences of poor adaptive coping mechanisms to regulate the intensity of affects experienced with a stress-inducing or traumatising caregiver is the impaired capacity for neurological, behavioural and emotional self-regulation (Shore 1994). Such poor capacity for regulating the intensity and duration of stress while experiencing poor care characterised by high anger or high fear states impacts healthy development and increases the risk for disorder.

Below we conceptualise aspects of parenting style, the child or adolescents attachment responses and the likely developmental impact (see Table 10.1).

Table 10.1 Speculative summary of parenting, child attachment and developmental impact

Parenting Style	Child or adolescent's characteristics	Developmental impact Potential disorder
Unreliable Unpredictable, Intrusive Critical/antipathy Intermittent rejection or separation	**Anxious ambivalence:** Enmeshed, Anticipation of unpredictable parental availability, worry about abandonment	**Behaviour:** Dependent/ clinging, ambivalence, disruptive behaviour **Disorder:** Separation Anxiety Disorder, school phobia, depression
Controlling Domineering Dismissive Rejecting Physical abuse Psychological abuse	**Angry Avoidance:** Angry-dismissive Difficulty in acknowledging and expressing feelings	**Behaviour:** Withdrawal with anger, mistrust **Disorder:** Conduct Disorder; Oppositional Defiant Disorder, deliberate self-harm
Helpless Neglect Role reversal	**Anxious Avoidance:** Fearful withdrawal and anxiety in relation to expectation of parent's incompetence and concern about harm to parent	**Behaviour:** Inhibition, isolation, fearfulness **Disorder:** Anxiety, panic attacks, social phobia, deliberate self-harm
Dangerous Domestic violence Multiple neglect and abuse in combinations	**Disorganised:** disorientated, or indiscriminate behaviour due to fear of parent alternating with anger. Dissociated anger	**Behaviour:** Alternating angry and fearful, contradictory need for independence and reliance **Disorder:** PTSD, substance abuse, personality disorder, self-harm, dissociation

PTSD = post-traumatic stress disorder.

10.1 Assessments in therapy

Assessment of parental attachment style can contribute important understanding of the attitudes guiding the parent's behaviour, with partner, close others and offspring, as well as providing a profile of relational characteristics that can predict how the child's behaviour, organised in response to parental caregiving, is likely to be perceived and responded to. Many of the available tools for assessment, while raising awareness of specific risk factors that may contribute to medium and high risk of disorder in the children or young people, have very brief questionnaire formats, and do not allow for assessment that more closely investigates the characteristics of the parent–child and family relationship. More specifically, attachment patterns that both adult and child have developed in response to their respective caregiving and more recent relational experiences are not investigated.

As described in Chapter 8, there is an overall absence of scales which can assess the child's interpersonal context and relating and Insecure attachment style. This includes the parent/carer–child relationship or the specific characteristics of the child's and parent's attachment style. This could provide crucial measurement of the way in which the child or young person's behaviour may reflect developmentally salient functions in terms of emotional, or even physical, self-protection. Thus no assessment is made of the emotional climate in which the child or adolescent negotiates daily interpersonal interactions. Furthermore, assessment of stress factors or attitudinal factors and characteristics that underpin difficulties in relating to family or within other social contexts can provide key information in relation to risks for disorder but are not routinely covered.

Parents engaged in therapeutic work, whether participating in individual or dyadic intervention, are by and large themselves victims of interpersonal trauma in which experience of rejection and emotional neglect will have predisposed them to a basic mistrust of others. This is likely to include the perception of others as unavailable, with anger as a ready response to the expectation of others as unaccepting and unsupportive leading to hostile and dismissive parenting style, social withdrawal and high conflict in the few relationships maintained. For such a parent, the child's cues are also likely to be perceived as threats, may cause high arousal and thus perpetuate the cycle of hostility, rejection, feelings of anger and aggression. Parents with high Fearfulness readily perceive rejection and rebuff and are likely to over-react to messages of negativity or ambiguity. Their sensitivity to the expectation of rejection involves avoidance of social relationships to avoid further hurt, even if they crave more intense engagement. For such parents the child's developing assertiveness and negativity is likely to be interpreted as being intended to wound, exclude and reject, and thus may cause withdrawal and an abdication of parental authority.

The parent whose style is characterised by an Anxious preoccupation with the availability of relationships and fears separation and loss, is suspicious of other's commitment, easily feels abandoned and does not believe their needs can be met. For this parent, the child's developing autonomy is a threat of abandonment and cues of need from others will be interpreted as betrayal in demanding attention that should be exclusively focused on the parent. Here also, as in the Angry-dismissive style, anger and aggressive feelings in relation to the child's perceived messages of threat and rejection are aroused and responded to with anger and hostility.

Case illustrations in this chapter highlight the benefits of using attachment style constructs to prevent the perpetuating of relationships that are experienced as rejecting and abusive or neglectful of need, and also identify the origins and treatment needs of the child's pattern of emotional expression or behaviour. In this way identification of the parental and child mechanisms can be directly targeted to improve parent–child relationships with healthier outcomes for all family members and breaking cycles of intergenerational risks for Insecure attachment.

10.1.1 Attachment-style assessment

Holistic assessments, as provided with the ASI, can serve to inform the level of support needed to prevent harm to the child and accelerate processes towards child protection services. They can also contribute key data to inform and support relationship-based treatments focused on the specific attachment tensions that both parent and child bring to the therapeutic process. Case study material is used here to illustrate the usefulness of working directly with the attitudinal and behavioural variables of each distinctive attachment style. The aim is to prevent further abuse and neglect, and treat the constructs contributing to psychosocial vulnerability to depression in adults and both anxious inhibited (internalising) and anti-social aggressive acting out (externalising) symptoms in children and young persons. With this approach ASI assessment sets in context the way in which attachment style can indicate risk of perpetuating abusive relationships and simultaneously identify the origins and treatment of the child's maladaptive patterns of behaviour. Elaboration of the ways in which Attachment Style assessment can inform service provision so that clinical work can be tailored to the need of specific attachment failures and their ensuing behavioural and emotional symptoms is offered. As discussed in Chapter 9 several authors note that adoptive and foster parents frequently express high need for support and that these needs are likely to be unrecognised and unmet in generic mental health services. Foster and adoptive parents, and those vulnerable to depression, feel inadequate or rejected when their children do not turn to them for comfort when distressed (Thoburn, Norford *et al.* 2000; Leiberman 2003; O'Connor and Zeanah 2003a).

This chapter will focus on Filial Therapy. This is a play-based approach to working with children and families in family therapy, and is a way of approaching the treatment of child and adolescent emotional and behavioural difficulties through the prism of family context and attachment categorisation. The ASI used as a pre-clinical measure before engaging the family can be used to assess the parents and the dyadic factors that contribute to the child's internalising or externalising symptoms associated with poor family and individual functioning. The case material below describes assessment and therapeutic work undertaken in response to referrals to psychological services indicating difficulties in the child's emotional state and behaviour suggestive of Insecure attachment. Assessment with the ASI highlighted risks for parental vulnerability and poor parenting. In some cases ASI assessment indicated that the referral was not appropriate as the parent's own fragility meant that they lacked the required security to be therapeutically supportive of change. When deemed sufficiently robust, the resilient characteristics of the primary carer's were used therapeutically to make significant changes in the relationships between parent and child and thus facilitate change in the child's behaviour. Identifying information about the cases are disguised to protect the privacy of the children and families.

10.1.2 The Filial Therapy approach

The Filial therapeutic approach described is used to facilitate change for families and children referred for behavioural, social or emotional difficulties, by helping address the relational conflicts that contribute to difficulties within the parent–child relationship. Such difficulties can further challenge the parent's attachment style and leave them feeling inadequate and out of control. Such difficulties may also amplify the risks of their parenting style. By providing parents with insight and understanding of their own relational style and the fear, anger or blunted emotions that underpin this, enables the parent to address the experiences which are likely to have contributed to the child's poor functioning within the context of the 'therapeutic' family. In elucidating the parent's attachment style before therapy they are helped to acquire self-awareness of their attachment style and the risks associated with their inability to get support, their propensity to problems with interactions, trusting or relying on others, marital or partner difficulties and barriers to responding to their children. With such enhanced awareness they are freed to learn the skills that enable them to grow in understanding and acceptance of the child, as well as to sensitively and empathically respond to the child's communications. This also facilitates the creation of a transparently communicated understanding of how the child's fears, anxieties and anger may be related to earlier experience which can then be explored and expressed within a new special parent–child alliance.

Feedback is given to parents or carers following assessment necessarily avoids a technical emphasis on categorisation. The strengths-based principles of the Filial approach in which feedback is at least three-quarters positive on skills development enables the parent to assimilate information about the quarter that can be improved. Attachment style characteristics, in terms of both strengths and vulnerabilities, need to be communicated in such a way that they do not interfere with the relationship formation between therapist and parent nor challenge the developing trust in the therapist. However, the aim of sensitive feedback is to enhance the therapeutic alliance by helping family members develop awareness of their relational weaknesses through transparently shared understanding and acceptance of vulnerabilities that can be made digestible when understood in the context of earlier care experiences and subsequent life events.

Thus as therapist and parent embark on a genuine and honest approach to reduce or eliminate the problems which brought the family to therapy, labelling is avoided in favour of highlighting strengths followed by a focus on what impedes more secure functioning. Such a focus is both in terms of behaviour as well as in the exaggerated negative attitudes that lead to anger, emotional withdrawal or high dependency needs that may contribute to how they perceive and react to their children.

10.1.3 Identifying parental Insecure attachment style

In identifying the parent as being highly Insecure in terms of the ASI, the inherent inability to access effective support, difficulties with interactions and problems in trusting or relying on others will be openly noted from the outset. In relation to the specific core characteristics of each style, strengths such as perceptiveness, thoughtfulness and commitment which can accompany Fearful attachment style are acknowledged along with risks for isolation feelings of unworthiness and sensitivity to slights. Strengths for those who are Angry-dismissive are identified as assertiveness, strong advocacy and motivation with the negatives including angry and critical interactions, lack of empathy and risk of hierarchical, punitive and controlling relationships. The strengths of Enmeshed styles are perceived as warmth, inclusiveness and sociability, with the negative aspects involving diffuse boundaries, over-dependency and intrusiveness likely to be experienced by the child suffocating and controlling. For the Withdrawn style, strengths are acknowledged in unflappability, consistency and self-sufficiency while the negatives of isolation and emotional coolness may prevent closer emotional engagement, playfulness and warmth. The following chart (Figure 10.1) has been found useful to aid such feedback.

LEVELS OF INSECURITY

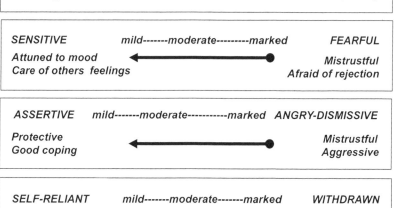

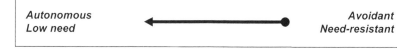

Figure 10.1 Example of client feedback on attachment style

Summary

- Core characteristics of neglecting and abusive parenting were described as they impacted on the emotional climate of the care environment. Also in relation to developmental impacts and internalising and externalising difficulties or disorders in children.
- In therapeutic contexts, assessment of parental attachment style can contribute important understanding of the attitudes guiding the parent's behaviour. It can also provide a profile of relational characteristics that can predict how the child's behaviour is likely to be perceived and responded to. Many of the available tools for assessment are self-report or limited in information provided.
- Holistic assessments, as provided with the ASI, can serve to inform the level of parental support needed for family resilience to prevent harm to the child and accelerate processes towards child protection services. The ASI can also contribute key data to inform and support relationship-based treatments focused on the specific attachment tensions that both parent and child bring to the therapeutic process.

- The ASI assessment can be used as a pre-clinical measure before engaging the family in Filial Therapy, a play-based approach to working with children and families in family therapy. It is a way of approaching the assessment of child and adolescent emotional and behavioural difficulties through the prism of family context and Attachment categorisation.
- The ASI can be used to assess the adult family characteristics and dyadic factors that contribute to the child's internalising or externalising symptoms associated with poor family and individual functioning.
- The Filial therapeutic approach described is used to facilitate change for families and children referred for behavioural, social or emotional difficulties, by helping address the relational conflicts that contribute to difficulties within the parent–child relationship. Such difficulties can further challenge the parent's attachment style and leave them feeling inadequate and out of control. Such difficulties may also amplify the risks presented by their parenting style.
- In identifying the parent as being highly Insecure in terms of the ASI, the inability to access effective support, difficulties with interactions and problems in trusting or relying on others can be openly noted from the outset of therapy. In relation to the specific core characteristics of each style, strengths as well as weaknesses are identified.

10.2 Case examples

In the following three cases, the child has been referred for psychological assessment and treatment, and in each case the mother has psychological disorder and two have a Dual/disorganised attachment style and one Fearful. All three are single parent families. The examples serve to highlight the impact on the child of the mother's state of mind, clinical disorder and behaviour.

10.2.1 Mother Daphne's Dual/disorganised style and alcohol abuse

Daphne was a single mother, looking after her daughter Sally aged nine, and had a history of alcohol abuse from when Sally was born. Daphne was aged 48, did not work and had been separated on and off from Sally's father since her birth. She had for some time stopped drinking alcohol and following a period of rehabilitation was determined to resume full-time care of Sally following a period of temporary foster care. However, Daphne's health was fragile as a result of many years of alcohol abuse.

Referral information described her daughter Sally's emotional difficulties as including phobias, fears and behavioural difficulties, such as frequent temper tantrums, screaming, shouting and attempts to hit and hurt her mother. Whilst living with Daphne, Sally had taken on a 'young carer' role and had been pushed to attend to Daphne's needs, which left her resentful of her mother. Daphne in turn alternated between being intrusive with her daughter as well as punitive and controlling, and at other times unresponsive when self-absorbed and depressed. The parental support advisor recognised Sally's need for a private and safe place where she could express the feelings she struggled to manage in trying to cope with her mother's alternating coerciveness and helplessness. This was with a view to involving Daphne in the therapy at a later date to help her develop better understanding of Sally's feelings and needs. ASI assessment indicated that Daphne had a Dual/disorganised attachment style having both Fearful and Enmeshed features.

Daphne's support: Acknowledging a very poor ongoing relationship with her own mother with ongoing high antipathy, Daphne's view of her family was divided. She saw her father as supportive and loving but her mother as dismissive, critical and rejecting and threatening towards her. Daphne only named her father as Very Close, but on further probing reported being unable to either confide or elicit emotional support from him. Although she did have a non-live-in boyfriend Ben, they were not close and she did not confide in him or seek support. She had no other support figure and no close friends. With no close supportive relationship she was rated as 'little/none' in terms of ability to make and maintain relationships, and therefore markedly Insecure.

Daphne's markedly Fearful and Enmeshed Attachment attitudes: Daphne expressed her mistrust and wariness of others' motives: *'I trust Lou, my parent support advisor, but I doubt she will be there for the long term. I don't know why she has referred Sally for therapy. I guess she must be making plans to get rid of me.'* She also voiced her belief that others might betray her or reject her: *'Yes, because I know in the end they all let you down. Like my neighbour. I thought that she and I had a good relationship. But without saying anything to me I saw her talking to Sally's social worker and I just knew that she was telling her things I had told her. Probably also that I had shouted at Sally. She really let me down. I feel really betrayed by my neighbour. She and all the others are one thing to your face, quite another behind your back.'*

Her self-reliance and desire for company were both contradictory, showing the push and pull in approaching or avoiding. About her desire for company she said: *'I am really a sad and lonely person aren't I? If Sally were any older I would definitely have a closer relationship with Ben, because I would like to have someone, you know, have someone to be with, I need a life too. But I certainly wouldn't want him there all the time, no not at all. He'll have his place and I'll have* mine because I wouldn't want him around all the time, only when I need him to be there. Not that I really need him, just sometimes when I feel lonely and need someone to look after me.'

Her self reliance was also contradictory. She said *'It depends really. I couldn't manage without Lou and Sally, and my dad's advice, but I like to make up my own mind. When I get really muddled I need to ask Lou, and Sally, but I don't rely on their advice, because I know what I need to do and I like making decisions alone . . . but when I can't decide of course I do feel I need them.'* On her need for others and fear of separation: *'Yeah. Sally now wants to go out and play with her friends but I told her she can't. But she nagged me so much I finally gave in and bought her a telephone, so she can call me every half hour. I really don't know why she wants to go out so much. But when she gets home I will get angry at her. I get very anxious not knowing what she is doing.'* Daphne also had high anger, harbouring a number of resentments to her mother, her neighbour and to Sally. *'They drive me mental at times, and sometimes I just feel like telling Mum to p*** off. I never have though, but I just scream at her "enough is enough".'*

Comment: ASI assessment indicated that Daphne had a Dual/disorganised attachment style having both Fearful and Enmeshed features with high anger when her needs were not met. This contributed to clarifying the contribution of Daphne's attachment insecurity, to her poor parenting skills. It confirmed that Sally would need to be placed on the Child in Need list to provide her with the necessary Safeguarding. In the meantime an intensive package of direct work without her mother's involvement was offered first and a referral for individual psychotherapy for Daphne to help her deal with her own anger and need before she could cope with Sally's high anger and feelings of neglect and unmet need. Figure 10.3 summarises the features in this dyad with the parenting involving role reversal, antipathy and high control and the child in return exhibiting over-concerned behaviour for her mother along with unpredicatable hostility. It was considered that the mother's attachment style involved high need for attention from her daughter combined with fear of loss and separation. This was suffocating for the child alternating with high rejection. Sally in turn was required to service the mothers need for company and support. The elements in this case are shown in Figure 10.2.

10.2.2 Mother Debbie's Dual/disorganised attachment style, her Depression and Anxiety

Background: Danny was a six-year-old boy and the eldest of two children. He lived with his mother Debbie (aged 33) and his younger sister Cordelia (4), and from infancy had often been left in the care of his mother's many partners. An allegation of physical abuse of Cordelia by one of Debbie's many partners had been made when Danny was four, and it was then that

Single mother Dual/disorganised
Fearful and Enmeshed

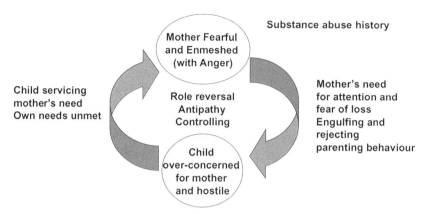

Mother Fearful
and Enmeshed
(with Anger)

Substance abuse history

Child servicing
mother's need
Own needs unmet

Role reversal
Antipathy
Controlling

Mother's need
for attention and
fear of loss
Engulfing and
rejecting
parenting behaviour

Child
over-concerned
for mother
and hostile

Figure 10.2 Diagram of Daphne's Disorganised attachment and Sally's behaviour

concerns about Debbie's parenting had led to both children being given a Child in Need status.

Debbie had a history of depression and anxiety. She was also known to the many professionals she regularly accessed for seeking medical diagnoses for Danny. The extensive log showed her frequent visits to mental health clinics, hospitals or family centres where she demanded medication for Danny's ADHD, enuresis and encopresis as well as strategies for his anger management. Following earlier involvement with mental health services Danny underwent assessment and was diagnosed with only mild ADHD. When Danny was six, therapy was proposed as a last resort in an attempt to meet his psychological and relational needs with the aim of eventually progressing the work to Filial Therapy.

Reasons for referral included Danny's mother's reports of his hyperactivity, persistent attention seeking with extreme anxiety if left in a room alone, but with dislike of being comforted when he was upset. She also described his risk-taking, such as running into the street, destructive behaviour, temper tantrums, swearing and hitting in the playground at school which indicated extreme externalising behaviours associated with distress. In addition his bed wetting, soiling and fear of the dark further contributed to a picture of extremely poor emotional and behavioural functioning suggestive of attachment and behavioural difficulties. Hyperactivity, a short-attention span and difficulty with staying in one place contributed to his diagnosis of ADHD and 'communication disorder'. His behavioural difficulties, which included impulsiveness, rage and explosiveness as well as intense fears, depression and poor self-regulation, suggested Danny's Disorganised attachment with both fearful and angry elements and his persistent difficulties were associated with ongoing family problems, maternal depression and external psychosocial stress. As a result, Debbie underwent ASI assessment to gain understanding of the emotional climate in which Danny was cared for.

Debbie's support: Debbie named only one close support figure, a friend in whom she had little confiding and no support. Her only other contacts were superficial with other mothers in internet chat rooms, whom she had never met face to face. ASI assessment of Debbie's ability to make and maintain relationships was 'little/none' and therefore her attachment insecurity as 'marked'. Her family relationships with her mother and sister were hostile and not close.

Debbie's markedly Angry-dismissive and Fearful Attachment attitudes: Debbie had high levels of mistrust and was suspicious of most people. She felt people were against her. *'They all say they will help you but I know they're thinking something else. They're just waiting to see how they can trip me up.'* She was particularly mistrustful of men. *'They chat you up and then they're off – they're out to get from you what they need – and then they're off.'* Of her only VCO, she said *'She says she can sort things out for me but I know she will let me down.'* She was also fearful of rejection, and cited the lack of professional validation of her many concerns about Danny's difficulties as a source of being let down. *'I'll never listen to anyone again so there's no one I go to at the moment – I come here because I have to but I am not going to open up because whatever I say will never be good enough. So I don't ask for help unless I am desperate.'* She had also felt let down in her personal life, by Danny's father and her many other partners. She was also very angry in relationships: *'I hate my sister. Where is she when I need her? And Danny, well, he's just a troublemaker, always winding me up, and he knows how.'* She had high negative interaction with her mother, argued with her current partner and expressed many resentments with her family: *'Well, they did and still do annoy me.'* She caused rows in many contexts, blaming others for her situation and being particularly aggressive towards Danny. ASI assessment of Debbie showed her to have a Dual/disorganised style (Angry-dismissive and Fearful), with high ratings for both anger and fear of rejection.

Debbie's parenting: Her parenting of Danny was unpredictable, frightening and chaotic. Debbie admitted to shouting frequently and reluctantly acknowledged an incident when she had shaken Danny. She complained that parenting her children raised her blood pressure and also that she often felt unable to cope. Debbie acknowledged her fearfulness of saying anything to Danny, as this would unleash even more of his anger. She also felt fearful of her own voice and felt that whatever she said would be inadequate. As she spoke of her ongoing feelings of despair, Debbie was referred for psychiatric assessment of depression. As she refused medication for her low mood she was referred for therapy to address her own mental health needs. An initial six sessions were provided as an assessment of Danny's needs, with recommendations for therapy to follow.

Danny's behaviour: Danny's play revealed the anxious and urgent sense of alarm that pervaded his highly aroused and distressed emotional state. When he was playing, he raced toy ambulances to scenes of high emergency and his play sequences included a high incidence of chaos, conflict, punishment and harsh victimisation. In role play he told the therapist she was bad because she hit little boys and in imaginary play Danny was able to show how he feared his mother's anger and hostility. The smallest transgression caused Danny to panic, anticipating a punitive response. When overwhelmed by feelings of vulnerability he would run out of the room to seek access to his mother in the waiting area where he was invariably greeted with a mixed reception as Debbie kissed him while also calling him 'horrible'. Danny also demonstrated a need to be seen and valued, as shown in his tireless display of skills, his feelings of loss and needing to be found.

In the waiting room Danny struggled to gain his mother's attention, but she could only denigrate him with unrestrained hostility. In the playroom Danny was easily overwhelmed by his own expressions of negative emotion and when unable to soothe himself became fearful, sad and angry. He also often panicked at any noises heard outside the playroom. Danny's overwhelming anxiety and expressed need for his mother led to Debbie joining Danny in the playroom for the final 15 minutes of the session. As he explored his access to his mother he was only rarely able to elicit a warm and caring response. When in need of soothing, Danny sat close to Debbie and engaged her in a joint activity. Debbie clearly enjoyed these moments and began to recognise Danny's growing expression of attachment to her and was able to acknowledge her pleasure in the acceptance and need he showed her. However, Debbie's warmth and responsiveness were short-lived. Danny's play soon reverted to highly agitated and chaotic sequences and hyper-aroused behaviour. His bid for emotional safety was seen in the way he quickly became highly anxious, running out of the waiting room as he anticipated his mother's anger and punitive threats. Debbie was unable to make the link between Danny's worsening behaviour and the sudden arrival of a new partner in her life. She claimed that even though they had only just met, Danny really loved this new partner.

Therapeutic work: The therapist worked with Debbie to help her anticipate triggers such as her feelings of anger and her perceptible fear of Danny's angry feelings that contributed to Danny's hyper-arousal and heightened anxiety. A crucial point was the attempt to redirect Debbie's focus onto

Danny's relational needs, thereby inviting her to reflect on her own inattention to Danny and his expression of need for her. Recognition of the emotional meaning behind Danny's play and the importance of themes that indicated attachment need proved even more difficult. So did developing an awareness of Danny's low threshold for stress-reactions and recognising early indicators of potentially frightening cues. Unable to elicit any acknowledgment that Debbie valued her child and the increasing need to accept that Danny above all feared Debbie's anger and punitive threats, meant the case was referred to Child Protection because of abuse and neglect risks to Danny. Debbie was referred to another team to address her own mental health needs. Figure 10.3 illustrates this mother's inconsistent parenting and physical abuse, the child's response with panic and aggression, the mother's need for attention but fear of threat from her son and the child's intermittent desire to please and anxiety for his mother.

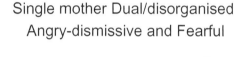

Single mother Dual/disorganised
Angry-dismissive and Fearful

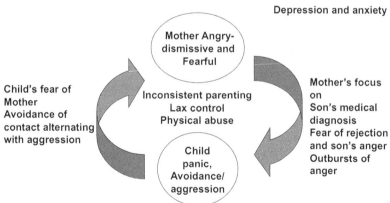

Figure 10.3 Debbie's Dual/disorganised style

10.2.3 Freddy's developmental impairment; mother Faith's Fearful style and depression

Background: Freddy was referred with reported developmental impairment which resulted in behaviour suggestive of autistic spectrum symptomatology, including social disability, impairment in communication and restricted play and interpersonal activities. His mother Faith (aged 29), a single mother, looked after Freddy alone. Faith had spent most of her early childhood in care and following the birth of her son her marriage had ended in an acrimonious divorce. Faith was open about her periods of depression. She had used drugs when she was younger. The ASI was used to provide insight into Faith's attachment style so that she could be supported to increase her empathy with her child and reduce his behavioural and social difficulties both of which contributed to her stress levels and challenged her parenting of Freddy.

Freddy, aged nine, was described as having few social skills, was difficult to manage and often appeared to be cut off and lost in a 'world of his own', so that he was often unable to follow instructions. His mother Faith and other professionals engaged with supporting the family, believed him to be mildly autistic, a label welcomed by his mother. Faith frequently emphasised this aspect of his functioning, and in his mother's presence Freddy did appear to be cut off and emotionally restricted. His play indicated a limited range of emotions, lacked spontaneity and his behaviour suggested withdrawal and inhibition. Freddy seemed to have little anticipation that play could be a cooperative and a shared experience. He occasionally glanced at Faith but as she looked into the distance he also turned away and withdrew into his own emotional world seemingly blocking all further expression of feeling.

Mother Faith's support: Faith had little support. She had no current partner and was not able to name any close family or friends in whom she confided or from whom she received support. She relied on professionals and her church for practical support, but was effectively socially isolated. She was rated as having 'little or no' ability to make and maintain relationships and therefore rated markedly Insecure.

Faith's markedly Fearful Attachment attitudes: Faith's attachment attitudes showed high intensity of negative feelings. Her fearfulness and high mistrust was clearly reported: *'I have no reason to trust. I wish I could but I am always let down. I was left to sort things out from an early age and there is no way I will do things differently now. I have these feelings about people. I know straight away if I have this feeling or not. And yes, I am always waiting to find out why someone really wanted to do this – so I never ask for help. I am sure it will be thrown back at me that I needed to ask for something because I was so helpless and sad. There are my friends at the church but they are not really friends, I couldn't tell them personal things. I wouldn't tell anyone personal things. I used to talk to my neighbour but then she moved away and I thought maybe I could call her but she would probably not be too keen to hear from me. She has moved on I'm sure and has a new life in which I do not belong.'*

Faith showed evidence of strong psychological blockages preventing her from getting close to others or asking for help as well as fear of rejection: *'Since my mother betrayed me the way she did, and my father allowed her to do this,*

I cannot let anyone know what I am thinking or feeling. As a matter of fact I ended up in care as a result, so I know how much showing your vulnerable side can hurt you. I prefer to try and sort things out alone because if I show any weakness I am sure people will let me down. People don't like to help people who need help. Anyway, with me I'm sure they will find a reason to turn me down. It isn't easy raising a boy alone but I have only myself to do it. That way I don't have to rely on anyone else. It is hard enough when he goes and sees his dad. I am sure everything he does is done to undermine me. I have a lot of reasons for feeling this way. When I started to take drugs it was because I knew I couldn't ask anyone to help or tell them how low I felt.'
Faith displayed no anger towards others, not even towards her parents, and had no dependency characteristics such as fear of separation or desire for company.

ASI assessment of Faith's Fearful style and behaviour and attitudes provided important insight into how frightened she was of others' views of her, how easily slighted and rejected she felt and importantly how crucial it was to be an ally. This involved not challenging her view of her son as being autistic without sensitively reframing his behaviour as threatening her own feelings of being rejected by him.

Interactions in therapy: During the Family Play Observation the therapist was struck by how quickly Freddy and Faith turned away from each other. Freddy seemed unaware of his mother's presence and showed no enthusiasm for engaging her in his play. He made no eye-contact with her and absorbed himself with repetitively opening and closing the doors of a toy ambulance. The joylessness of this activity and Faith's silent withdrawal painted a picture of fearfulness, mis-attunement and disconnection. Freddy played in a solitary and silent way, further fuelling Faith's feelings of rejection and exclusion by her son. Following this observation the therapist discussed the observed dynamic with Faith. Faith felt embarrassed that Freddy had been so uninterested in her but quickly attributed this to his autism; *'That is what Freddy is like, so cut off and remote, it's as if he doesn't see or hear anything when he goes into that place.'* The therapist was able to touch on Faith's feelings of being excluded from Freddy's play and the hurt and feelings of rejection it engendered, causing her to turn away to avoid further pain. The therapist was also able to empathically relate what she had observed to what Faith had openly discussed in the ASI interview, specifically her feeling that she could never do well enough to gain approval or interest. Also that she had learnt to do things her way as she had no anticipation of a relationship, even with her own son, in which she was valued and appreciated.

In understanding how Faith's mistrust and anticipation of rejection and disapproval guided her perception of others and the way she believed herself to be judged, the Filial therapist was given an indication of how important approval was to Faith. In Filial Therapy, parental feelings of empowerment are paramount and in post-play session discussions the therapist provides high levels of positive feedback. Because of Faith's high fear of rejection and need for non-critical acceptance it was clear that Faith struggled to absorb even the quarter of feedback that suggested areas for improvement as she heard these as failures and shortcomings. In Faith's own words: '*There always seems to be more that I should be doing – always things I am never getting right.*'

During the Filial training phase Faith and the therapist were scheduled to meet on a weekly basis and Faith's Fearfulness was shown in the sudden cancellations and absences. She would call to say that she could not face being in the room as she worried that her skills were likely to be inadequate and she feared the unacceptability of her every utterance. ASI assessment contributed in important ways to the therapist's way of engaging Faith, emphasising at all times her understanding of Faith's reluctance to ask for help and how past experiences of rejection were not about her unworthiness or lack of lovability but the result of the illness, and hostile cruelty of those who had failed to care for her. In this way each of the sessions was approached with an added understanding that Faith applied brakes as soon as she felt uncomfortable with her son's expression of aggression and anger as these were perceived as directed at wounding her and threatened her most basic feelings of emotional safety.

The therapist's ability to help Faith explore and understand her emotional reactions to her child based on her experience of rejection helped challenge her belief that her son disliked her and rejected her. In the final observed play session Freddy playfully engaged his mother's attention. Faith, no longer fearful of all the aggression and hostility she had felt threatened by, was able to permit her son to express himself. Freddy, was now perceived as a young boy whose experience of his mother's withdrawal and fearfulness had caused him to turn inwards. Faith in being helped to link the feelings Freddy's internalising behaviour engendered in her related to earlier relationship experiences, was able to see how feeling rejected and inadequate as a parent had required her to exonerate herself through viewing her son as autistic.

The Filial Therapy intervention led to important changes in Faith and Freddy's relationship. Becoming aware of her own sensitivity to rejection and able to see this as a reflex to the hostile and rejecting parenting she had experienced, Faith was able to re-establish a healthy parent–child relationship. In this she could be responsive to Freddy's needs and wishes but also authoritative without feeling that Freddy would push her away. Faith also became more able to tolerate not only the positive feelings but the more negative emotions expressed by her son. Importantly she was able to think about him as a nine-year-old boy with emotional and relational needs whose fears no longer threatened her and to whom she as a mother could respond to with equanimity. These elements are illustrated in Figure 10.4.

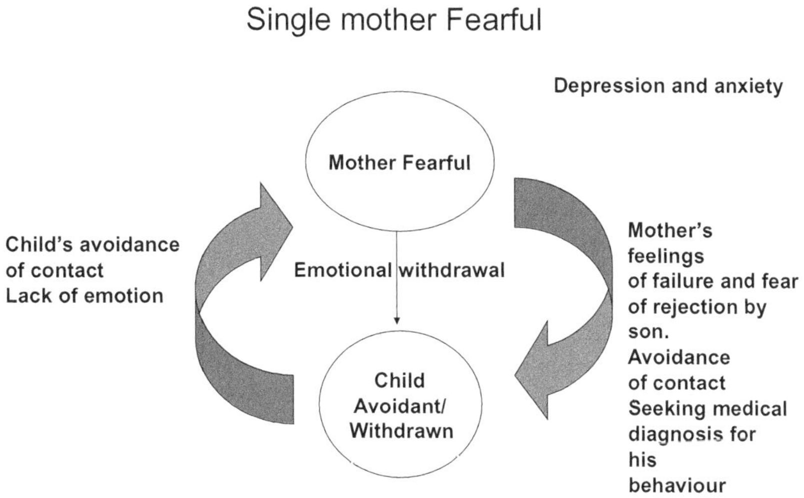

Single mother Fearful

Figure 10.4 Faith's Fearful style

Summary of cases

- Cases are presented where children are referred because of psychological disorder and in each case the parent has both Insecure attachment style and clinical disorder. The patterning of the various vulnerabilities is examined in terms of impact on the child, and in relation to therapeutic intervention.
- The cases show how the parents often project their own unmet need on to the child, at times involving role reversal where the child is expected to act as parent, and find interpretations of the child's behaviour which is overly medicalised and which blocks out their own contribution to failed interactions.
- These mothers were all single and very isolated, coping with their own psychological disorders as well as with a child for whom they expressed little attachment and experienced as burdensome.
- Identifing sources for mother's fear and anger, and her interactions with her child in play helped to identify, and in some cases improve such interactions.

10.3 Presentation of attachment style to therapist

In the next section we aim to highlight the way in which children in particular present themselves in therapy, with reference to the behaviour characteristic of their parent's different attachment styles. We further examine the potential role of such parental features impacting on the child and on the organisation of the child's emotional, social and behavioural development. These are cases where there is no overt clinical disorder in the mother, and include some cases where both mother and father are present, and are included to consider how the parent's attachment styles can impact on the family interaction.

10.3.1 Amy living with Enmeshed mother Eleanor

Amy was aged eight and lived alone with her mother Eleanor (35). Her parents were separated. Amy presented with anxiety, over-compliance and need to please her mother, but avoided contact when Eleanor's neediness became too great. Amy presented herself to her first session for the purpose of assessment before transferring to Filial Therapy sessions by running into the playroom before her mother could engage the therapist with immediate disclosure of things deeply personal. Once in the room, Amy expressed her shame and embarrassment at being late. Looking anxiously at the clock she delivered her apology which became a weekly refrain: '*Mummy wasn't very well this morning, she was really ill, and then she bumped her head and she had to go to the doctor's surgery before we came here,*' cataloguing a long list of exonerating situations in an effort to make her mother look less culpable for her serial lateness and chaotic lack of organisation. Once she had unburdened herself Amy wasted no time in engaging in the therapeutic work she had come to do. Embarking on her weekly session Amy announced, as she always did, that she had a score to settle and unleashed the full range of the anger and frustration that she had withheld from her mother on the playroom inflatable punch bag. In releasing her anger in a physically unrestrained way her shouting gradually escalated into a high-decibel rage.

Amy's mother Eleanor, who on assessment was shown to have a markedly Enmeshed attachment style with anger, presented as needy and demanding. For Amy, her mother's self-pitying helplessness in the reception area contrasted sharply with the unpredictable controlling and shouting rages at home and left her feeling powerless and defeated. Alert to Eleanor's emotive diatribes, she would flee from the room as soon as yet another catastrophic tale of accident, or injury, would be recounted. In her mother's absence, Amy told these stories as if they were her own, emphasising the hurt or the insult her mother had endured, always speaking in her defence against the onslaught of prying social workers or demanding teachers.

In the therapy room Amy's play, unmasking her real preoccupations, demonstrated her feelings of vulnerability, unmet infantile need and emotional hunger. 'Caring for the baby' was a recurrent theme in play, in which the baby's safety and care were threatened when a returning mother was shown to rant and rage, during which the baby is eventually hurled aside and forcefully ejected in a maelstrom of unfettered anger and high anxiety.

When Eleanor gradually came to join Amy and the therapist in the room for the last 15 minutes of the therapeutic hour, Amy, mindful of what her mother could tolerate, reduced the intensity of her own need and showed Eleanor less-threatening play. Curtailing her own need to a level she believed her mother could manage, she instead focused her attention on her mother's need. This was the protective strategy Amy was constrained to adopt. In Eleanor's presence she smiled placidly, her voice becoming small as she called out for 'mummy' to be on her team. But when alone with the therapist Amy's own anger blunted all other emotions. As an eight-year-old girl she bore the hallmarks of years of mute rage borne silently to placate her mother and to keep the social workers at bay. She had little confidence in her own sense of agency and requested permission for every choice she made, apologising for every toy not cleared up and every spillage caused. Above all she needed to loudly express her rage and her anguish as the therapy room was the only place where she could be heard.

In attachment terms, Amy's compliance provided a useful strategy for protecting herself against her mother's alternating neglect and hostile neediness, and in masking her own feelings of anger and ineffectiveness. At home Amy had little trust in the availability of care and felt rage against her powerlessness in securing this. Now in middle childhood, therapy helped her develop the self-esteem required to feel motivated and competent at school and to engage in positive peer relationships. But at home she still felt unable to express the needs of an eight-year-old girl. Worn out by the need to disguise her frustration and deep anger, Amy would show defiance and pleasure in attacking her mother verbally and at times even physically.

Amy's mother's deep anxiety about her own lovability and low self-value meant that she was obsessively preoccupied with the interest others had in her and worried endlessly about other's attention being lost. Amy experienced Eleanor's suffocating behaviour as demanding and insistent with no real sense of interest in her. When Eleanor felt threatened with the loss or abandonment she anticipated at all times, she became coercive in her control of Amy, forcing her to attend to her. In processing the 15 minutes witnessed sessional content with the therapist, she was unable to accept and acknowledge Amy's feelings of frustration and despair in relation to her chaotic environment. Eleanor had little capacity to concentrate on any subject not directly focused on her own endless struggles, feigned illnesses or exaggerated dramas. The expectation of oscillating anger and suffocating need, punitive control, unboundaried intimacy coupled with rejection from her Enmeshed mother led Amy to find control, and some safety, through compliance and role-reversed caregiving. Figure 10.5 illustrates these elements in the interaction.

Single mother Enmeshed

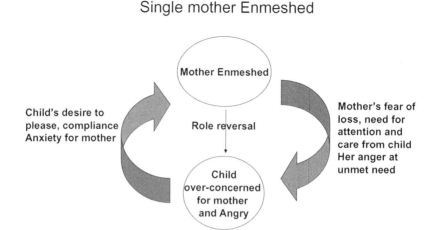

Figure 10.5 Eleanor's Enmeshed style

10.3.2 Milo Living with Angry and Avoidant parents

Milo, aged eight, was living with two battling parents, his mother Annette (aged 36) and father William (aged 42). Milo's behaviour was subdued, minimally expressive and pared down. In the school playground this was harder to control and his often anxious, depressed and detached behaviour would give way to sudden outburst and attacks on peers in the playground when in moments of heightened stress and arousal he could no longer control his anger. Milo's play was initially solitary and his repertoire limited. He would turn his back to the therapist as he played alone and silently with the cars and the soldier figures allowing her to hear the sounds of the bombs dropping and the guns firing while soldiers and tanks engaged in a battle in which there could be no victory. A recurrent theme in Milo's play was Hitler and the struggle to live in a hierarchical dictatorship in which there was no escape from hostility and control.

Milo's behaviour was understandable in terms of his parents' styles and relationship. Annette was markedly Angry-dismissive: '*I feel really resentful of my husband. Whenever I ask him to back me up with the kids all I get is a sneer. He says "You're so tough, what's all the need for support now?"*'Always vigilant to the expectation of disapproval and fearful of not ever meeting his mother's expectations, Milo had difficulty expressing his need for approval and acceptance, or his wish for time spent with his mother that was not exclusively focused on his achievements at school and less critical of his endeavours. Milo usually kept his distance and denied any feelings of distress. He also anticipated that any negative feelings shown would lead to further rejection. He distracted himself from any interaction or expression of emotion that would challenge the successful inhibition of his negative feelings and in the therapy room seldom allowed himself any activity other than the relentless demonstration of his football skills to gain the therapist's admiration and approval.

His father William, despite having support outside of the marriage, said*: 'I don't think I've ever relied on anybody's help in making decisions. I just manage. I like to be independent and I can cope well without others getting involved.'* This meant that he could seldom overcome his imposed self-reliance to ask for help or to voice any distress when in need of support. Whilst he did not engage with the therapy, his interaction with Milo was distant and disengaged. Unlike Annette he was not hostile or critical, but had difficulties in showing warmth and affection to his son. He was dominated by his wife and did not interfere with her parenting style. Therefore, Milo received no support from his father. However, whilst William did have better adaptation outside of the marriage (he confided in his mother and had a work colleague) he was unable to cope with Annette's anger without withdrawing, and thus offered no help to his child. He was rated as mildly Withdrawn.

Behaviour in the therapy room: When Annette joined Milo in the playroom he would try to engage his mother in his play, but her criticism of his approach, her confrontational style and her own wish for victory in competitive games denied Milo his chance for gaining her approval. He would quickly divert his attention elsewhere and direct her to the board games where she also found it hard not to express her disdain for Milo's limited gains. She became confrontational and humourless when it looked as if Milo might beat her at a game. Annette found it hard to hear the therapist tell her she should play fairly but not so competitively that Milo would never have a chance to win. Annette believed that in real life there were no soft options and he would have to overcome his own weakness to survive. No matter what strategies were offered for empathic listening or less criticism, Anette always considered herself to be in the right including her insistence that the play sessions would only feed into Milo's more infantile needs, something she wished at all cost to avoid. She was quick to devalue the benefits of therapy for Milo and the offer of a more family systems approach to include Milo's brother and father were summarily dismissed as 'rubbish' and out of the question.

Therapy revolved around getting William more involved, encouraging him to show greater warmth to his son, and learning more assertiveness with Annette. She in turn was encouraged to modify her critical behaviour, and to recognise the anxiety which lay beneath it. Figure 10.6 illustrates the dynamics involved with the anger from mother and withdrawal by father resulting in Milo's anxiety and defeat.

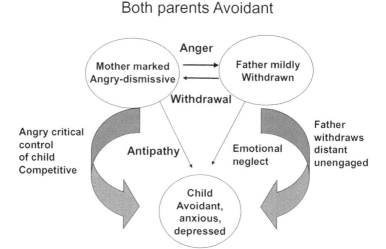

Figure 10.6 Living with avoidant/hostile parents

10.3.3 Louis living with two Fearful parents

Frieda (aged 32) and Finn (aged 35), both previously divorced, struggled to parent Louis, aged seven. They described him as being at times good and at others very, very bad and were clearly frightened of his temper tantrums and of his controlling and demanding behaviour. They had difficulty in recognising that his highly ambivalent behaviour reflected a need for firm boundaries, acceptance and containment of his strong feelings and showing robustness and authority in the face of his high-pitched demands.

Both Frieda and Finn were rated moderately Fearful and each acknowledged that their experience of rejection and betrayal in previous marriages continued to influence the way they approached others now. Following two miscarriages Frieda had finally carried Louis to term and she and Finn had been delighted by his arrival. Now Louis was a worry due to his angry, defiant and oppositional behaviour. He was described as bossy and controlling and if he didn't get his way he would scream the house down. Both parents were terrified of him and convinced themselves that Louis much preferred his own company as he was much more interested in watching his DVDs and was happier to play on his own.

Louis's behaviour: Louis experienced his parents as inconsistent, at times rewarding of his oppositional behaviour, vulnerable and sensitive to slights. Aware that he held inappropriate power at home he was able to turn on his anger and controlling behaviour at will thus cowing Frieda and Finn into agreeing to his every demand. Their loss of authority as parents further fuelled their sense of inadequacy and Louis was able to perpetuate his terrorising. Finn and Frieda's Fearful attachment style and anxious parenting, due to fear of confrontation and fear of eliciting rejection as limit setters contributed to Louis's lack on internal control and poor self-mastery. In usurping authority from his fearful parents with most of his effort focused on feeling empowered by pushing the buttons that would make Finn and Frieda jump, Louis had little confidence in his own capacity for appropriate mastery and was left feeling perpetually out of control. Feeling rejected by his parents as they withdrew to lick their wounds Louis would worry and ask repeatedly about how Frieda was feeling. Hyper-vigilant to his mother's feelings of rejection and vulnerability Louis's own need to express his feelings was further and further inhibited and he had difficulty in accepting comfort when sustaining a bump or small injury.

Unable to express feelings except through the release of pent-up emotions in explosive temper tantrums, Louis's emotional development was impacted by strong feelings of insecurity related to his pseudo-adult power. Lacking trust in authoritative care that could ensure his emotional safety Louis developed guilt, shame and doubt about his ability to ever 'get it right'. His tendency to seize power from peers also impeded his ability to make positive peer relationships and as a result he was at risk of becoming increasingly isolated and lonely and only able to communicate his feelings through solitary fantasy play. Figure 10.7 shows the dynamic between Louis and his parents.

Therapeutic interaction: The Filial Play sessions showed that Frieda and Finn were both frightened of the intensity of Louis's play. Their levels of energy were no match for his and their Fearfulness made them passive when he challenged them with aggressive and competitive play. Both had difficulty setting limits. Louis subjected Frieda to humiliating challenges in which '*she could never get it right*' and while she showed willingness to do exactly as he instructed her, her fears of rejection made her feel that he enjoyed seeing her fail. With Finn, Louis's emotionally charged anger play was equally threatening and, unable to respond to the intensity of his feelings, Finn would try to set a limit and responded with a resounding '*NO, you can't do that.*' However, when the same unacceptable action was repeated Finn chose to ignore it. In one session Finn even ventured to follow the three-step sequence of stating the limit, giving a warning and enforcing the consequence used during Filial play sessions but, anticipating Louis's protest and angry outburst at the perceived injustice of this, he backed off before Louis uttered a word. '*OK then, if you're a good boy you can have 10 more minutes.*'

Both parents worried that Louis would not like them if they set boundaries. The same reluctance to be firm when Louis challenged limits in his play sessions inhibited their ability to stand firm when Louis screamed and shouted that he needed to be carried to bed, wanted more food or required another DVD immediately. Fear of rejection made both parents anxious about Louis rebuffing them. Resistance to become active participants in the sessions was evident and both parents insisted that the therapist would be better equipped to do this as Louis would probably prefer someone else and was likely not to accept them as playmates.

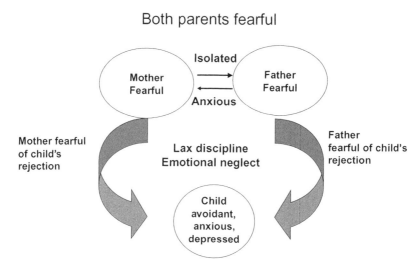

Figure 10.7 Living with Fearful parents

Summary of Insecure attachment presentations at therapy

- The way in which parents and children present themselves in therapy, with behaviour characteristics of the different attachment styles was examined in relation to the potential role of such features impacting on the child and in the organisation of the child's emotional, social and behavioural development. Cases are presented where there is no overt clinical disorder in the mother, and cases with both parents present.
- Features of Insecure attachment style were readily observable in early stages of parents interaction with their children, and in presenting to the therapy sessions. Maternal neediness and child over-compliance and need to please were very evident outside of the play sessions.
- When both parents had Insecure styles this led to patterning of the parental response to the child with parents at times forming a pact against the child.

- When both parents had Avoidant styles, with an admix of anger, fighting between parents and hostile or avoidant behaviour towards the child resulted in very avoidant behaviour in the child. The lack of external support for parents led to an intensity in the expression of parents Insecure style with no outlet or modification by other involved adults.
- When both parents had Anxious styles, their fear of rejection from their child lead to angry controlling behaviour from the child who held a dominant role. Again lack of support outside the nuclear family led to an intensity in the parents clinging to each other with no respite from external influence.

10.4 Discussion

Emphasising the child-parent relationship is an accepted prerequisite of child protection, family support or clinical work assessment. Current assessment procedures, however, fail to capture important characteristics of the family systems around the child and adolescent. Knowledge of the parent's inability to be responsive to the child's cues if they themselves have Insecure attachment styles, at best are passively neglectful and at worst prone to hostile, controlling and violent parenting. Understanding adult styles can provide integrated understanding of environmental variables that contribute to both internalizing and externalizing symptoms and disorders in the child. This can be key in the planning and selection of appropriate treatment interventions, family work and child protection decisions. Assessment of parental attachment style thus contributes important information related to those attitudes guiding the parent's style of responding to the child's behaviour, which in turn is organised in reaction to the parental caregiving style.

In addition to highlighting risks for psychological vulnerability and poor parenting, the ASI scale which measures negative interactions with partner and close others can provide assessment of risk for conflict in the home as well as predict depression for the victims of domestic violence. While conflict and negativity add additional stressors to the emotional environment, victims of violence in the home are known to have more difficulty in maintaining non-distressed relationships with children (van der Kolk, Pelcovitz *et al.* 1996). In acknowledging the nature of emotional development as intimately related to the developing child's attachment to those who care for him, the following aspects around child care, parenting and children's vulnerabilities are relevant for the development of emotions and the strategies needed to protect against vulnerability in childhood: Children who are parented in an emotional environment defined by high anger, hostility and over-control live with daily stressors that contribute to the over-regulation of stress responses. The lack of predictability in the capacity to mediate fear-related behaviour means that the child lacks the means to find a resolution to distress and is forced to develop a strategy for self-protection that requires inhibiting emotional needs so that they do not risk further rejection, anger or injury. Shared understanding through sensitive feedback of the attachment characteristics that underpin potentially corrosive family dynamics can contribute to enhanced insight into family support and therapeutic needs and also contributes to accelerating therapeutic change in guiding parental insight and shifts in expectations and perceptions.

Viewing child and adult functioning across of a range of difficulties through an attachment lens can refocus understanding of emotional and behavioural difficulties and their development into disorders as variations in attachment related developmental outcomes. The evidence that children and young people exposed to problem care by those with highly Insecure attachment style are at risk for a legacy of difficulties both personal and interpersonal with impaired functioning across emotional, social and behavioural domains. Difficulties, in the offspring include increased risks of emotional and developmental disorders, hyperactive disorders, depression and substance abuse. What is not yet understood are the direct pathways leading from the parent's style, in which mediators are coerciveness, hostility and love withdrawal or dependency, intrusiveness and psychological control, to specific behavioural and disorder outcomes. These trajectories of risk are known to have different developmental outcomes for each family member but what is less well-understood is what specific factors contribute to diverse psychopathology outcomes in both parent and child.

Approaching child and adolescent emotional and behavioural difficulties through the prism of the Attachment categorisation is proposed as a way of assessing the adult family and dyadic factors that contribute to the child's internalising or externalising symptoms of poor family and individual functioning. The case material describes therapeutic work undertaken in response to referrals indicating difficulties in the child's emotional state and behaviour suggestive of an Insecure attachment. Pre-intervention assessment with the ASI highlighted risks for parental vulnerability and poor parenting. The core characteristics of the primary carer were, when not indicative of child protection needs, used therapeutically to make significant changes in the relationships between parent and child and thus facilitate change in the child's behaviour.

The final chapter will attempt to bring together the accumulated learning in this book and return to issues raised in the introduction in order to encompass different models of adult attachment style as seen through both social-psychological and clinical lenses.

11 Conclusion

11.0 Introduction

In the introductory chapter, different models were outlined to underpin different aspects of adult attachment style, for example showing its relationship to self-esteem, affect-regulation, couple and family models and biological stress factors as well as a lifespan approach. Varied aspects correlated with adult attachment style have been explored throughout this book through reviewing relevant research literature and analysis of a programme of research which yielded both quantitative findings and illustrative case material. This final chapter will summarise key findings as well as study limitations and will identify further developed models of adult attachment style as well as discuss additional clinical implications.

11.1 Ten key findings

We here contribute to conceptual and model-development as a result of the analyses provided. First we summarise 10 key findings related to the different chapters and topics in relation to the organisational diagram (Figure 11.1) which was presented at the beginning of the book:

1. **Measurement:** Measuring adult attachment style by categorising the quality of partner and family or friend support as a basis for insecurity provides a behavioural as well as attitudinal basis for attachment categorisations with attention to context. Grounding the assessment in the here-and-now, as in the ASI, gives greater facility for monitoring change over time as well as providing independent assessment of its relationship to early life experience.
2. **Clinical disorder:** Attachment styles at marked or moderate levels of insecurity (Dual/disorganised, Enmeshed, Fearful or Angry-dismissive) relate to emotional disorder in the 12-months of study (major depression and anxiety states) among adult women as well as lifetime recurrent depression and teenage episodes. The Anxious styles (Enmeshed or Fearful) similarly relate to emotional disorder in young people. However, in young people Angry-dismissive style only relates to

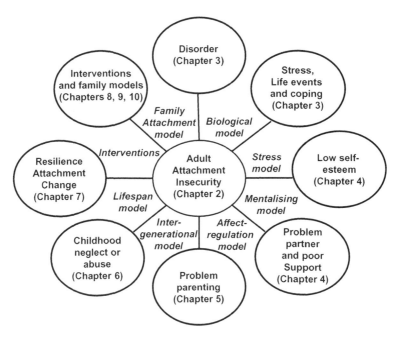

Figure 11.1 Diagram of attachment themes explored

DSH behaviour and Dual/disorganised style only relates to substance abuse. Withdrawn style is unrelated to disorder in either sample.

3. **Self-esteem:** Insecure attachment style is related to low self-esteem or NES which is highly related to Enmeshed and Fearful styles, categorised as Anxious, in both adult women and the younger offspring. However, in adult women only, those with Angry-dismissive style also have high rates of NES. This may relate to their high anxiety rates and suggests anxious and self-critical substrata to the angry and blaming exterior presentation. Withdrawn style is unrelated to low self-esteem.

4. **Stress and coping:** Clinical disorder such as depression is provoked by severe life events, many of which are interpersonal, with partner relationships having particular prominence. Individuals with Insecure attachment style are more prone to severe life events, particularly those in close relationships, and to financial events. They are also prone to high rates of lifetime adult adversity, as well as having poorer coping skills to deal with such stressors. There is some patterning of attachment style to type of coping. Those with Anxious styles (Enmeshed or Fearful) showed more avoidant strategies (cognitive avoidance or denial) as well as helplessness and self-blame. Angry-dismissive style was linked with externalising the stress for example with blame of others and anger, although also exhibiting helplessness and emotional

distress. Those with Dual or disorganised styles used an array of negative coping responses.

5. **Partner relationships:** Insecure attachment style is related to problem partner relationships as well as to single parent status in the samples described. Those with Fearful styles are less likely to be in a partnership, and more often single parents, with Enmeshed and Angry-dismissive most often with a partner. Those Dual/disorganised are more likely to have been separated from partner. Problem partnerships with no support and either conflict or apathy correspond to different attachment styles. Those with Enmeshed or Withdrawn styles were most likely to lack partner support. This related to conflictful and apathetic relationships, respectively. Those with Angry-dismissive styles also had a high rate of partner conflict. Evidence of a history of poor partner relationships is evident in many women with Insecure adult styles. Those with Enmeshed style were more likely to have been in a violent partner relationship whilst those Dual/disorganised were more likely to have had partners with antisocial behaviour, disorder or criminality. Those with Angry-dismissive styles also had high rates of antisocial partners and those Fearful had partners with disorder or criminality. Improvement in partner relationship, or change to a new supportive partner was a factor in positive attachment change.

6. **Family and friends support:** Having Very Close confidants contributes to ratings of ability to make and maintain relationships and hence to Security. These can include family members or friends. Withdrawn style is the most likely to lack any close confidant and Enmeshed the least likely of the Insecure styles. Acquiring a new close confidant was a factor in positive attachment change.

7. **Childhood adversity:** Neglect or abuse is a major early life factor associated with adult Insecure attachment styles, apart from Withdrawn style. Insecure attachment style is shown to mediate between early adversity and adult emotional disorder. Whilst the overlap of different neglect or abuse experiences make differentiation difficult, evidence is presented in adults of lack of care experiences relating to Anxious (Enmeshed or Fearful) and Disorganised styles, with abuse relating to Angry-dismissive style. In the young sample, there was a similar pattern although less sexual and psychological abuse was evident. Here there was a significant relationship between maternal antipathy, neglect or physical abuse and emotional disorder. There was some association of fathers' antipathy and Angry-dismissive and Dual/disorganised style in relation to behavioural disorder such as substance abuse.

8. **Problem parenting:** Mothers with Insecure styles have higher levels of incompetent parenting and this is associated with offspring accounts of maternal neglect or abuse. There is, however, no direct link between mother's attachment style and offspring neglect or abuse other than through her estimated incompetent parenting. Fathers/substitute

fathers also play a role and problem partners (if criminal, disordered or violent) increase the likelihood of mother showing incompetent parenting, with marital adversity contributing to the child's neglect/abuse context. Attachment elements highlighted are hostile and helpless parenting styles. Enmeshed and Angry-dismissive styles had the highest rates of incompetent parenting.

9. **Resilience and Attachment change:** Secure, mildly Insecure and Withdrawn style were all related to lower rates of emotional disorder, even when childhood adversity was present, indicative of resilience factors. Positive childhood and teenage experience contributed to Secure outcomes. Around a quarter of adult women changed attachment style significantly over a three-year follow-up period, half in a positive direction. An increase in support was associated with positive change to more security.

10. **Attachment and services:** the use of the ASI in child and family services has shown its utility in assessing adoption carer suitability, in conceptualising family and parent–child problem interactions in attachment terms and in identifying attachment difficulties in young people in residential care. Case examples highlight patterning of different attachment styles and behaviours drawing out the implications for family disruption and conflict and pointing to ways in which these might be helped or repaired in different interventions.

11.2 Study limitations

The research component of this book, while drawing on research findings from a wide array of studies in this area to inform the knowledge developed, is also based on findings from interconnected community-based studies undertaken in London, UK. These were ambitious studies in terms of the range of experience encompassed including narrative interview elements as well as quantitative findings. As such, the output is rich in generating further hypotheses and in incorporating context into an understanding of adult attachment. However, as with all studies, these have a number of limitations which need to be acknowledged for the reader to judge the weight of the findings described.

These are listed below:

* The samples are mainly of women, and these in inner city London, and thus not representative but selected high-risk individuals, and so the issue of generalisability needs to be considered. In terms of representativeness, the samples are repeats of earlier studies of lifespan risk extended intergenerationally, suggesting findings can be interpreted more widely. The extension to males needs to be the subject of further investigation. Other work undertaken on this model in male series, both in London and in continental Europe, and the findings of the young

males in the Offspring study suggests the model is applicable to both genders.

- Whilst use of retrospective methods is embraced as one of the only means of researching adversity in the past successfully, it is used with care to maximise reliability and validity. This is done through detailed questioning about factual circumstances, using dates and calendars to scaffold recollection of timing of experience, questioning in chronological sequence. It is impossible with the passage of long periods of time to reproduce the fine detail of timing and experience which can inform how internal working models are developed in childhood.

- The study lacks detail on childhood clinical disorders and associated early life developmental problems or educational or learning difficulties. In this it takes an intentional adult (or young adult) perspective exploring in detail disorders occurring in teenage years and later adulthood.

- Whilst encompassing self-esteem, it makes no assessment of mentalising function nor of affect-regulation, nor of any biological correlates of different styles or different childhood adverse experience. All of these would throw further light on how early adversity can affect adult functioning according to attachment principles and we hope future research will utilise the measurement approaches described here to link projects with such elements and hope that research funding may develop the vision to encompass large programmes covering such scope in investigation.

- The studies are presented here only briefly and the number of variables investigated may well seem disproportionate to sample sizes. However, the samples and studies are only presented in summary. Each had a different aim in testing the lifespan and intergenerational attachment models and therefore focused on particular types of variables. These are described in more detail in the appendix. By using contextual narrative data, there is always the danger of over-working the quantitative variables utilised because of the rich detail available. This constitutes a difficult balancing act between confirming hypothesised relationships and exploring new linkages. We hope the analyses have stayed within acceptable bounds, but are also aware of our responsibilities with such a unique and costly data set to use it to its full potential.

We will now further explore the attachment models outlined in the course of this book.

11.3 Attachment models

In the introduction to this book, a variety of approaches to investigating adult attachment style were outlined, with potential for developing different models around lifetime development, social experience, stress and parenting. All of these are shown in the findings and clinical cases presented to be relevant to the development and influence of Insecure attachment styles. However, these are varied and complex and operate at different levels of functioning and in different time scales and thus cannot be subsumed in a single attachment model. Below we look at three models of attachment style in relation to clinical disorder, which have been a focus of the analysis presented. Each is limited in its perspective, but selecting three allows for an outline of the three most important aspects of adult attachment style. First a lifespan model to show experience over time whereby Insecure adult attachment is a mediator for adult clinical disorder, second an interactive model focused on an individual's functioning at a single point in time and finally a parenting model to inform intergenerational transmission.

11.3.1 Lifespan model

The approach presented in this book has followed the lifespan in showing how early life experiences relate to those in adolescence and then in later life. In addition it subsumes the stress model with the more detailed differentiation of vulnerability, stress, coping and disorder. A key step in developing a lifespan model is testing for the mediating role of Insecure attachment style between early life maltreatment and later adult disorder. This has been confirmed in prospective study by showing the Insecure styles mediating between a general index of neglect/abuse and emotional disorder (depression or anxiety) outcomes. Whilst additional mediation models with more specificity have not been tested, the general findings from the analysis suggest other pathways from aspects of lack of care or abuse through Anxious, Angry-dismissive or Dual/disorganised styles to a wider range of disorder outcomes. These are shown in Figure 11.2.

The full lifespan model presented in the introduction to this book can be elaborated to include attachment style as a key linking experience for a range of social and psychological risks for clinical disorder. These are represented as different strands, spread across life stages. The model does not differentiate specific experiences through the life course, nor is it tailored to different styles, although this would be an important line of research to further investigate. However further differentiation in the stress part of the model identified on the right-hand side is now possible from this analysis. This has important implications for preventions, interventions and clinical work.

11.3.2 An interactive adult attachment model

From the information contained in this book, an overall model of adult attachment style in relation to levels of functioning is proposed. The model includes four aspects of ongoing functioning: psychological, affect-regulating, social and interpersonal as its cornerstones. These in turn are

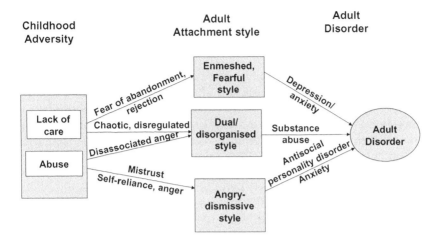

Figure 11.2 Potential attachment style mediating pathways

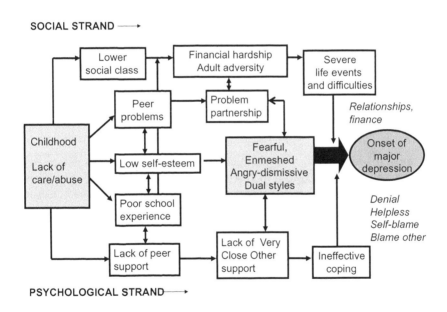

Figure 11.3 Lifespan model of attachment style

informed by specific longer-term childhood maltreatments, biological impairments, social adversity and relationship difficulties. The specific psychological relating biases derived from the internal working model, representing reporting patterns, trust, recognition of need and autonomy together drive the momentum to clinical disorders. The model is represented for each style, beginning with those more resilient. Speculative elements are added from other research approaches, including the biological factors and mentalising function. Here only the most basic acknowledgement to biological function is made, since there are complexities in terms of differentiating forms of system dysfunctions. For example cortisol response to stress is differentiated from cortisol response to awakening, these negatively associated with each other and the former relating to attachment anxiety alone (Quirin, Pruessner *et al.* 2008). Similarly in examining oxytocinergic and dompaninergic systems it is argued that in Insecure Avoidant attachment and prior neglect, there is reduced activation of both systems in response to infant facial cues and to mother–infant contact (Strathearn 2011). Therefore these labels are added to the models as a reminder of the likely contributions once more about biological underpinnings but are not given greater specificity.

We now summarise the key information developed from the analysis for each style with the integrated model presented. We begin with those styles most resilient:

Secure style

The majority of the population have Secure style as healthy attachment development. When combined with those mildy Insecure who share similar characteristics this would account for about three-quarters of the population. The following attributes can be summarised for Secure and mildly Insecure styles and are shown in Figure 11.4:

- Most will also have low levels of **childhood adversity,** although a proportion will be Secure or mildly Insecure despite early life neglect or abuse, due to parallel positive experience in childhood or adolescence (such as support, close to a parent, good school experience). Secure style may also emerge somewhat later due to adult positive relationships.
- Those with Secure/mildly Insecure style have lower rates of **lifetime adversity** and recent severe life events, attain higher social class positions and are thus less exposed to stress.
- These individuals manage to create positive supportive **relationships** both with partners and with close others, with low levels of conflict.
- They show effective coping with stress.
- They have very low rates of NES, and **self-esteem** is in the normal range. It is expected that those Secure will have good mentalising skills.
- Their **parenting** style is generally competent, and expected to be sensitive and attuned.
- **Biological** development is normal with none of the impairments associated with the other styles in HPA or other functions arising from childhood adversity or problem relationships.

- **Reporting style** for those Secure is clear and insightful, suggestive of coherence in their internal working models.
- **Disorder levels** are low for all the above reasons.

Secure Attachment style (and mildly insecure)

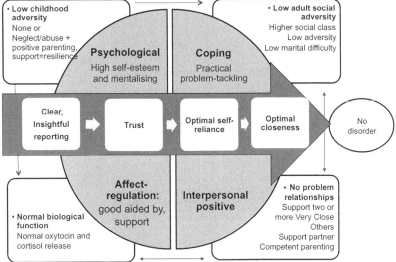

Figure 11.4 Model of Secure Attachment style

Withdrawn style

This is identified as the most detached Insecure attachment style, but actually shows few of the vulnerabilities associated with the other styles (see Figure 11.5). Findings show:

- The key feature is poor ability to make relationships, shown as either a **lack of relationships** or those characterised by indifference.
- There is also evidence of **lower adversity** levels, either in childhood through poor parenting, or in adulthood with fewer difficulties and higher social class position.
- **Coping** is characterised by high self-reliance and practical problem tackling with no negative coping strategies evident.
- There is low perception of personal need and low emotionality with less stated need for confiding with probable deactivated **emotion-regulation**.
- **Self-esteem** is not differentiated as either negative or positive, and may indicate lack of reflective self-function and thus poor mentalising skill.

- **Parenting** behaviour is competent although it would be expected to be distant at times, but also 'unflappable' and calm.
- **Biologically** those Withdrawn may represent those with genetic differentially low susceptibility to the environment and would be expected to have low cortisol levels due to low expression of stress and fewer external stressors but also low oxytocin due to lack of relationships and social contact.
- **Disorder:** They have low disorder levels, little different from those Secure.

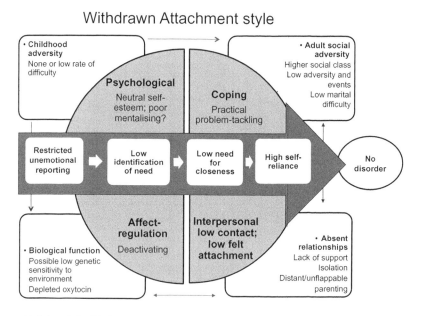

Figure 11.5 Model of Withdrawn attachment style

Enmeshed style

This is categorised as an Anxious style, and is also known as an anxious-ambivalent style in other measurement approaches, to reflect the combined dependency and hostility which can be part of the profile (see Figure 11.6). Findings show:

- In terms of **childhood adversity**, those Enmeshed experience lack of care in childhood, specifically Antipathy often from mother, and experience father separation, but do not report abuse. They experience high levels of **adult adversity** relating to finances, lower social class position, problem partner relationships including domestic violence and more separations/divorces.

- In terms of ongoing **relationships** they are more likely to be married or cohabiting and to be in conflictful partner relationships. They are more likely to have a confidant than any other Insecure style, but their typical description of having many support figures usually involves idealised elements. They have high levels of **parenting incompetence** and anxiety.
- Their **self-esteem** reports tend to be mixed, often fluctuating between negative and very positive statements, but not categorised here as negative. They are likely to be poor mentalisers given their idealised views of others and inattention to important negative aspects of relationships involving danger.
- Their **coping** involves inferred denial but also self-blame and helplessness and thus is not effective at dealing with stressful situations. Often there is an 'over-bright' aspect of being falsely optimistic about change in what appear to be very destructive relationships or situations.
- They have **under-regulated** emotions with hyperactivating in relation to stress and support-seeking. There is likely to be fluctuating oxytocin levels with high cortisol due to stress.
- In terms of **reporting styles,** those with Enmeshed style provide more emotional accounts, and interviews tend to be lengthy, with full narrative, often rambling and switching between time periods and with little spontaneous factual content.

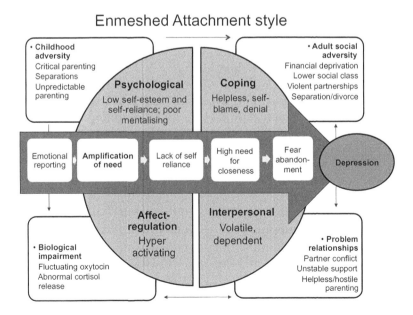

Figure 11.6 Model of Enmeshed adult attachment style

- Key biases arising from the distorted internal working model are amplified in fear of separation/abandonment and low levels of self-reliance, with child-like characteristics.
- **Disorder:** Those with Enmeshed style are prone to depression although rates are not as high as for Fearful styles.

Fearful style

This is also classified as an Anxious style in certain analyses due to the distinctive fear of rejection involved but could equally be considered Avoidant because of behavioural avoidance and mistrust (see Figure 11.7). Findings show:

- **Childhood experiences** indicate the highest rate of both neglect and abuse experiences of all the individual styles. In the younger sample neglect and abuse from mothers was more common than from fathers.
- Those Fearful, also have high rates of **adult adversity** due to lower social class position, higher rates of single parenthood and previous partners having antisocial behaviour.
- In terms of ongoing **relationships** they are less likely to be in a partner relationship and to be single parents but do not have high rates of partner conflict or indifference.
- **Parenting** shows poor competence levels but with helplessness and anxious rather than hostile parenting.
- They have the lowest **self-esteem** of all the styles and present as underconfident and pessimistic. Despite expressing loneliness and greater desire for closeness, their isolation involves a 'harm-reduction' strategy.
- They have high rates of stressful events and their **coping** involves cognitive avoidance as well as helplessness.
- **Emotion-regulation** is noted as deactivating in relation to behavioural avoidance, but coupled with hyperactivating in relation to the anxiety associated with relationships. Biological underpinnings are considered to be the low dopamine associated with abusive childhoods, fluctuating oxytocin associated with the deactivation together with high social need, and high cortisol levels due to stress levels.
- **Reporting style** shows reluctance in reporting and stated inability to recall the past. The biases arising from the internal working model are those involving fearful–mistrust framed as fear of rejection, with behavioural avoidance and suppression of need. Autonomy levels are usually in the normal range.
- In terms of the biases arising from their distorted internal working model, these individuals will be driven by fear of rejection suppression of need and behavioural avoidance.
- **Disorder:** Those with Fearful styles have high rates of depression as well as social anxiety.

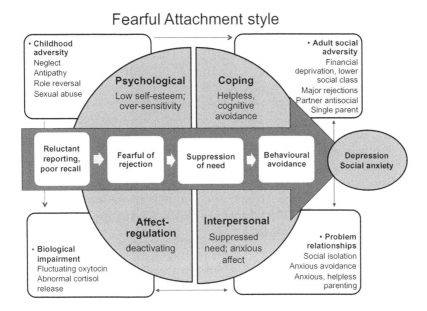

Figure 11.7 Model of Fearful attachment style

Angry-dismissive style

This is an Avoidant, but mistrustful, style with high levels of self-reliance accompanied with high anger towards others (see Figure 11.8). These individuals see the outside world as dangerous, and react with blame and anger. Findings show:

- High rates of **childhood abuse**, particularly physical and psychological abuse.
- **Adult adversity** levels are high, as are ongoing severe life events, and those matched to chronic difficulties.
- Their **coping** styles involve blame of others, anger but also sadness and distress at events.
- **Relationships** involve partnerships with high rates of conflict. Previous partnership involve high rates of separation or divorce and antisocial partners which includes those substance abusing.
- **Self-esteem** was low in the midlife women, which is unexpected since the external attributions of blame could have served to keep self-esteem high. However, this finding did not hold in the Offspring sample suggesting either age or gender effects.

- They had the highest rates of incompetent **parenting** of any of the styles with hostility being a key element although they also rated highly on anxious parenting.
- In terms of **biological** aspects of the style, it was speculated that they would have lower oxytocin levels due to low levels of positive support, low dopamine levels and high levels of cortisol related to their life stressors.
- **Reporting style** is not reluctant, nor emotional, but there is some insistence on inability to recall the past. This does not seem to have influenced the actual reporting of childhood or early life adversity.
- In terms of key biases arising from distorted working models, their view of others is angrily-mistrustful, with over-self-reliance and behavioural avoidance in relationships.
- **Disorder:** Midlife women showed high rates of both Depression and GAD. In the younger sample Angry-dismissiveness was associated with DSH, also with conduct disorder as evidenced by the young people in residential care.

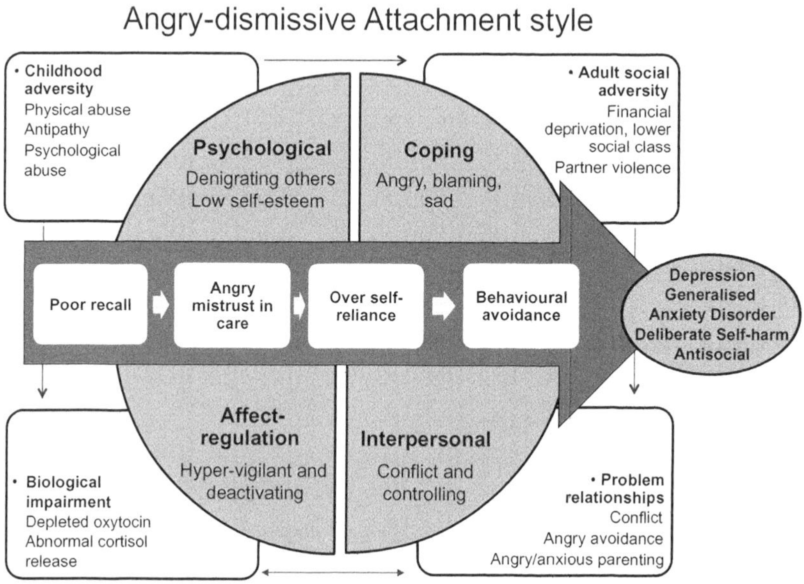

Angry-dismissive Attachment style

Figure 11.8 Model of Angry-dismissive attachment style

Dual or disorganised style

These styles usually contain elements of both Anxious and Avoidant attachment style and are taken to indicate a more disordered attachment strategy (or lack of strategy) when interacting with other people (see

Figure 11.9). The most common combination of style in the analysis reported is Angry-dismissive and Fearful with alternating angry and fearful responses. However, Angry-dismissive and Enmeshed is also found, often denoting possessive and jealous control of close others. Enmeshed and Fearful, although both anxious styles, are also included as Disorganised because of the potential conflict between the Enmeshed desire for closeness and Fearful avoidance. Whilst rare, Enmeshed and Withdrawn is also a possible combination – one observed in other studies of adolescents using the ASI showing problems in individuating from parents with whom they show excessive need for closeness, despite withdrawal from the outside world. Another scenario in adults is Enmeshed dependence on a partner with avoidance of the outside world, this seen in some learning disabled clients. Occasionally there maybe three styles involved with individuals effectively reporting all the negative attitudes with contradictory ratings on self-reliance and desire for company.

Therefore interpreting Dual or disorganised styles can be difficult, and the category itself may mask different types of problem attachment. Thus case material presented earlier supports both unresolved loss issues (for example around death of a child) as well as dissociated anger potentially linked with antisocial personality disorder observable in a few of the young men in the younger sample, as well as adolescents in residential care. At other times when three styles are evident it is possible that no discernible style is present and that 'Can't Classify' or truly disorganised patterns are evident. Those with Dual/disorganised styles tend to have all the negative features in terms of poor relationships, conflict, low self-esteem, stress and poor coping associated with all the other vulnerable attachment styles. Findings show (see Figure 11.9):

- In terms of **childhood adversity**, both lack of care and abuse are present, but in logistic regression models it is the former which takes precedent.
- Their **adult adversity** levels are high and they have lower social class position, high financial difficulties, previous partner separations and partners with antisocial behaviour and substance abuse. They have the highest rates of recent severe life events of all styles.
- Their **coping** is not differentiated by any particular strategy, perhaps due to contradictory elements arising from the style combinations.
- Partner **relationships** are often conflictful and parenting is highly incompetent. This is viewed in the research literature as both 'frightened and frightening' which encompasses the combined angry and fearful styles.
- They also have low **self-esteem** and are speculated as having very poor mentalising skills with dissociated anger which can be explosive.
- In **biological** terms it is expected that there is greater fluctuation of different contributing elements including oxytocin and dopamine, with high cortisol levels due to stress.

- Their **reporting style** is contradictory.
- Similarly their cognitive biases in relating derived from distorted working models include which involve intermittent approach/avoidance and contradictory reports of self-reliance.
- They have higher rates of comorbid, or combined **disorders**, although their rates of depression are no higher than those with singly Insecure styles. In the young sample, this style was uniquely associated with substance abuse.

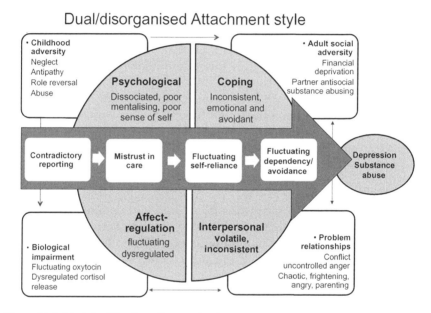

Figure 11.9 Model of Dual or disorganised attachment style

Therefore it can be seen that each style has specific 'doses' of childhood or adult adversity, of biological impairment as well as differential relationship and coping styles. The emotion-regulation also differs with extremes of Withdrawn being most highly regulated to Dual/disorganised the least regulated.

One of the issues that arises from such model development and detailed information in this book, is that the simplified Anxious/Avoidant dichotomy is not sufficient to explain the patterning of behaviours and attitudes involved in adult Insecure attachment styles. Whilst at one extreme Withdrawn can be said to be truly Avoidant, and at the other Enmeshed to have truly anxious-ambivalent elements, the two remaining styles, which carry higher levels of risk for disorder and childhood adversity (Fearful and Angry-dismissive) both have avoidant, emotional and even ambivalent characteristics which do not perfectly fit in to Anxious and Avoidant categories. Thus Fearful style has anxious attitudes and behaviourally avoidant characteristics but if a clear strategy for harm-avoidance easily distinguishable from the more chaotic Dual/disorganised style. Angry-dismissive style has behavioural avoidance, but the anger and need for control in relationships and distressed coping suggests more ambivalent underpinnings. Differential social experience in relation to neglect or abuse, to type of partner relationship and type of parenting, are shown to illustrate different attachment style categories. Anger and fear are key components, in addition to the approach-avoidant dimensions.

11.3.3 Intergenerational models

Poor experiences in partnership, parenting, attachment style and clinical disorder are all implicated in the intergenerational transmission of risk for neglect/abuse of children, children's Insecure attachment style and their disorder. Research around parenting of infants and attachment insecurity has argued that the transmission of insecurity across generations is through maternal insensitivity, intrusive or detached interaction and poor emotional regulation when engaging with the child (De Wolff and van Ijzendoorn 1997). Further research using a family systems approach has shown that mother and father's attachment representations, quality of relationships and parenting style provide the best fit for explaining internalising and externalising behaviour in offspring respectively but with the quality of the partner relationship proving central in models of women's affective disorder. The mechanisms through which this occurs can be due to an absent partner through the increased burden of sole parenting, or the added burden of a partner with unpredictable behaviour related to alcohol use, antisocial disorder or poor work history. Family discord, domestic violence from the father and physical abuse from father are as key for disorder in the offspring as the direct parenting behaviour of the mother (Bifulco, Moran *et al.* 2009).

To indicate how Insecure attachment styles can transmit risk across the generations through parenting and care of children, the model in Figure 11.10 sums up information covered in this book. It shows that mechanisms of transmission are through problem parenting which is the result of the confluence of Insecure style from both parents, conflict or indifference in their relationship, social adversity and parental psychological disorder. The insensitive parenting known to arise from Insecure styles is shown to escalate into neglect or abuse of the child when the other factors are present in families under stress and suffering disorder. Thus all aspects need ideally to be assessed when calculating dangers to children living in such households.

A positive aspect, however, is that there is no direct link between an individual's own neglect/abuse in childhood and that of their children – associations only develop through updated risk and adult vulnerability,

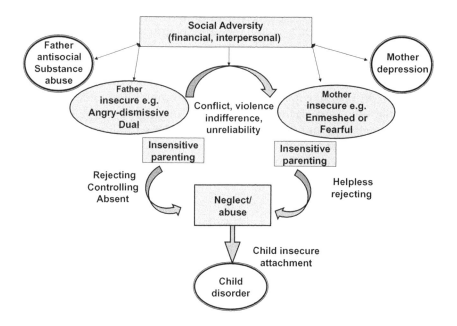

Figure 11.10 Intergenerational model

including Insecure attachment style, partner relationships (see earlier Figures 6.1 and 6.2). The other positive factor is that only a proportion of individuals with Insecure attachment style have problem parenting behaviour. There is substantial scope for resilience in choice of partner as well as in averting the stress conditions under which parenting becomes abusive.

Finally some implications of the material presented in this book are addressed.

11.4 The importance of Fear and Anger in attachment

The ASI is unique in not only questioning about relationships with romantic partners and close support figures but also questioning closely about attitudes such as anger, fear of rejection, fear of separation and low self-reliance indicative of Insecure attachment to arrive at categorisation of attachment style. Unlike other measures it has the capacity not only for keying into the attitudes but also for determining the intensity with which such attitudes come to determine the degree of insecurity. The intensity of attitudes thus indicates the degree to which marital interaction difficulties and poor support access can contribute to the level of insecurity with impacts for the whole family and thus indicate risk for family discord and offspring disorder. Key behavioural markers are high conflict in partner and other close relationships, and attitudes underpinned by high anger or fear states. Such emotional states in relation to others hold high risks for parental psychological disorder, social isolation, marital conflict and family break-up. In the analysis reported earlier, marked and moderate levels of Insecure styles were categorised together, partly because of low numbers in the former, but also because of similar associations with risk and disorder variables. However, differentiating those most impaired within such styles may prove important for differentiating other disorders such as personality disorders. To date there has been no investigation of the ASI and personality disorder, but it may well prove to constitute a 'subclinical' threshold for such disorders, useful in community study and practice.

The opportunity to identify intensity of anger and fear states is not similarly presented in other measures of adult attachment. Transmission of attachment insecurity through maternal insensitivity, as emphasised in research related to other measures of adult attachment, highlights an inability to be optimally cooperative and collaborative in responding to infant and childhood developmental need but it fails to capture a more fine-grained understanding of how such insensitivity is behaviourally expressed and experienced by the child. Key is how such intense attitudes not only guide behaviour but also contribute to an emotional environment in which anger and fear may become inextricably interwoven into a climate of hostility and harsh and punitive care that perpetuates fearfulness and anger in partner and offspring. The category of Dismissiveness in the AAI for example is arrived at when the respondent minimally acknowledges negative affect or denies any personal sense of agency in relationships, whereas Preoccupied reflects an ongoing preoccupation with early parental attention and care accompanied by anger and ambivalence related to past relationships. By contrast, categorisation of attachment style by way of ASI assessment provides a here-and-now profile of vulnerability, lack of support and isolation or conflict. In highlighting the corrosive presence of high anger or high fear or both, potentially in two parents, as contributing to an emotional climate characterised by conflict, or fear in the home, it points to increases in risk for abuse, neglect discord and, family breakdown and transmission of risk for disorder outcome.

Identification of the intense attitudes, specifically heightened fear and anger states, which contribute to increased risks of conflict and volatility in the home environment and thus have a direct causal relationship to poor parenting and to perpetuating cycles of familial dysfunction and disorder, offers an opportunity for breaking the cycle of poor environmental management and regulation. The parent whose early life is characterised by poor care and instability, with no network of support, and whose subsequent relating style is characterised by anger or fear states is not able to effectively parent. The scope for assessment of the behavioural and attitudinal factors that influence parenting capacity which in more extreme conditions lead to early abuse and neglect holds promise for intervening with the perpetuating cycles of early deprivation of care, insensitive responsiveness to expressed need, abuse, neglect, domestic violence, marital breakdown and social instability. Anger and fearfulness add further risks for depression which further blunts the capacity for responding to the child. Increasing awareness in the child of parental vulnerability consequently necessitates the development of a strategic response of need to emotionally withdraw or behaviourally control so as to maintain a basic level of environmental safety leading to attachment insecurity and so the cycle continues.

The implications such inadequate care has for children's neurological development and physiological regulation have been the focus of the work of neuropsychological attachment scientists such as Alan Shore, Bruce Perry and Bessel van der Kolk, and has highlighted poor development of empathy as an outcome of impaired early development with further risks for maltreatment and traumatising environments in which developmental windows to develop healthy attachments and emotion regulation abilities may be lost forever.

Inability to access support networks due to heightened withdrawal and isolation resulting from high fear or anger states, with high mistrust as a dominant emotion, indicates a trajectory leading to dysfunction, poor mental health and disorder with inevitable risks for the perpetuation of further cycles of damage.

Assessment of the behavioural and psychological functioning of adults in terms of attachment relationships, in social work as well as in psychological health contexts, offers scope for breaking such a cycle in which poorly regulated emotional environments dominated by anger, fear, hostility and withdrawal form the cornerstones for poor developmental outcome, neurological impairment and poor mental health.

11.5 Attachment style in parents and child disorders

The analysis and discussion presented in this book has not covered child disorders. Whilst adolescent disorders have been discussed, there are additional disorders prevalent in younger children, notably ADHD but also anxiety disorder associated with separation anxiety and school refusal. Assessment of parental attachment style may contribute important information about the parental style used to help the infant or child regulate their emotions to avoid such symptoms. In the UK 10–20% of school-aged children experience emotional and behavioural difficulties (Meltzer, Gatward *et al.* 2000). Pre-pubertal boys are more likely to have problem behaviours than girls, and the prevalence of mental illness is greater among children living within disrupted families and those in disadvantaged areas (op cit). With such prevalent disorders as ADHD for example, the contribution of parental attachment style may be better understood when the relational style of the dyad is approached in the light of parental rejection, avoidance or dependency and capacity for positive and negative quality of interactions. The attitudes parents draw on in relationships and whether these are likely to be guided by highly negative attachment attitudes and whether mother–infant transactions are likely to be coloured by maternal avoidance, or high dependency needs add to them. Understanding of maternal attachment style and may help to better target prevention and intervention efforts.

ADHD is defined on the basis of developmentally inappropriate inattention, motor activity and impulsivity, causing impairment in social and academic functioning and is one of the most frequently diagnosed forms of externalising psychopathology in child psychiatry with prevalence rates ranging from 3–9% in normal populations (Spencer, Biederman *et al.* 2002). Its frequency has led to controversy regarding aetiology, pathological validity and treatment. One study to date has examined the distribution of attachment quality in children with ADHD (Clarke, Ungerer *et al.* 2002) and only one has looked at parental attachment representations (Kissgen, Krischer *et al.* 2009). Clinical findings emphasise similitude between attachment disorders and ADHD. Parental caregiving, including maternal sensitivity and positive parenting practices has been shown to be associated with better outcomes in ADHD children.

Empirical research is growing in investigating the association between attachment insecurity and ADHD, with a focus on where impairment in self-regulation in ADHD children may have its roots in strained early caregiver–child interactions and disrupted primary attachments (Olson, Roese *et al.* 1996; Clarke, Ungerer *et al.* 2002). Deficits in self-regulation, including impulse control, self-soothing, patience, and inhibition, feature prominently in ADHD symptomatology and involve a generalised difficulty in integrating cognitive, affective and motor functions (Barkley 1997). Similarly, many childhood emotional and behavioural problems are rooted in dysregulation difficulties leading to externalising and internalising emotional and behavioural manifestations. Most children referred during the primary school age are referred for difficulties that are likely to be associated with parenting style associated with parental attachment style.

11.5.1 Attachment, child development and education

Research investigating the link between children's emotional and developmental performance at school has highlighted the association between poor scholastic performance and insecurity of attachment to mothers (Barrett and Trevitt 1991). The basic tenets of attachment theory, as elaborated and illustrated in the previous chapters, hold that inconsistent, uncaring or hostile parenting in the early years of life have long-lasting consequences for future relating style and adjustment (Fraley and Waller 1998; Fraley, Davis *et al.* 1998). We now also know how influential they continue to be throughout life in the formation of social relationships and, importantly, how behaviour outside the family continues to reflect relationship expectations developed in early parent childcare experiences.

Not only are children who experience insensitive care likely to develop little capacity for anticipating help in regulating their negative arousal and have corresponding difficulty in regulating their emotions, there is evidence that insensitive parental behaviours can themselves be negatively arousing and interfere with the child's developing capacity to regulate arousal (Cummings and Davies 2002).

Reasons for referral in the primary school years may include difficulty with school work, concentrating and remembering but often such impairments are underpinned by anxiety, nervousness, agitation, easily aroused anger, verbal or physical aggressiveness, defiance and oppositionality. More extreme behaviours are also seen in hyper-vigilance, startle reactions, lying, stealing, breaking things, disregard for rules, difficulty with friendships, detachment, non-engagement and inappropriate behaviours. Each of these also reflects aspects of Avoidant, Anxious or Disorganised attachment strategies developed to ensure a sense of safety and protection in an unstable context. In approaching work with such emotional and behavioural manifestations of attachment-related difficulties, assessment of the degree of security of the parental attachment style may help to better target prevention and intervention efforts.

Most referrals to services are for six- to ten-year-old boys who present with disruptive and angry behaviours, who regularly become embroiled in playground fights, and have poor peer relationships. Angry ambivalent 'externalising' behaviour, characterised by negativity, hostility and defiance, including hyperactivity, non-compliance and aggression, represents the largest reason for referring boys who exhibit acting out behaviours (Offord, Boyle *et al.* 1992). 'Internalising' behaviours in which emotional arousal in situations of fear or anger is inhibited, results in anxiety, depression and withdrawal. Most referrals for those who are overly silent, nervous or withdrawn tend to be for girls. Nevertheless, withdrawn children equally experience difficulties with peer relationships (Rubin and Mills 1988). Both threaten the ability to access the curriculum and, more importantly, get in the way of educational achievement as part of healthy emotional development.

On the positive side, research findings presented earlier show that when children from adverse family backgrounds do well at school this can have considerable positive impact on their subsequent functioning and life course. This works not only through structure provided by well-run schools, but also through learning experience and the impact of this on the child's self-esteem. The school environment can provide a lot of opportunities which can be missing from home life. This includes opportunities for friendships, adult support, developing social roles and the confidence from achieving. Clearly if the inhibitions which can arise from Insecure attachment styles and poor emotional functioning in early years can be overcome in the school environment then the benefits for later development can be substantial.

11.6 Attachment style in child and family services

We have also aimed to highlight the highly valuable contribution of assessment of attachment style to the adoption and fostering field and child Safeguarding. Identification of characteristics of prospective carers in terms of both stable supportive relationships and parenting capacity is viewed as critical in practice guidelines (DfES 2006) The former is required to provide a consistent caring context for the child being placed, as well as to sustain the carers under the stress often induced by the demands of the carer role. The latter is to ensure adequate parenting capacity in caring for, and relating to, the child being placed, who will often have specific and complex developmental needs. Accurate assessment of support networks and quality of relationships is not only relevant for suitability for placement. It is also an assessment of likely support requirements post-placement in those accepted as adoptive parents. Thus where support networks or individual relationships, or support-seeking capacity looks fragile, these elements can be aided through additional service provision through direct social work intervention, support groups, befriending or other schemes. Supportive context is relatively fluid, and amenable both to erosion under change in context, but also to enhancement through use of appropriate intervention. Being forewarned about such likelihoods makes for better provision and utilisation of service-based support during future crises.

11.6.1 Matching for adoption

Much of the focus in the adoption–fostering field has been on the potential parenting capacity of the new carers and the psychological 'match' between their characteristics and those of the child to be placed. The preoccupation with matching has at times considerably delayed the adoptive process with the result that the parental candidates have been intrusively if not exhaustively assessed and the children have missed important developmental windows for attachment. Yet attachment style in parents provides those in search of an as yet elusive-matching tool with considerable material for hypothesising about a best-fit match.

In addition to the well-established findings that the ASI accurately measures supportive contexts and ability to access support among parents, its role in matching (for example to child attachment style or type of behaviour) or to the carer's relationship with the child post-placement is not currently established. But the information about the parental contribution to the family climate already serves to potentially add further to the measures usefulness. While the ASI does not measure parenting styles, research has firmly established that moderately and markedly Insecure attachment styles are associated with more problematic parenting. In addition the PRI, is now increasingly used alongside the ASI in identifying parenting incompetence to show this mechanism in operation and to help services to identify not only where problems in parenting may lie but also importantly how parents see themselves in their parenting role. Often there is clear lack of insight into the parenting difficulties.

More specific is the ability to infer parenting aspects from the attachment style characteristics. It is likely that high levels of anger are problematic for all relationships, however, those with highly Angry-dismissive features will likely also be overly controlling, punitive, hostile and too critical with children. Children who have been in care and who are required to accommodate to new adoptive environments in which they will need to gradually develop trust in the care they are offered, will be already sensitive to anger, critical parenting and hostility. If these are re-experienced, they are likely to trigger highly aroused and fearful reactions and activate severe behavioural responses, indicative of the parents not being experienced as safe, with the added risk that the child may be re-traumatised.

For highly Insecure Enmeshed styles, lack of autonomy and fear of separation in the parent may give cause for concern with regard to role reversal and parentification, with the child having to attend to the parent's needs. For highly Insecure Fearful styles, parenting that is overly anxious and preoccupied with rejection and the parent's own worries and sensitivities rather than a more appropriate involvement with the child's issues can be expected. Such parents may also be over protective and stifling. With those markedly Insecure Withdrawn there may be lack of affection and insistence on privacy and boundaried space, making the parent inaccessible and distant with the child while also expecting too much autonomy in the child and giving too little nurturance. All styles will have an issue about providing suitable emotion regulation and appropriate soothing when distressed.

When the ASI is used in child and family or therapeutic services, feedback to clients would usually emphasise resilient aspects such as sociability, sensitivity or authoritativeness as positive elements of the style. The negative aspects have already been outlined. Thus one aim of therapy or intervention would be to move individuals with a 'moderately' Enmeshed style, to one at least 'mildly' Enmeshed since this does not hold the same risk. In other words the individual does not have to abandon all characteristics of the style which may be in part temperamentally based but needs to modify them such that relationships are more stable and supportive and fear of separation is modified with autonomy aspects (desire for company and low self-reliance) adjusted. There has been speculation among practitioners working in adoption or fostering care, that for purposes of matching the carer with child, those with mild levels of Enmeshed style may be suitable for caring for children who require high levels of nurturing and who may not experience this as intrusive. For example children with disabilities who may not develop age-appropriate levels of autonomy which can be seen by the carer as rejecting. This premise needs further development and testing.

Each of the style characteristics will also have specific sensitivity and reactivity to the child's style. A Fearful parent, sensitive to rejection is unlikely to be robust enough to stand up to an angry and controlling child. An Enmeshed parent with high dependency needs and fear of separation will find a withdrawn and isolating child a very great challenge and will find an older child's developmental need for autonomy and preference for peer relationships both provocative of anger and anxiety.

11.6.2 Working with the different styles

Some general points can be made about working with clients with the different styles in child and family or therapeutic practice. Since Secure styles are those with the best relating style, have best coping with stress and clarity in their reporting and descriptions of stress, these are not separately differentiated. However, for a practitioner to acknowledge that an individual undergoing adversity and difficulties does have a Secure style is likely to aid good adjustment and appropriate intervention.

Withdrawn styles: This has proved to be a generally resilient style despite having remoteness from close others with low need for both company and support. Such styles may be more common in men than in women. Discussion with practitioners about their role as prospective adopters, whilst acknowledging their resilience to stress, sometimes invokes concerns about potential lack of warmth in parenting and the lack of a social network to create stress-buffering effects and practical support. However, when a couple present for adoption with the main carer Secure and the second carer Withdrawn, this is frequently seen as an acceptable combination for further exploration of adoption suitability. In terms of feedback to clients, the detached nature of the style is also described in terms of the associated independence and good coping. Direct work would be around increasing sensitivity to others emotional states and developing more social contact.

Enmeshed styles: In terms of working with individuals with Enmeshed styles in services, feedback involves emphasising more reality-orientated view of relationships and stressors in an attempt to counter-act the idealising which is common. This also requires bolstering of self-esteem likely to plummet when the reality of a negative situation is realised. Interventions will also involve increasing autonomy and reducing dependence, improving coping strategies around self-blame and denial. It will also involve working on partner relationships to reduce conflict and increase communication. In terms of parenting it will require asserting authority rather than wanting to be 'friends' with the childen. In terms of matching such carers with children in adoption services, it is considered best to match with children who are needy, such as babies or those with disability, and who will not have strong needs for independence and separation.

Fearful styles: In terms of working with individuals with Fearful styles in services, feedback involves emphasising positive characteristics of sensitivity to others' moods and feelings. Interventions will often be around raising self-esteem as well as assertiveness and moderating levels of fear of rejection. It should be noted that those with Fearful styles are very aware of their own fearfulness which may make engagement in interventions easier. In terms of matching such carers with children in adoption services, it is considered important not to match with children who are hostile and rejecting since this will be very difficult and punishing for such carers.

Angry-dismissive styles: In terms of working with individuals with Angry-dismissiveness in services, feedback can emphasise positive characteristics of assertiveness and authority. However, they can present with a lack of insight into their own anger, often presenting as victims rather than people who can be quite frightening to others, particularly children. Therefore, challenges in intervention can be around increasing insight into their own aggression. As parents they can be very hostile and punitive. In terms of matching carers to children for adoption purposes with mild levels of Angry-dismissive style, children who require structure and authority from parents may fit best.

Dual/disorganised styles: In terms of services and interventions it is considered that those with Dual/disorganised styles are not suitable as carers for children in adoption or fostering, and this style occurs commonly amongst abusive parents who are being assessed in child protection services. In terms of engagement, there is likely to be a lack of insight into their own aggression and their inability to relate to others or to parent. This style is likely to require substantial intervention to move to higher functioning attachment. In residential care some of the young people assessed changed over time to a single Insecure style which was taken as improvement and potentially more amenable to further intervention.

11.6.3 Feedback to clients

Sharing therapeutic formulations with the prospective carers in adoption–fostering services, or more widely in clinical services can act as a psycho-educational tool. This can help develop awareness of how thoughts, feelings and behaviours are related to beliefs about the self, others and the world and to identify, evaluate and challenge cognitive biases and those emerging from Insecure attachment styles. In this way it is possible to share with the client both strengths and vulnerabilities for each style and demonstrate how strengths are linked to increasing access to support. Importantly sharing the findings with the client which are derived from evidence provided to transparent questions about support, behaviour and attitudes, offers scope for the forging of a strong therapeutic alliance in the process of joint formulation, further enhancing a trusting therapeutic partnership in which beliefs and thoughts can be challenged. In identifying the absence of supportive relationships, access to these can be facilitated through group work and network based activities which may be lacking due to behavioural avoidance.

11.7 New opportunities for clinical assessment

Assessment of Attachment Style in adults and adolescents also contributes critical understanding of personal, interpersonal and family functioning to support evaluation of therapeutic need and enlighten therapeutic assessment and practice.

Current pre-clinical assessment for depression and for informing obstacles to therapeutic success for instance relies on a Cognitive Behavioural model of depression (Beck 1967) to formulate the client's difficulties. In proposing that early life experiences lead individuals to form assumptions or schemas about themselves in the world, which in turn influence how they perceive and respond to their experiences (Hawton, Salkovskis *et al.* 1989) draws on approaches stating that early adaptive schemas remain open to development during childhood, but may become rigid and maladaptive in later life. Critical incidents can trigger unhelpful schemas, and activate Negative Automatic Thoughts (NATs) about the self, the world, and the future and may contribute to symptoms of depression which, in turn, reinforce these same NATs. Depressed individuals show cognitive biases in their information processing which are likely to confirm unhelpful beliefs (Beck *et al.* 1988). The negative cognitive triad involving the self, the world and the future (low self-esteem, helplessness and hopelessness) in persistent depression is underpinned by unconditional beliefs, tacitly held as unquestionable truths, which guide the processing of information in a prejudicial fashion and which cluster around two common themes: weakness ('I am inadequate') and unacceptability ('I am unlovable') (Padesky 1994).

An attachment perspective on such themes as 'I am inadequate' and 'I am unlovable' would demonstrate such feelings to be linked to Fearful attachment style in which confidence is lacking due to a belief that the self is not likeable or lovable. This leads to the belief that once the individual's true self is exposed rejection is inevitable. Closeness to other is avoided because of feelings of inadequacy and inferiority and the anticipation that rejection and betrayal of trust is imminent. Trust in relationships, therefore, is low and closeness avoided, not by choice but by necessity, as a means of protecting the self from further hurt. For other attachment styles the patterning is more complex. For those Enmeshed, feeling unlovable oscillates with feeling special, and for those Angry-dismissive feelings of being unlovable is masked by denigration of others to moderate self-esteem levels.

In both approaches early life experiences are hypothesised to have contributed to the development of schema that influence such negative appraisals, however, the Fearfulness that colours the schema can remain unidentified. Whereas a CB model identifies how parental verbal abuse or disorder will have contributed to the client's beliefs about him or herself as inferior and incompetent and as contributing to the patient shying away from confrontations, a support-based attachment perspective will contribute to a perspective on behavioural vulnerability and risk in highlighting core avoidant constructs: constraints on closeness and inhibition of feelings for fear that the client would be rejected or high negative attitudes: fear of rejection meaning that needs cannot be met as a result of withdrawal

In the CB model the client is likely to demonstrate compensatory Safety-Seeking Behaviours (SSBs) such as not expressing his or her own needs and avoiding social situations and work in order to prevent negative core beliefs being confirmed. Thus the client avoids social situations to avoid being rejected. By avoiding social situations anticipated feelings of humiliation are avoided. Such a client is likely to become increasingly isolated seeking access to a limited social group. Identification of the fear that contributes to the harm-avoidance strategy for those Fearful involving mistrust and constraints on closeness and fearing rejection, can aid therapeutic processing of the precursors of this attachment style and can illustrate how the inability to trust in particular, can lead to further withdrawal, isolation, low self-esteem and depression.

Combating a world seen as hostile with anger, is an alternative strategy to protect the self from harm and rejection. There are two Insecure styles which use anger: Angry-dismissive and those ambivalent Enmeshed. Differences between the two are related to the radically different sense of autonomy – for Angry-dismissive there is only reliance on the self; for Enmeshed there is solely reliance on others. So the level of need for others is different, but conflict arises similarly in those relationships considered close. In both cases the anger proves to be linked to anxiety. For those Angry-dismissive the high risk of anxiety disorder suggests the anger masks deeper feelings of anxiety, particularly around loss of control and is likely to have its origins in childhood experience of powerlessness, leading to vulnerability and victimisation in abusive contexts. For the Enmeshed it is when needs are not met that the anger shows itself linked to high and unfulfilled neediness. For those Dual/disorganised, the hostility shown is often dissociated from cognitive processing of feelings of anger, and can appear as impulsive and violent. Anger is thus a critical aspect of attachment style running parallel to fear and needs identifying in CB models.

Obstacles to accessing treatment often impede the ability to overcome the depressed individual's overwhelming sense of hopelessness and belief that nothing will change. Enhanced understanding of the behavioural constraints on closeness to others, lack of trust and fear of rejection will contribute to understanding of the client's reluctance or inability to engage in and trust the relational process implicit in therapeutic intervention.

Assessment of attachment style enables detailed understanding of the core constructs that contribute to the clients' profile and whether this is coloured by anger or fear, or by unmet high dependency needs. Identification of feelings in relation to victimisation can usefully address how such feelings do not reflect a reality of the self as being unworthy and unlovable but that such feelings can be attributed to the experience of the cruelty and inadequacy of others and how early templates or internal working models developed in response to inadequate care continue to contribute to the view of the self as not being worthy to receive love, care and attention.

The often unconscious conflicts and defences that develop in response to attachment difficulties and failures are often beyond the scope of cognitive behavioural work. As has been demonstrated in the previous chapters, abusive parental relationships contribute to disturbances of mood and self-identity and the capacity to deal with emotional arousal. Lack of adequate caregiving contributes to the experience of the subsequent loss of an attachment bond in a way that further impedes the formation of adaptive and mutually supportive and security-enhancing attachments. The experience of profound helplessness arises as a result of a bias in interpreting loss as a failure to make stable relationships that reinforces a sense of failure and inadequacy. A model of the self as unlovable and inadequate and the expectation of others as rejecting, hostile and punitive becomes rigid and unchallengeable. The actual loss of a relationship confirms the belief that the individual cannot remedy the situation and is doomed to failure (Bowlby, 1980). Avoidance of such emotional issues through fear is difficult to work with unless this is tackled from a knowledge base that is shared by the therapist and client. Transparent assessment reduces the need for cognitive avoidance of such key constraining emotions and can usefully contribute to challenge a client's NATs and enhance therapeutic work with their core beliefs. In this way assessment of attachment style contributes a much-needed dimension to other existing clinical interviews aimed at assessing the client's or patient's current functioning in terms of risks and resilience. In addition, such assessment aids clear understanding of the lifespan and relational factors that have contributed to poor self-identity, low self-esteem and mood disturbance with an enhanced perspective on how such templates have become established as well as on the psychological impairments that continue to drive behavioural avoidance or over-dependence.

There is scope for adding adult attachment assessments into a range of individual and family interventions and therapies. The linkage to child maltreatment, whether in the early years of the adults concerned or in the recent experience of children in services is a critical part of both understanding Insecure attachment styles and in effecting interventions. The Common Elements Framework is a new approach to conceptualising clinical practice in terms of generic components cutting across different treatment protocols to focus on clinical procedures common to evidence-based practice (Chorpita and Daleiden 2009). Its premise is that common or non-specific features of treatment (such as therapist personal qualities, therapeutic alliance, client's expectations) have equally beneficial effects. An integrative framework is used to help encapsulate relevant elements to improve therapeutic treatment practice across different models. In a similar way common elements of assessment for different outcomes can be utilised, with measures of adult attachment style for example being used effectively in a range of intervention modes.

11.8 Conclusion

Since the earliest efforts several decades ago, to observe, classify and understand attachment security and insecurity and their psychological and behavioural manifestations, both theory and practice have undergone directional change and conceptual revision. Since Bowlby's original observations on the impact of maternal deprivation and felt security, and Ainsworth's work on classifying patterns in children, more than half a century of rigorous research and clinical application has required a refocusing of the lens through which attachment is viewed, assessed and analysed. This has led to important investigation of attachment styles in adults and how this affects functioning in relationships and increases vulnerability to psychological disorder as well as its impact on parenting and intergenerational transmission, as developed in this book. Further linkages can be made to cognitive-emotional responses, for example in the capacity for mentalisation and self-reflective function in the recognition and awareness of separate mental states (Allen and Fonagy 2006). Also, the importance of affect-regulation in response to stress and the soothing effects of positive support in adults have been shown to be key attachment benefits, these contrasted to the problematic impacts of either avoidance or anxious approach to others resulting in further amplifying emotion or shutting it off to the detriment of coping, both also having implications for help-seeking in general and service-utilisation. The field has expanded to examine physical health outcomes of those with Insecure styles to the experience and control of diabetes (Ciechanowski, Russo *et al.* 2006) including doctor–patient communication, recognition of the seriousness of the condition and following treatment regimes. Significant further developments have been in the biological domain, such as revealing mechanisms by which early attachment experience may contribute to behavioural genetics and epigenetics (Suomi 2005; Meaney 2001), HPA axis regulation, shape of brain structure and function (van der Kolk 2003; Perry 2008). Attachment theory is now more than ever a truly integrative theory, an umbrella under which detailed bio-psychosocial models can be developed and elaborated.

Measurement of attachment phenomena has also undergone change and innovation, and has expanded to encompass the manifestations of different aspects of attachment behaviour to develop more complex models about development and experience at different life stages and at bio-psychosocial levels. From the earliest assessments of infant and maternal behaviour, measures of adult attachment style have contributed to an increasingly expanding understanding of the social and behavioural correlates and effects, and the way in which early relationships play a part in the causation of family, social and psychiatric problems. Such measures use a range of techniques, those behavioural (such as the classic SST but also the Global Rating Scales of mother–infant interaction), projective (such as the children's Story Stem measure), verbal (through interviews including the AAI, which is also the basis for Self-Reflective function and the ASI outlined in this book) or self-report and cursory measures.

Whilst all these measures tackle different manifestations of attachment behaviour at different ages, key underlining elements of attachment style manifestation are the basic Secure, Insecure-Anxious, Insecure-Avoidant and Disorganised classifications. These have somewhat different definitions and labels in various measures, are more or less dimensional and vary in their incorporation of interpersonal anger and fear in addition to autonomy and approach-avoidance issues. But all adult measures seek associations with childhood adverse relationships, concurrent problems in self-esteem or self-identity and seek to show adult repetitions of dysfunctional childhood relationship patterns in later close attachments with partners, close friends and children. This book has sought to introduce the ASI to a wider audience as a practical assessment tool which can be used to aid future development of both research and practice through a social and lifespan approach to clinical disorder.

Attachment style and behaviour are now understood to encompass aspects of interpersonal functioning that range from relatively simple observable dyadic behaviours and narrated attitudes, to complex interpersonal interactions and neurobiological transactions, each of which has far-reaching implications for the formation and perpetuation of optimal or dysfunctional patterns of relating. Its reach is extensive, for example in further outlining risky or protective contexts to which genetics and behaviour may respond with divergent biological sensitivity (Ellis and Boyce 2008). With each strand of research new insights have emerged into the origins of behaviours in early relationships as well as predictive understanding of the ongoing implications for disorders at different ages or conversely in the ability to thrive in spite of adverse and challenging conditions.

Thus recent attachment and psycho-biological research (Bakermans-Kranenburg and van IJzendoorn 2007; Ellis and Boyce 2008; Suomi 2008) has contributed to the 'genetic vulnerability model' proposing that certain gene variants increase susceptibility to clinical disorders potentially through mechanisms related to attachment development and insecurity. A transactional model has been proposed in which genetic risk is understood as genetic sensitivity to environmental adversity. In reviewing genetic vulnerability within the context of negative environmental experience, a new 'plasticity' hypothesis is proposed for genetic sensitivity (Belsky, Bakermans-Kranenburg *et al.* 2007). Whereas in the context of toxic environments and poor parenting genetic sensitivity dooms the child to failure and poor behavioural and mental health outcomes, in the context of more positive and nurturing environments 'genetic risk' can be reconceptualised as 'possibility' for developing successful and optimal outcomes. However, such lack of plasticity may also incur resilience as seen in those with Withdrawn styles who may lack the permeability in relation to adverse environments which helps protect them from the negative impact.

The implications for attachment theory, and assessment of its dynamic and environmental shortcomings, are potentially far-reaching in such an adaptive and evolutionary model. There is scope for identifying factors that cause genetic frailty and those that can contribute to optimal environments suited to the particular genetic needs of those who have responded negatively to their early experience of adversity. It has been argued that heightened genetic sensitivity to early adversity, leading to symptoms of pathology, may in fact be critical to resilience in other challenging situations. The 'plasticity' hypothesis thus argues that vulnerability can in fact be strength given the right environment. The role of 'risk alleles', gene variants responsible for an increased likelihood of developing certain behaviours, is already being used to investigate responsivity of ADHD children to different environments (Bakermans-Kranenburg and van IJzendoorn 2007). Already critical has been research demonstrating that intervention is more efficacious with those who have risk alleles than with those who have protective alleles, thus reinforcing the hypothesis that what constitutes risk in one environment may in fact constitute possibility and strength in another.

Thirty years ago, attachment theory was seen to have come of age with authoritative publications and handbooks of attachment, as well as diverse academic and professional courses of study. Today, in its maturity, new levels of understanding of attachment invites reflection and acceptance that, indeed, attachment is multi-layered and has many meanings. Such reflection is particularly necessary in light of new methods of enquiry into neurobiological processes and genetic underpinnings of attachment and mechanisms in regulating physiological and neurological processes which underlie the behavioural manifestations familiar to psychosocial researchers and clinicians.

The method of enquiry that has guided the writing of this book has followed a particular strand of social and lifespan psychology, focused on adult attachment style as exhibited through constraints in relating in both partner relationships and wider social support access and clinical disorder outcomes, and relies on research that continues to emphasise the need for examining the part Insecure attachment style plays in causing family dysfunction and increased risk for intergenerational transmission of psychopathology. Central to this has been the development of the ASI, an easily undertaken interview that takes around an hour to administer and around two hours to score from the recorded interview, as a relatively user-friendly tool capable of reliably categorising adult attachment style as well as descriptive categorisation of partner, family and close friendships and their supportiveness. It gives a clear assessment of the current context and behaviour in relationships, has shown associations with adverse childhood experiences and has proved predictive of future disorder and relationship difficulty.

Unlike the 'state of mind' or neuropsychological approaches that guide assessment of attachment, the approach elaborated in this book focuses on identifying factors that contribute to the individual's capacity to achieve good support, close partner relationships and effective parenting. In doing so it points to a pathway to assessment that seeks to make enquiry into attachment practicable and to make a tool accessible to researchers, clinicians and practitioners with the aim of sharing a practical language around identification of risk and resilience, facilitating both quantitative and qualitative analysis and informing choices for effective intervention.

In each of the chapters we have aimed to elucidate vulnerability and resilience pathways in the adult, adolescent and child, as well as family relationships. We have also highlighted how Insecure attachment style categorisation can contribute to identifying increased risks for social isolation, negative affective states, poor interpersonal functioning and high conflict.

Each of these personal or interpersonal risks has implications for volatile and violent home environments, inadequate and high-risk parenting and poor developmental outcomes for children and young people as well as psychopathology in different family members. Assessment of specific support contexts and quality of close relationships leading to categorisation of attachment style can thus contribute to understanding of need for urgent intervention or can be used for preventing onset of family dysfunction and breakdown. Conversely it also elucidates protective factors that can aid resilience and help resist adversity.

Thus the purpose of this book is to provide a social and lifespan approach to the understanding of adult attachment style, exploring partner and support relationships, childhood experience and parenting experience and common psychological disorders. The findings point to the range of implications of Insecure style in terms of adult functioning, including issues around resilience. The combinations of experience which lead to adult style at any one point of time are complex and depend on negative and positive mixes of experience. However, Secure styles and those only mildly Insecure incur greater protection from disorder.

Attachment, as has been shown, is no longer merely a dyadic construct but takes place in family and wider relationship settings. It is a complex network of neurological, biological and psychological functioning that has social and behavioural and also genetic expression. Assessment of the social, behavioural and psychological functioning of family contexts will have an important role to play in the future shaping of environments where those previously doomed to cycles of adversity and failure can come to thrive.

Appendix 1:
The research sample

The research analysis presented in this book is taken from two consecutive MRC-programme grants over a 10-year period in the 1990s. It consists of community-based families and subsumes five separate interconnected studies. The sample questionnaire screening and numbers are given in Figure A.1. More details can be found in the published papers referred to, but a summary is provided here for the research reader to follow the analyses in the body of the book more easily. The beginnings of the sample selection were a questionnaire-screened sample of 303 midlife women selected through their registration at local GP practices in London, who were selected according to either childhood or adult vulnerabilities (sample 1 and 2). This was later extended to a follow-up of half the women (sample 3). From this follow-up and from a second smaller screening 146 mother–offspring dyads were interviewed (sample 4 and 5). These are described below with prevalences of main risk factors and disorders given.

A1.1 Sample 1 – Adult Risk sample (n=105)

Aims: (i) To confirm the vulnerability-provoking agent model prospectively among women selected for vulnerability, (ii) investigating the role of attachment style as a vulnerability factor and (iii) coping with life events as an additional risk for onset of major depression (Bifulco, Brown *et al.* 1998).

Sample selection: One hundred and five mothers were screened from GP surgeries for having ongoing vulnerability for depression and were free of clinical depression. The sample selection followed the same procedure as an earlier representative study of women in the same area with the same remit (Brown, Bifulco *et al.* 1990). However, the study described here only selected vulnerable women, included more lifespan data and used the ASI for the first time. The women were aged 25–55 and selected for adult vulnerability by questionnaire (Moran, Bifulco *et al.* 2001) to include women with: (a) high negative interaction with partner or (b) high negative interaction with child in household, or, (c) if single parent, lack of close confiding support or (d) NES. Those with probable clinical depression as indicated by the General Health Questionnaire (GHQ) were excluded. The women were interviewed at first contact for vulnerability and attachment style characteristics and then followed up on three occasions over the next 12 months, to look at emerging life events, coping and onset of major depression. Prevalence of risk and disorder are shown in Table A1.1.

Measures:
Vulnerability interviews: ASI, Self Evaluation and Social Support (SESS) for NES.
Disorder: SCID for 12 month and lifetime clinical disorder.
Life Events: LEDS interview and Crisis Coping.
Childhood and adult adversity: CECA for childhood neglect/abuse experience, ALPHI for adult lifetime stressors and previous partner relationships including previous partner violence.

Main findings: The previously published main findings from this study were:

- Confirmation of vulnerability factors in predicting new onset of depression.
- Insecure attachment style shown to predict depression.
- Childhood neglect and abuse shown to relate to both Insecure attachment style and depression.

New findings presented in this book include:

- Analysis of severe life event and coping behaviour in the follow-up in relation to both attachment style and depression; and
- Adversity in adult life shown to relate to childhood experience, attachment style and depression.

A1.2 Sample 1A – Childhood Risk sample (n=198)

Aims: (i) To explore childhood experience among a group mainly selected for adversity looking at both risk and resilience aspects and to include sister-pairs in order to corroborate childhood experience. (ii) To look at adult adversity as a lifespan risk factor and Insecure attachment style as an outcome and (iii) to develop an attachment-based lifespan model of recent and lifetime major depression.

Sample: The women aged 25–55 were selected through GP screening for the presence of childhood adversity and the presence of a sister within five years of age (Bifulco, Brown *et al.* 1994; Bifulco, Moran *et al.* 2003; Bifulco, Bernazzani *et al.* 2000). Forty of the index women were consecutive responders to the questionnaire, but also fulfilled the sibling requirement and were included as a comparison group. For each of the index women, one or more sisters were selected for study (Bifulco, Brown *et al.* 1997). Two groups were selected and interviewed: (i) **high childhood-risk:** 59 women who reported adverse childhood experience were interviewed, as was a sister for each (n=118) and (ii) **comparison group:** 40 women unselected for risk were interviewed, as was a sister for each (n=80). The women were interviewed at one point in time and given long life-history interviews, sometimes on more than one sitting. Sisters were interviewed independently, with interviewers blind to the information of other sister.

Measures:
Vulnerability: ASI, SESS for NES.
Disorder: SCID for 12 month and lifetime depression.
Lifetime adversity: CECA for childhood neglect/abuse experience including positive experience, ALPHI for adult lifetime stressors and previous partner relationships.

Main findings:
Note: Sisters were included as separate respondents after checks that (a) there was no significant association of sisters' clinical history and (b) that the same findings held when sister status controlled in the analysis.

- Severe levels of neglect, physical abuse or sexual abuse confirmed as childhood risk factors for adult depression, tripling risk. Other risk factors such as antipathy from parent, role reversal and psychological abuse explored and confirmed as risk factors (Bifulco, Moran *et al.* 2003).
- Childhood reports showed high level of corroboration between sister accounts (Bifulco, Brown *et al.* 1997).
- Childhood adversity significantly related to Insecure attachment style, negative evaluation of self and poor support at interview.
- Childhood adversity increased risk of high adult adversity score and both contributed to depression outcomes (Bifulco, Bernazzani *et al.* 2000).
- Problem pregnancy experience and parenting increased risk of depression (Bifulco, Bernazzani *et al.* 2000).

New findings presented in this book include:

- The differentiation of childhood neglect and abuse experience (use of the Lack of Care and Severe Abuse indices), analysis of childhood positive factors and Security for resilience and analysis of adult adversity and partner violence in relation to attachment styles.

Table A1.1 Prevalence of risk and disorder variables in midlife sample 1

Risks and disorder prevalence	Sample 1A High adult risk	Sample 1B High childhood risk	Sample 1C Comparison	Total
	n=105* %(n)	n=119 %(n)	n=80 %(n)	n=303** %(n)
Demographics				
Working class	54% (56)	33% (39)	19% (15)	36% (110)
Married/cohabiting	70% (73)	51% (61)	63% (50)	61% (184)
Parent	100% (104)	50% (60)	54% (43)	69% (207)
Single parent	30% (31)	16% (19)	14% (11)	20% (61)
Separated/divorced	44% (46)	56% (66)	56% (44)	52% (156)
Black or minority ethnic group	11% (11)	7% (8)	0	6% (19)
Vulnerability				
Negative Evaluation of Self	60% (63)	50% (59)	42% (33)	52% (156)
Marked/moderate Insecure attachment style	60% (62)	50% (59)	19% (15)	45% (136)
Lifetime Adversity				
Childhood neglect or abuse	55% (57)	77% (92)	20% (16)	55% (165)
Adult adversity score 4+	43% (45)	59% (70)	38% (30)	48% (145)
Adult adverse change points 2+	48% (50)	29% (35)	29% (23)	36% (108)
Severe life event (provoking event) 12 months	71% (74)	–	–	–
Problem partner	27% (28)	37% (44)	17% (23)	28% (85)
Disorder				
12-month major depression	38% (39)	31% (37)	17% (13)	30% (89)
Lifetime chronic or recurrent depression	32% (33)	50% (59)	27% (21)	37% (113)

* One value missing on attachment style so total used is 104;
** One missing value on attachment style, so total used in the analysis is 302.

A1.3 Sample 2 – Follow-up midlife women (n=154)

Aim: (i) To examine the relationship of ASI to new episodes of disorder prospectively, including anxiety states; (ii) to establish ASI as mediating factor between childhood adversity and onset of emotional disorder;

(iii) to look at changes in attachment style at follow-up; (iv) and to question retrospectively about parenting for those paired in the intergenerational sample.

Sample: Half of the original women interviewed were followed-up an average of three years later (range 2 to 5). The women were selected for follow-up equally from three groups in samples 1 and 2: i) 57 mothers (sample 1) who had previously been selected for poor ongoing relationships and had offspring aged 16–25; ii) 55 women (sample 2 chidhood risk) selected for adverse childhood experience under age 17; and iii) 42 comparison women (sample 2 comparison). No paired sisters were included in this follow-up (Bifulco, Kwon *et al.* 2006)

Measures:
Vulnerability: The ASI was measured again to look at stability/change, as well as SESS for NES.
Adversity: The ALPHI to look at stressors in the follow-up period.
Disorder: SCID for clinical disorder (Depression or Anxiety disorder) in the intervening follow-up period.

Main findings:
* Insecure attachment style was related to new onset of depression and anxiety at follow-up and played a mediating role in relation to childhood adversity (Bifulco, Kwon *et al.* 2006).

New findings reported in this book:

* Attachment style changed for a quarter of women. Positive change occurred more for some styles and was related to positive change in partner and VCO support.

Table A1.2 Prevalence rates new variables in follow-up midlife women sample 2

Risks and disorder prevalence	n=154 % (n)
Depression in follow-up	40% (62)
Anxiety disorder in follow-up	36% (56)
Depression or anxiety in follow-up	55% (85)
Marked/moderate Insecure attachment style at follow-up	47% (72)
Positive attachment change including minor change	30% (19)
Positive change in support	17% (26)
Negative Evaluation of Self at follow-up	46% (71)
Childhood neglect/abuse	59% (91)

A1.4 Sample 3 – Mother–offspring dyads (146)

Aim: To look for intergenerational transmission of risk to male and female offspring in 'emerging adulthood' between the ages of 16 and 30. To test mother's Insecure attachment style, her parenting behaviour and her partner characteristics as potential drivers of transmission.

Sample: One hundred and forty-six mothers from sample 1 and 2 who had one or more offspring in the relevant age range where both agreed to re-interview (Bifulco, Moran *et al.* 2009). A new screening for vulnerable mothers in the community, identical to sample 1, through GP surgeries in the same area of London, yielded a further 41 mother–offspring pairs to supplement the sample. These had the same demographic and risk factors as the main sample dyads. Offspring were 146 young people aged 16–30 (average age 20) half of whom were male. Mother and offspring interviewed independently by different interviewers blind to information about the other in the pair.

Measures used for the mothers:
Vulnerability: ASI, SESS for NES.
Parenting: PRI retrospectively.
Disorder: SCID for major depression and Anxiety disorder at follow-up (GAD, Social Phobia, Panic/Agoraphobia) but lifetime disorder from previous interviews used.

Main findings:
- Mothers' Insecure attachment style significantly related to her estimated incompetent parenting. Partner problem behaviour related to her parenting.
- Mothers' incompetent parenting was associated with offspring reports of her neglect, antipathy or physical abuse in parenting. Mother's depression did not add to the model.
- Chronic marital difficulties of mother contributed to offspring report of neglect/abuse from mother.
- Neglect/abuse from mother related to offspring emotional disorder (depression or anxiety).

Table A1.3 Prevalence rates in mother intergenerational sample 3

Prevalence	n=146 % (n)
Vulnerability	
Insecure attachment style	53% (77)
Negative Evaluation of Self	44% (64)
Mother estimated incompetent parenting	41% (60)
Adversity	
Mother's problem partner behaviour	36% (52)
Mother's chronic marital difficulty	59% (86)
Disorder	
Mother's 12-month depression	23% (34)
Mother's chronic, recurrent lifetime depression	46% (67)

A1.5 Sample 4 – Offspring sample (n=146)

Aim: (i) To examine the relationship between childhood adversity and clinical disorder in an 'emerging adult' sample. Emotional disorder (depression and anxiety) as well as substance abuse, deliberate self-harm and conduct disorder examined and childhood care and abuse differentiated by mother and father/substitute father. (ii) To examine attachment style in this age group in relation to clinical disorder and childhood experience.

Sample: One hundred and forty-six community-based young people aged between 16 and 33 (average age 20.63 years, standard deviation = 4.46), were the offspring of women in sample 1 and 2 originally studied for susceptibility to depression and the same individuals as in sample 3, but utilised an unpaired analysis (Bifulco 2008; Schimmenti and Bifulco 2008).

Measures:
Vulnerability: ASI, SESS for NES.
Childhood adversity: CECA extended to include peer and school experience in mid-teenage years,
Disorder: SCID for emotional disorder and substance abuse in 12 months and lifetime. Additional questions for DSH lifetime, both suicidal and non-suicidal.

Main findings:
- Childhood neglect and abuse related to different clinical disorders in the young people. Specifically, neglect, antipathy or physical abuse from mothers related to emotional disorder and deliberate self-harm.

The same experience from father/substitute fathers related to substance abuse and conduct disorder.

- Insecure attachment style related to disorder. Anxious styles (Enmeshed or Fearful) related to emotional disorder.
- A model showing mother's neglect/abuse, Offspring's Anxious attachment style, and negative eveluation of self provided a good fit for offspring emotional disorder.
- Positive experiences in teenage years related to Secure style and this acted as a resilience factor for lack of disorder outcome.
- Role reversal had a specific relationship with deliberate self-harm (odds ratio 11).

New findings:
Dual/disorganised styles related to substance abuse and to deliberate self-harm. Angry-dismissive style related to deliberate self-harm.

Table A1.4 Prevalence risk and disorder – Offspring sample 4

Risks and disorder prevalence	n=146 % (n)
Demographics	
Working class	44% (64)
In education	38% (56)
Living at home	64% (93)
Vulnerability	
Insecure attachment style (marked or moderate)	47% (68)
Anxious attachment (marked or moderate)	28% (41)
Avoidant attachment (hi)	18% (27)
Negative Evaluation of Self	32% (47)
Problem peer group age 16	32% (46)
Parental violence	21% (31)
Disorder	
Emotional disorder 12 months	27% (40)
Substance abuse 12 months	21% (30)
Deliberate self-harm (lifetime)	21% (30)
Any case 12 months	41% (60)
Emotional disorder ever	45% (65)
Behavioural disorder ever	32% (46)
Childhood adversity	
Neglect, physical or sexual abuse	35% (51)
Neglect, antipathy, physical abuse mother	27% (39)
Neglect, antipathy, physical abuse father	28% (41)

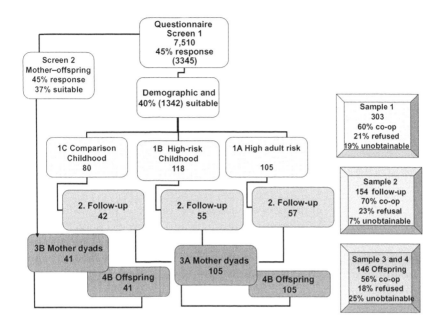

Figure A.1 Total sample

Appendix 2:
Summary of research case examples

The table overleaf summarises the research cases presented in the text of the book with a brief summary of their risk and disorder characteristics.

Note: Cases have been anonymised, and the names chosen use the same initial as the ASI style. Family identification numbers are consistent across generations and relate to the sample. Source – Sample 1b: Family id 1-60; Sample 1C Family id 60-100; Sample 1A: family id 101-210

Table A2.1 Midlife cases sample 1

Name	Sample ID Family (subject)	Age	Chapter	Negative Evaluation of Self	Depression 12 month	Chronic/ Recurrent depression	Childhood
Susan Secure	015 (1)	26	2	No	No	No	LC
Faye Moderate/ Fearful	022 (1)	24	5	Yes	No	Yes	LC, SA
Wendy Moderate/ Withdrawn	025 (1)	35	6	Yes	No	Yes	LC, SA
Alexa Mark/ A–D	041 (1)	32	2, 3	Yes	No	Yes	LC, SA
Sheila Secure	059 (2)	29	7	No	No	No	LC, SA
Eloise Moderate/ Enmesh	102 (0)	43	5, 7	Yes	No	No	LC
Ellie Moderate/ Enmesh	113 (0)	40	2, 3, 4	No	Yes	Yes	LC, SA
Fiona Moderate/ Fearful	120 (0)	43	2, 3	Yes	Yes	Yes	None
Deirdre Dual (AD–E)	122 (0)	36	2, 3	Yes	Yes	Yes	LC, SA
Emma Moderate/ Enmesh	130 (0)	30	6	Yes	Yes	Yes	LC, SA
Alma Moderate/ A–D	147 (0)	37	4, 5, 6	No	Yes	Yes	LC, SA
Whitney Moderate/ Withdrawn	164 (0)	46	2, 7	Yes	No	No	SA

Family numbers consistent in the Offspring sample. A–D=Angry-dismissive;
AD–E=Angry-dismissive and Enmeshed; LC=Severe lack of care; SA=Severe abuse.

Table A2.2 Offspring sample cases (sample 4)

Name and style	Sample Identifi- cation	Age	Chapter	Emotional disorder 12 months	Substance abuse ever	DSH ever	Problem parenting	NES
Donna Dual (AD–F)	025 (21)	24	4, 6	Yes	Yes	Yes	Father	No
Eric Moderate/ Enmeshed	067 (21)	23	4	No	Yes	No	None	No
Dean Dual (AD–E)	067 (22)	29	3, 5	Yes	Yes	Yes	Mother and father	No
Ethan Mild/ Enmeshed	106 (2)	25	7	No	No	No	Father	No
Felicity Moderate/ Fearful	147 (3)	19	3, 6	Yes	No	Yes	Mother and father	Yes

Poor parenting=Severe antipathy, neglect or physical abuse.
AD–E=Angry-dismissive and Enmeshed; AD–F=Angry-dismissive and Fearful;
DSH=Deliberate Self-harm, lifetime; NES=negative evaluation of self.

Table A2.3 Summary of service-based cases

Family member	Attachment Style (Level)	Chapter	Age	Disorder	Partner difficulty	Parenting difficulty
Erin	Mild/Enmeshed	9	35	None	No	High expectations unmet
Frank	Moderate/Fearful	9	37	None	No	High expectations unmet
Fern	Marked/Fearful	9	25	Learning disabled Post-natal depression	Yes	Child protection
David	Dual Marked Fearful/Enmeshed	9	35	Anxiety/ Substance abuse	Yes	Child protection
Warren	Markedly/ Withdrawn	9	53	None	Yes, separated	Custody issues
Darren	Dual Marked Angry-dismissive and Fearful	9	14	Hyperactive	N/A	Residential care
Daphne	Dual Marked Fearful and Enmeshed	10	48	Substance abuse	N/A	Controlling parenting
Debbie	Dual Marked Angry-dismissive and Fearful	10	33	Depression/ Anxiety	N/A	Seeking medical diagnosis for child
Faith	Markedly Fearful	10	29	Depression	N/A	Feelings failure; fear rejection
Eleanor	Markedly Enmeshed	10	35	Anxiety	N/A	Over-protective, Role reversing
Annette	Markedly Angry-Dismissive	10	36	None	Yes	Antipathy to child
William	Mildly Withdrawn		42	None	Yes	Distant parenting
Frieda	Moderately Fearful	10	32	None	No	Anxious parenting
Finn	Moderate Fearful	10	35	None	No	Anxious parenting

N/A=Not applicable.

References

(1989) Children Act. London, HMSO.

(2004) Children Act. London, HMSO.

Ainsworth, M. D. S., Blehar, M., Waters, E. and Wall, S. (1978) *Patterns of attachment: A psychological study of the Strange Situation.* Hillsdale, NJ, Lawrence, Erlbaum.

Allen, J. G. and Fonagy, P. (2006) *Handbook of Mentalization-based Treatment.* Chichester, UK, John Wiley & Sons Ltd.

Andrews, B. and Brown, G. W. (1988) 'Marital violence in the community: A biographical approach.' *British Journal of Psychiatry*, 153: 305–12.

Andrews, B., Brown, G. W. and Creasey, L. (1990) 'Intergenerational links between psychiatric disorder in mothers and daughters: The role of parenting experiences.' *Journal of Child Psychology and Psychiatry*, 31: 1115–29.

Asen, E. and Fonagy, P. (2012) 'Mentalisation-based Family Therapy.' In A. Bateman and P. Fonagy (eds). *Handbook of mentalising in mental health practice.* Washington DC, American Psychiatric Publishing, pp. 107–28.

Asendorpf, J. B. and Wilpers, S. (2000) 'Attachment security and available support: Closely linked relationship qualities.' *Journal of Social and Personal Relationships*, 17: 115–38.

Bakermans-Kranenburg, M. J. and van IJzendoorn, M. H. (2007) 'Research review: genetic vulnerability or differential susceptibility in child development: the case of attachment.' *Journal of Child Psychology and Psychiatry,* 48 (12): 1160–73.

Bakermans-Kranenburg, M. J., van Ijzendoorn, M. and Juffer, F. (2003) 'Less is more: meta-analyses of sensitivity and attachment interventions in early childhood.' *Psychological Bulletin*, 129: 195–215.

Baldwin, M. and Fehr, B. (1995) 'On the stability of attachment style changes.' *Personal Relationships*, 2: 247–61.

Barkley, R. A. (1997) 'Behavioral inhibition, sustained attention, and executive functions: Constructing a unifying theory of ADHD.' *Psychological Bulletin*, 121 (1): 65–94.

Barrett, M. and Trevitt, J. (1991) *Attachment Behaviour and the Schoolchild: An Introduction to Educational Therapy.* London, Routledge.

Bartholomew, K. (1990) 'Avoidance of intimacy: An attachment perspective.' *Journal of Social and Personal Relationships*, 7 (2): 147–78.

Bartholomew, K. (1994) 'Assessment of individual differences in adult attachment.' *Psychological Inquiry*, 5 (1): 23–7.

Bartholomew, K. and Horowitz, L. M. (1991) 'Attachment styles among young adults: A test of a four-category model.' *Journal of Personality and Social Psychology*, 61 (2): 226–44.

Bartholomew, K. and Shaver, P. R. (1998) Methods of assessing adult attachment - do they converge? In J. A. Simpson and W. S. Rholes (eds). *Attachment Theory and Close Relationships*. NY, London, Guilford Press.

Bartholomew, K., Henderson, A. J. Z. and Dutton, D. G. (2001) 'Insecure attachment and abusive intimate relationships.' In C. Clulow (ed.). *Attachment and Couple Work: Applying the 'Secure Base' Concept in Research and Practise*. London, Brunner-Routledge.

Bateman, A. and Fonagy, P. (2004) *Psychotherapy for Borderline Personality Disorder: Mentalization-based treatment*. Oxford, Oxford University Press.

Bateman, A. and Fonagy, P. (2012) Handbook of mentalizing in mental health practice. Washington, DC: American Psychiatric Publishing.

Beck, A. T. (1967) *Depression: clinical, experimental and theoretical aspects*. New York, Hoeber.

Becker-Weidman, A. and Hughes, D. (2008) 'Dyadic Developmental Psychotherapy: An evidence-based treatment for children with complex trauma and disorders of attachment.' *Child & Adolescent Social Work*, 13: 329–37.

Belsky, J. (2002) 'Developmental origins of attachment styles.' *Attachment and Human Development*, 4 (2): 166–70.

Belsky, J., Bakermans-Kranenburg, M. J. and van Ijzendoorn, M. H. (2007) 'For better and for worse: Differential susceptibility in child development: the case of attachment.' *Current Directions in Psychological Science*, 16 (6): 300–4.

Belsky, J. and Nezworski, T. (1988) *Clinical Implications of Attachment*. Hillsdale, NJ: Lawrence Erlbaum Associates.

Belsky, J. and Pluess, M. (2009) 'Beyond diathesis-stress: Differential susceptibility to environmental influences.' *Psychological Bulletin*, 135 (6): 885–908.

Belsky, J. and Vondra, J. (1989) Lessons from child abuse: the determinants of parenting, a process model. In D. Cicchetti and V. Carlson (eds). *Child maltreatment – theory and research on the causes and consequences of child abuse and neglect*. Cambridge, Cambridge University Press, pp. 153–203.

Bentovim, A. and Bingley Miller, L. (2001) *The Family Assessment: Assessment of Family Competence, Strengths and Difficulties*. York, Child and Family Training.

Bentovim, A., Cox, A., Bingley Miller, L. and Pizzey, S. (2009) *Safeguarding children living with trauma and family violence. Evidence-based assessment, analysis, and planning interventions*. London, Philadelphia, Jessica Kingsley Publishers.

Bifulco, A. (2008) Risk and resilience in young Londoners. In D. Brom, R. Pat-Horenczyk and J. Ford (eds). *Treating traumatised children: Risk, resilience and recovery*. London, Routledge, pp. 117–31.

Bifulco, A., Bernazzani, O., Moran, P. M. and Ball, C. (2000) 'Lifetime stressors and recurrent depression: preliminary findings of the Adult Life Phase Interview (ALPHI).' *Social Psychiatry and Psychiatric Epidemiology*, 35: 264–75.

Bifulco, A., Brown, G. W., Moran, P. M., Ball, C. and Campbell, C. (1998) 'Predicting depression in women: the role of past and present vulnerability.' *Psychological Medicine*, 28: 39–50.

Bifulco, A. and Brown, G. W. (1996) 'Cognitive coping response to crises and onset of depression.' *Social Psychiatry and Psychiatric Epidemiology*, 31: 163–72.

Bifulco, A., Brown, G. W. and Harris, T. (1994) 'Childhood Experience of Care and Abuse (CECA): A retrospective interview measure.' *Journal of Child Psychology and Psychiatry*, 35: 1419–35.

Bifulco, A., Brown, G. W., Lillie, A. and Jarvis, J. (1997) 'Memories of childhood neglect and abuse: Corroboration in a series of sisters.' *Journal of Child Psychology and Psychiatry*, 38: 365–74.

Bifulco, A., Figueirido, B., Guedeney, N., Gorman, L., Hayes, S., Muzik, M., Gatigny-Dally, E., Valoriani, V., Kammerer, M., Henshaw, C. and the TCS-PND group (2004) 'Maternal attachment style and depression associated with childbirth: Preliminary results from a European/US cross-cultural study.' *British Journal of Psychiatry (Special supplement)*, 184 (46): 31–7.

Bifulco, A., Gunning, M.. Figueiredo, B., Glatigny-Dally, E., Klier, C., Muzik, M., Kammerer, M. and Murray, L. (2006) Attachment style in pregnancy and inter-action with baby at 6 months – a cross-cultural finding. *Marce Society*. Oxford University.

Bifulco, A., Kwon, J-H., Jacobs, C., Moran, P. M. and Bunn, A. (2006) 'Adult attachment style as mediator between childhood neglect/abuse and adult depression and anxiety.' *Social Psychiatry & Psychiatric Epidemiology*, 41 (10): 796–805.

Bifulco, A., Mahon, J., Kwon, J-H., Moran, P. M. and Jacobs, C. (2003) 'The Vulnerable Attachment Style Questionnaire (VASQ): An interview-derived meas-ure of attachment styles that predict depressive disorder.' *Psychological Medicine*, 33: 1099–110.

Bifulco, A. and Moran, P. (1998) *Wednesday's Child: Research into women's experience of neglect and abuse in childhood and adult depression.* London/New York, Routledge.

Bifulco, A., Moran, P. M., Baines, R., Bunn, A. and Stanford, K. (2003) 'Exploring psychological abuse in childhood: II Association with other abuse and adult clin-ical depression.' *Bulletin of the Menninger Clinic*, 66: 241–58.

Bifulco, A., Moran, P. M., Ball, C. and Bernazzani, O. (2002a) 'Adult attachment style I: Its relationship to clinical depression.' *Social Psychiatry & Psychiatric Epidemiology*, 37: 50–9.

Bifulco, A., Moran, P. M., Ball, C., Jacobs, C., Baines, R., Bunn, A. and Cavagin, J. (2002) 'Childhood adversity, parental vulnerability and disorder: examining inter-generational transmission of risk.' *Journal of Child Psychology and Psychiatry*, 43: 1075–86.

Bifulco, A., Moran, P. M., Ball, C. and Lillie, A. (2002b) 'Adult attachment style II: Its relationship to psychosocial depressive-vulnerability.' *Social Psychiatry & Psychiatric Epidemiology*, 37: 60–7.

Bifulco, A., Moran, P. M., Jacobs, C. and Bunn, A. (2009) 'Problem partners and parenting: exploring linkages with maternal insecure attachment style and adolescent offspring internalizing disorder.' *Attachment & Human Development*, 11 (1): 69–85.

Bonanno, G. A. (2004) 'Loss, Trauma and Human Resilience: have we underesti-mated the human capacity to thrive after extremely aversive events?' *American Psychologist*, 59 (1): 20–8.

Bond, S. B. and Bond, M. (2004) 'Attachment styles and violence within couples.' *Journal of Nervous and Mental Disorder*, 192 (12): 857–63.

Booth, C. L., Rubin, K. H. and Rose-Krasnor, L. (1998) 'Perceptions of Emotional Support from Mother and Friend in Middle Childhood: Links with Social-Emotional Adaptation and Preschool Attachment Security.' *Child Development*, 69 (2): 427–42.

Borman-Spurrell, E. (1996) Patterns of adult attachment and psychotherapy outcomes for patients with binge-eating disorder. Yale University. PhD.

Bowlby, J. (1969) *Attachment and loss: vol 1. Attachment.* New York, Basic Books.

Bowlby, J. (1973) *Attachment and loss: vol 2. Separation: Anxiety and anger.* New York, Basic Books.

Bowlby, J. (1977) 'Aetiology and psychopathology in the light of attachment theory.' *British Journal of Psychiatry,* 130: 201–10.

Bowlby, J. (1980) *Attachment and loss: vol 3. Loss; sadness and depression.* New York, Basic Books.

Bowlby, J. (1982) *Attachment (2nd edition) Attachment and Loss.* London/New York, Hogarth Press, Basic Books.

Bowlby, J. (1988) *A secure base: Clinical application of attachment theory.* London, Routledge.

Bradley, R., Heim, A. and Westen, D. (2005) 'Transference patterns in the psychotherapy of personality disorders: Empirical investigation.' *British Journal of Psychiatry,* 186: 342–9.

Bratton, S. and Landreth, G. (1995) 'Filial Therapy with single parents: Effects on parental acceptance, empathy and stress.' *International Journal of Play Therapy,* 4: 61–80.

Brennan, K. A., Clark, C. L. and Shaver, P. R. (1998) Self-report measurement of adult attachment: An integrative overview. In J. A. Simpson and W. S. Rholes (eds). *Attachment theory and close relationships.* New York/London, The Guilford Press, pp. 47–76.

Bretherton, I. (1985) 'Attachment Theory: Retrospect and Prospect.' *Monographs of the Society for Research in Child Development,* 50 (1/2): 3–35.

Bretherton, I., Ridgway, D. and Cassidy, J. (1990) 'Assessing internal working models of the Attachment relationship: an attachment story completion task for 3 year olds.' In M. T. Greenberg, D. Cicchetti and E. M. Cummings (eds). *Attachment in the pre-school years.* Chicago, Chicago University Press, pp. 273–308.

Bronfenbrenner, U. (1979) *The Ecology of Human Development: Experiments in nature and design.* Cambridge, MA: Harvard University Press.

Brown, G., Craig, T., Harris, T., Handley, R. and Harvey, A. (2007) 'Validity of retrospective measures of early maltreatment and depressive episodes using the Childhood Experience of Care and Abuse (CECA) instrument – A lifecourse study of chronic depression-2.' *Journal of Affective Disorders,* 103 (1–3): 217–24.

Brown, G. W. (1974) Meaning, measurement, and stress of life events. In B. S. and B. P. Dohrenwend (eds). *Stressful life events, their nature and effects.* New York, NY: John Wiley & Sons.

Brown, G. W., Andrews, B., Bifulco, A. T. and Veiel, H. O. (1990) 'Self esteem and depression: I. Measurement issues and prediction of onset.' *Social Psychiatry and Psychiatric Epidemiology,* 25: 200–9.

Brown, G. W., Andrews, B., Harris, T. O., Adler, Z. and Bridge, L. (1986) 'Social support, self-esteem and depression.' *Psychological Medicine,* 16: 813–31.

Brown, G. W. and Bifulco, A. (1985) Social support, life events and depression. In I. Sarason (ed.). *Social Support: Theory, Research and Applications.* Dordrecht, Martinus Nijhoff.

Brown, G. W., Bifulco, A. and Harris, T. O. (1987) 'Life events, vulnerability and onset of depression: Some refinements.' *British Journal of Psychiatry,* 150: 30–42.

Brown, G. W., Bifulco, A. T. and Andrews, B. (1990c) 'Self-esteem and depression: III. Aetiological issues.' *Social Psychiatry and Psychiatric Epidemiology,* 25: 235–43.

Brown, G. W., Bifulco, A. T., Veiel, H. O. and Andrews, B. (1990) 'Self-esteem and depression: II. Social correlates of self-esteem.' *Social Psychiatry and Psychiatric Epidemiology*, 25: 225–34.

Brown, G. W. and Harris, T. O. (1978) *Social Origins of Depression: A study of psychiatric disorder in women*. London: Tavistock.

Brugha, T. S. and Cragg, D. (1990) 'The List of Threatening Experiences: the reliability and validity of a brief life events questionaire.' *Acta Psyciatrica Scandinavia*, 82: 77–81.

Buchsbaum, H. K., Toth, S., Clyman, R., Cicchetti, D. and Emde, R. (1992) 'The use of narrative story stem technique with maltreated children: implications for theory and practice.' *Development and Psychopathology*, 4: 603–25.

Cameron, R. and Maginn, C. (2008) 'The authentic warmth dimension of professional childcare.' *British Journal of Social Work*, 38: 1151–72.

Carter, C. S. and de Vries, A. C. (1999) Stress and Soothing: An endocrine perspective. In M. Lewis and D. Ramsey (eds). *Soothing and Stress*. Mahwah, NJ: Lawrence Erlbaum Associates, pp. 3–18.

Caspers, K., Yucius, R., Troutman, B. and Spinks, R. (2006) 'Attachment as an organizer of behavior: Implications for substance abuse problems and willingness to seek treatment.' *Substance Abuse and Treatment Prevention Policy*, 1 (1–10).

Caspi, A. (2002) 'Role of genotype in the cycle of violence in maltreated children.' *Science*, 297: 851–4.

Cassidy, J. (1994) Emotion-regulation: Influences of attachment relationship. *The development of emotion-regulation. Biological and behavioural consideration*. N. Fox, Monographs of the Research in Child Development, 59: 228–49.

Cawson, P., Wattam, C., Brooker, S. and Kelly, G. (2000) Child maltreatment in the United Kingdom. *Cruelty to children must stop. FULL STOP. NSPCC*.

Chaffin, M., Silovsky, J. F., Funderburk, B., Valle, L. A., Brestan, E. V. and Balachova, T. (2004) 'Parent–child interaction therapy with physically abusive parents: efficacy for reducing future abuse reports.' *Journal of Consulting and Clinical Psychology*, 72: 500–10.

Chamberlain, P., Price, J. M., Reid, J. B., Landsverk, J., Fisher, P. A. and Stoolmiller, M. (2006) 'Who disrupts from placement in foster and kinship care?' *Child Abuse and Neglect*, 30 (4): 409–24.

Chappel, K. D. and Davis, K. E. (1998) 'Attachment, partner choice and perception of romantic partners: An experimental test of the attachment-security hypothesis.' *Personal Relationships*, 5: 327–42.

Chorpita, B. and Daleiden, E. L. (2009) 'Mapping evidence-based treatments for children and adolescents: application of the distillation and matching model to 650 treatments from 322 randomised trials.' *Journal of Consulting and Clinical Psychology*, 77: 566–79.

Cicchetti, D. and Barnett, D. (1991) 'Attachment organisation in maltreated preschoolers.' *Development and Psychopathology*, 4: 397–411.

Cicchetti, D. and Valentino, K. (2006) An ecological-transactional perspective on child maltreatment: Failure of the average exectable environment and its influence on child development. In D. Cicchetti and D. J. Cohen (eds). *Developmental Psychopathology: Vol 3, Risk, disorder and adaptation*. Hoboken, NJ: Wiley, 3: 129–201.

Ciechanowski, P. and Katon, W. (2006) 'The interpersonal experience of health care through the eyes of patients with diabetes.' *Social Science & Medicine*, 63: 3067–79.

Clarke, L., Ungerer, J., Chahoud, K., Johnson, S. M. and Stiefel, I. (2002) 'Attention Deficit Hyperactivity Disorder is Associated with Attachment Insecurity.' *Clin Child Psychol Psychiatry*, 7: 179–98.

Coan, J. A. (2008) Toward a neuroscience of attachment. In J. Cassidy and P. R. Shaver (eds). *Handbook of Attachment: Theory, research and clinical applications*. New York/London, Guilford Press, pp. 241–65.

Cohen, N. J., Muir, E., Lojkasek, M., Muir, R., Parker, C. J., Barwick, M. B. and Brown, M. (1999) 'Watch, wait and wonder: Testing the effectiveness of a new approach to mother-infant psychotherapy.' *Infant Mental Health Journal*, 20: 429–51.

Cohen, Y. (1996) 'Physical and Sexual Abuse and their Relation to Psychiatric Disorder and Suicidal Behavior among Adolescents who are Psychiatrically Hospitalized.' *Journal of Child Psychology and Psychiatry*, 37 (8): 989–93.

Cohn, D. A., Silver, D. H., Cowan, C. P., Cowan, P. A. and Pearson, J. (1992) 'Working models of childhood attachment and couple relationships.' *Journal of Family Issues*, 13: 432–49.

Collins, N. and Read, S. (1994) 'Cognitive representations of attachment: The structure and function of working models.' *Advances in Personal Relationships*, 5: 53–90.

Collins, N. L. and Feeney, B. C. (2000) 'A safe haven: An attachment theory perspective on support seeking and caregiving in intimate relationships.' *Journal of Personality and Social Psychology*, 78: 1053–73.

Collins, N. L. and Read, S. J. (1990) 'Adult attachment, working models, and relationship quality in dating couples.' *Journal of Personality and Social Psychology*, 58 (4): 644–63.

Colton, M. and Hellinckx, W. (1994) 'Residential and foster care in the European Community: Current trends in policy and practice.' *British Journal of Social Work*, 24: 559–76.

Condé, A., Figueirido, B. and Bifulco, A. (2011) 'Attachment style and psychological adjustment in couples.' *Attachment & Human Development*, 13: 271–92.

Cowan, C. P. and Cowan, P. A. (2005) 'Two central roles for couple relationships: breaking intergenerational patterns and enhancing children's adaptation.' *Sexual and Relationship Therapy*, 20 (3): 275–88.

Cowan, P., Cohn, D., Cowan, C. P., and Pearson, J. (1996) 'Parents' attachment histories and children's externalising and internalising behaviours: Exploring family systems models of linkage.' *Journal of Consulting and Clinical Psychology*, 64 (1): 53–63.

Cox, A. (2008) *The HOME Inventory: A guide for practitioners – the UK approach*. York: Child and Family Training.

Cozzarelli, C., Karafa, J. A., Collins, N. L. and Tagler, M. J. (2003) 'Stability and change in adult attachment styles: associations with personal vulnerabilities, life events, and global construals of self and others.' *Journal of Social and Clinical Psychology*, 22: 315–46.

Crittenden, P. (1988) 'Relationships at risk.' In J. Belsky and T. Nezworski (eds). *Clinical implications of attachment. Child psychology*. Hillsdale, NJ: Lawrence Erlbaum Associates, Inc, pp. 136–74.

Crittenden, P. M. (1985) 'Social networks, quality of child-rearing and child development.' *Child Development*, 56 (5): 1299–313.

Crittenden, P. M. (1995) Attachment and Psychopathology. *Attachment theory: Social, developmental and clinical applications.* S. Goldberg, R. Muir and J. Kerr. Hillsdale, NJ: The Analytic Press, pp. 367–406.

Crittenden, P. M. (1997) Toward an integrative theory of trauma: A dynamic-maturation approach. In D. Cicchetti and S. L. Toth (eds). *Developmental perspectives on trauma: Theory, research and intervention.* Rochester, New York: University of Rochester, pp. 33–84.

Crowell, J., Treboux, D., Gao, Y., Fyffe, C., Pan, H. and Waters, E. (2002) 'Assessing secure base behavior in adulthood: development of a measure, links to adult attachment representations, and relations to couples' communication and reports of relationships.' *Developmental Psychology,* 38 (5): 679–93.

Crowell, J. A. (1996) Current Relationships Interview. *Unpublished Manuscript.* State University of New York, Stony Brook.

Cummings, E. M. and Cicchetti, D. (1990) Toward a transactional model of relations between attachment and depression. In M. T. Greenberg, D. Cicchetti and E. M. Cummings (eds). *Attachment in the Preschool Years: Theory, Research, and Intervention.* University of Chicago.

Cummings, M. E. and Davies, P. T. (2002) 'Effects of marital conflict on children: recent advances and emerging themes in process-oriented research.' *Journal of Child Psychology and Psychiatry and Allied Disciplines,* 43 (1): 31–63.

Daniel, S. I. F. (2006) 'Adult attachment patterns and individual psychotherapy: A review.' *Clinical Psychology Review,* 26: 968–84.

Davila, J. and Bradbury, T. N. (2001) 'Attachment insecurity and the distinction between unhappy spouses who do and do not divorce.' *Journal of Family Psychology,* 15: 371–93.

Davila, J., Bradbury, T. N., Cohan C. L. and Tochluck, S. (1997) 'Marital functioning and depressive symptoms: Evidence for a stress generation model.' *Journal of Personality and Social Psychology,* 73: 849–61.

Davila, J., Karney, B. R. and Bradbury, T. N. (1999) 'Attachment change processes in the early years of marriage.' *Journal of Personality and Social Psychology,* 76(5): 783–802.

Davila, J. and Sargent, E. (2003) 'The meaning of life (events) predicts changes in attachment security.' *Personality and Social Psychology Bulletin,* 29 (11): 1383–95.

DCSF (2007) 'Impact assessment for White Paper on Children in Care.'

DCSF (2009) Children looked after in England (including adoption and care leavers) year ending 31 March 2009.

De Wolff, M. and van Ijzendoorn, M. (1997) 'Sensitivity and attachment: A meta-analysis of parental antecedents of infant attachment.' *Child Development,* 68: 571–746.

DfES (2006) Preparing and Assessing Prospective Adopters. www.everychildmatters.gov.uk adoption.

DfES (2004) Every Child Matters: next steps, Department for Education and Skills: 1–45.

DfES and DoH (2004) National service framework for children, young people, and maternity services: the mental health and psychological well-being of children and young people.

Diamond, D., Clarkin, J. F., Levine, H., Levy, K. N., Foelsch, P. and Yeomans, F. (1999) 'Borderline conditions and attachment: A preliminary report.' *Psychoanalytic Inquiry,* 19: 831–84.

Dobash, R. E. and R. P. Dobash (1992) *Women, Violence and Social Change.* London/New York, Routledge.

DoH (2000) Framework for the Assessment of Children in Need and their Families. *Quality Protects.* Department of Health.

DoH, Cox, A. D. and Bentovim, A (2000) *The Family Pack of Questionnaires and Scales.* London, The Stationery Office.

Domes, G., Heinrichs, M., Glascher, J., Buchel, C., Braus, D. F. and Herpertz, S. C. (2007) 'Oxytocin attenuates amygdala responses to emotional faces regardless of valence.' *Biological psychiatry,* 62 (10): 1187–90.

Dozier, C., Stovall-McClough, K. C. and Albus, K. (2008) Attachment and psychopathology in adulthood. In J. Cassidy and P. R. Shaver (eds). *Handbook of Attachment. Theory, Research, Clinical Applications.* New York/London, Guilford Press, pp. 718–45.

Dozier, M. (1990) 'Attachment organisation and treatment use for adults with serious psychopathological disorders.' *Development and Psychopathology,* 2: 47–60.

Dozier, M. (2003) 'Attachment-based treatment for vulnerable children.' *Attachment and Human Development,* 5 (3): 253–7.

Dozier, M., Lindheim, O. and Ackerman, J. P. (2005) Attachment and Biobehavioural Catch-up: An intervention targeting empirically identified needs of foster infants. In L. J. Berlin, Y. Ziv, L. Amaya-Jackson and M. T. Greenberg (eds). *Enhancing early attachments: Theory, research, intervention and policy.* Guilford Press, pp. 178–94.

Dozier, M., Lomax, L., Tyrrell, C. and Lee, S. (2001) 'The challenge of treatment for clients with dismissing states of mind.' *Attachment & Human Development,* 3: 62–76.

Dozier, M., Stovall, K. C., Albus, K. and Bates, B. (2001) 'Attachment for infants in foster care: The role of caregiver state of mind.' *Child Development,* 72 (5): 1467–77.

Dozier, M., Stovall, K. C. and Albus, K. (1999) 'Attachment and psychopathology in adulthood.' In J. Cassidy and P. R. Shaver (eds). *Handbook of Attachment: Theory, Research, and Clinical Applications.* New York, NY: The Guilford Press, pp. 497–519.

Dutton, D. G. (1995) *The domestic assault of women: Psychological and criminal justice perspectives.* Boston, MA: Allyn & Bacon.

Edwards, A. C., Nazroo, J. Y. and Brown, G. W. (1998) 'Gender differences in marital support following a shared life event.' *Social Science and Medicine,* 46: 1077–85.

Ellis, B. and W. Boyce (2008) 'Biological sensitivity to context.' *Current directions in psychological science,* 17 (3): 183–7.

Eng, W., Heimberg, R., Hart, T., Schneier, F. and Liebowitz, M. (2001) 'Attachment in individuals with social anxiety disorder: The relationships among adult attachment styles, social anxiety and depression.' *Emotion,* 4: 365–80.

Erikson, E. (1950) *Childhood and Society.* New York: Norton.

Farrington, D. P. (1990) Childhood aggression and early violence: Early precursers and later-life outcome. *The development and treatment of childhood aggression.* In D. J. Pepler and K. H. Rubin (eds). New Jersey, Lawrence Erlbaum Associates, pp. 5–29.

Fearon, P., Target, M., Sargent, J., Williams, L., McGregor, J., Bleiberg, E. and Fonagy, P. (2006) Short Term Mentalisation and Relational Therapy (SMART): An integrative family therapy for children and adolescents. In J. G. Allen and P. Fonagy (eds). *Handbook of mentalization-based treatment.* West Sussex, England, Jon Wiley & Sons Ltd, pp. 201–22.

Feeney, B. C. (2007) 'The Dependency Paradox in Close Relationships: Accepting Dependence Promotes Independence.' *Journal of Personality and Social Psychology,* 92 (2): 268–85.

Feeney, J. A. (1995) 'Adult attachment and emotional control.' *Personal Relationships*, (2): 143–59.

Feeney, J. A. (1996) 'Attachment, caregiving, and marital satisfaction.' *Personal Relationships*, 3: 401–16.

Feeney, J. A. (2003) 'The systemic nature of couple relationships: An attachment perspective.' In P. Erdman and T. Caggrey (eds). *Attachment and family systems: Conceptual, empirical and therapeutic relatedness.* New York: Brunner/Mazel, pp. 139–63.

Fergusson, D. M., Boden, J. M. and Horwood, J. L. (2008) 'Exposure to childhood sexual and physical abuse and adjustment in early adulthood.' *Child Abuse & Neglect*, 32: 607–19.

Fergusson, D. M., Lynskey, M. and Horwood, J. L. (1995) 'The adolescent outcomes of adoption: A 16 year longitudinal study.' *Journal of Child Psychology and Psychiatry*, 36: 597–615.

First, M., Gibbon, M., Spitzer, R. and Williams, G.(1996) *Users guide for SCID*, Biometrics Research Division.

Fisher, H., Bunn, A., Jacobs, C., Moran, P. and Bifulco, A. (2011) 'Concordance between mother and offspring reports of childhood adversity.' *Childhood Abuse and Neglect*, 35: 117–22.

Fisher, H. L., Jones, P. B., Fearon, P., Craig, T. K., Dazzan, P. and Morgan, K. (2010) 'The varying impact of type, timing, and frequency of exposure to childhood adversity on its association with adult psychotic disorder.' *Psychological Medicine*, 40 (12): 1967–78.

Fisher, P. A. and Chamberlain, P. (2000) 'Multidimensional Treatment Foster Care: A Program for Intensive Parenting, Family Support, and Skill Building.' *Journal of Emotional and Behavioural Disorders*, 8 (3): 155–64.

Fisher, P. A. and Kim, H. (2007) 'Intervention effects on foster preschoolers' attachment-related behaviors from a randomized trial.' *Prevention Science*, 8: 161–70.

Fisher, P. A., Stoolmiller, M., Gunnar, M. R. and Burraston, B. O. (2007) 'Effects of a therapueutic intervention for foster preschoolers on diurnal cortisol activity.' *Psychoneuroendocrinology*, 32: 892–905.

Fonagy, P. (2006) The mentalization-focused approach to social development. In J. G. Allen and P. Fonagy (eds). *Handbook of Mentalization-based Treatment.* Chichester, John Wiley & Sons Ltd, pp. 53–100.

Fonagy, P., Gergely, G., Jurist, E. and Target, M. (2002) *Affect-regulation, mentalisation and the development of the self.* New York, NY, Other Press.

Fonagy, P., Gergely, G. and Target, M. (2008) Psychoanalytic constructs and attachment theory and research. In J. Cassidy and P. Shaver (eds). *Handbook of Attachment: Theory, Research and Clinical Applications.* New York/London, The Guilford Press, pp. 783–810.

Fonagy, P., Leigh, T., Steele, M., Steele, H., Kennedy, R., Mattoon, G., Target, M. and Gerber, A. (1996) 'The relation of attachment status, psychiatric classification and response to psychotherapy.' *Journal of Consulting and Clinical Psychology*, 64 (1): 22–31.

Fonagy, P., Steele, H. and Steele, M. (1991) 'Maternal representations of attachment during pregnancy predict the organisation of infant-mother attachment at one year of age.' *Child Development*, 62 (5): 891–905.

Fonagy, P., Steele, M., Steele, H., Higgitt, A. and Target, M. (1994) 'The Emanuel

Miller Memorial Lecture 1992: The theory and practice of resilience.' *Journal of Child Psychology and Psychiatry and Allied Disciplines*, 35 (2): 231–57.

Fonagy, P., Steele, M., Steele, H., Leigh, T., Kennedy, R., Mattoon, G. and Target, M. (1995) Attachment, the reflective self and borderline states: The predictive specificity of the Adult Attachment Interview and pathological emotional development. In S. Goldberg, R. Muir and J. Kerr (eds). *Attachment theory: Social, Developmental and Clinical perspectives*. Hillsdale, NJ: Analytic Press, pp. 233–79.

Fonagy, P. and Target, M. (1997) 'Attachment and reflective function: Their role in self-organization.' *Development and Psychopathology*, 9 (4): 679–700.

Ford, T., Vostanis, P., Meltzer, H. and Goodman, R. (2007) 'Psychiatric disorder among British children looked after by local authorities: comparison with children living in private households.' *British Journal of Psychiatry*, pp. 319–25.

Forehand, R., Wierson, M., Thomas, A. M., Armistead, L., Kempton, T. and Neighbors, B. (1991) 'The role of family stressors and parent relationships on adolescent functioning.' *Journal of the American Academy of Child and Adolescent Psychiatry*, 30 (2): 316–22.

Fraley, C. R. and Shaver, P. R. (2000) 'Adult Romantic Attachment: Theoretical Developments, Emerging Controversies, and Unanswered Questions.' *Review of General Psychology*, 4 (2): 132–54.

Fraley, R. and Waller, N. (1998) *Adult attachment patterns: a test of the typological model*. New York, Guilford.

Fraley, R. C., Davis, K. E. and Shaver, P. (1998) Dismissing-avoidance and the defensive organization of emotion, cognition, and behavior. In J. A. Simpson and W. S. Rholes (eds). *Attachment Theory and Close Relationships*. New York/London, Guilford Press.

Garmezy, N. (1985) *Stress resistant children: The search for protective factors*. Oxford, Pergamon Press.

George, C., Kaplan, N. and Main, M. (1984) *Attachment Interview for Adults*. University of California, Berkeley.

George, C. and West, M. (1999) 'Developmental vs. social personality models of adult attachment and mental ill health.' *British Journal of Medical Psychology*, 72 (3): 285–303.

Gergely, G. and Watson, J. S. (1996) 'The social biofeedback theory of parent affect-mirroring. The development of self-awareness and self-control in infancy.' *International Journal of Psycho-Analysis*, 77: 1191–212.

Gerlsma, C. and Luteijn, F. (2000) 'Attachment style in the context of clinical and health psychology: A proposal for the assessment of valence, incongruence, and accessibility of attachment representations in various working models.' *British Journal of Medical Psychology*, 73 (1): 15–34.

Gianonne, F., Schimenti, A., Caretti, V., Chiarenza, A., Ferraro, A., Guarino, S., Guarnaccia, C., Lucarrelli, L., Mancuso, L., Mule, A., Petrocchi, M., Peuiri, D., Ragonese, N. and Bifulco, A. (2011) 'Validita attendibilita e proprieta pscyhometriche dela verdsione Italinana dell'intervesta CECA (Childhood Experience of Care and Abuse).' *Psiciatria e Psicoterapia*, 30: 3–21.

Glover, G. J. and Landreth, G. (2000) 'Filial therapy with Native American in the Flathead Reservation.' *International Journal of Play Therapy*, 9: 57–80.

Goldberg, S. (2000) *Attachment and Development*. London, Arnold.

Gottman, J. M. and Levenson, R. W. (2000) 'The timing of divorce: predicting when a couple will divorce over a 14 year period.' *Journal of Marriage and the Family,* 62 (3): 737–45.

Griffin, D. W. and Bartholomew, K. (1994) 'Models of the self and other: Fundamental dimensions underlying measures of adult attachment.' *Journal of Personality and Social Psychology,* 67 (3): 430–45.

Griffing, S., Ragin, D. F., Sage, R. E., Madry, L., Bingham, L. E. and Primm, B. J. (2002) 'Domestic Violence Survivors' Self-Identified Reasons for Returning to Abusive Relationships' *Journal of Interpersonal Violence,* 17 (3): 306–19.

Grskovic, J. A. and Goetze, H. (2008) 'Short-term Filial Therapy with German mothers: Findings from a controlled study.' *International Journal of Play therapy,* 19: 39–51.

Guedeney, M., Fermian, J. and Bifulco, A. (2009) 'La version Francaise du Relationship Scales Questionnaire de Bartholomew (RSQ: Questionnaire des echelees de relation): Etude de validation du construit. (Contruct validation study of the Relationship Scales Questionnaire (RSQ) on an adult sample.' *L'Encephale,* 218: 1–18.

Guerney, B. (1964) 'Filial Therapy: Description and rationale.' *Journal of Consulting Psychology,* 28: 303–10.

Gunning, M., Conroy, S., Figueiredo, B., Kammerer, M., Muzik, M., Glatigny-Daly, E. and Murray, L. (2004) 'Measurement of mother-infant interactions and the home environment in a European setting: preliminary results from a cross-cultural study.' *British Journal of Psychiatry,* 183: s38–s44.

Hammen, C. L., Burge, D., Daley, S. E., Davila, J., Paley, B. and Rudolph, K. (1995) 'Interpersonal attachment cognitions and prediction of symptomatic responses to interpersonal stress.' *Journal of Abnormal Psychology,* 104 (3): 436–43.

Hammond, J. R. and Fletcher, G. J. O. (1991) 'Attachment styles and relationship satisfaction in the development of close relationships.' *New Zealand Journal of Psychology,* 20 (2): 56–62.

Harkness, K. L. and Wildes, J. E. (2002) 'Childhood adversity and anxiety versus dysthymia co-morbidity in major depression.' *Psychological Medicine,* 32: 1239–49.

Harris, T. (2003) 'Depression in women and its sequelaé.' *Journal of Psychosomatic Research,* 54: 103–12.

Harris, T. O., Brown, G. W. and Robinson, R. (1999) 'Befriending as an intervention for chronic depression among women in an inner city. 1. Randomised controlled trial.' *British Journal of Psychiatry,* 174: 219–24.

Hawkins-Rodgers, Y. P. (2007) 'Adolescents adjusting to a group home environment: a residential care model of re-organizing attachment behaviour and building resiliency.' *Children and Youth Services Review,* 29: 1131–41.

Hawton, K., Salkovskis, P. M., Kirk, J. and Clark, D. M. (1989) *Cognitive Behaviour Therapy for Psychiatric Problems: A Practical Guide.* Oxford, Oxford University Press.

Hazan, C., Hutt, M. J. and Clark, D. M. (1991) 'Continuity and change in inner working models of attachment.' *Department of Human Development.* Cornell University.

Hazan, C. and Shaver, P. (1987) 'Romantic love conceptualized as an attachment process.' *Journal of Personality and Social Psychology,* 52 (3): 511–24.

Hazan, C. and Shaver, P. R. (1994) 'Deeper into attachment theory.' *Psychological Inquiry,* 5 (1): 68–79.

Hearn, B. (1995) *Child and family support and protection: A practical approach.* London, National Children's Bureau.

Heim, C., Young, L. J., Newport, D. J., Mletzko, T., Miller, A. H. and Nemeroff, C. B. (2009) 'Lower CSF oxytocin concentrations in women with a history of childhood abuse.' *Molecular Psychiatry*, 14 (10): 954–8.

Henderson, A. J. Z., Bartholomew, K, and Dutton, D. G. (1997) 'He loves me, He loves me not: Attachment and separation resolution of abused women.' *Journal of Family Violence*, 12 (2): 169–92.

Hesse, E. (2008) The Adult Attachment Interview: Protocol, method of analysis and empirical studies. In J. Cassidy and P. R. Shaver (eds). *Handbook of Attachment: Theory, Research and Clinical Applications*. New York/London, Guilford Press: 552–98.

Hill, E. M., Young, J. P. and Nord, J. L. (1994) 'Childhood adversity, attachment, Security and adult relationships: A preliminary study.' *Ethology and Sociobiology*, 15: 323–8.

Hill, J., Davis, R., Byatt, M., Burnside, E., Rollinson, L. and Fera, S. (2000) 'Childhood sexual abuse and affective symptoms in women: a general population study.' *Psychological Medicine*, 30: 1283–91.

Hodges, J., Steele, M., Steele, M., Hillman, S., Henderson, K. and Kaniuk, J. (2003) 'Changes in Attachment Representations Over the First Year of Adoptive Placement: Narratives of Maltreated Children.' *Clinical Child Psychology and Psychiatry*, 8 (3): 347–63.

Holmes, B. M. and Lyons-Ruth, K. (2006) 'The Relationship Questionnaire - Clinical Version (RQ-CV): Introducing a Profoundly-Distrustful Attachment Style.' *Infant Mental Health Journal*, 27 (3): 310–25.

Holmes, J. (1993) *John Bowlby and Attachment Theory*. London/New York, Routledge.

Howe, D. (2001) 'Age at placement, adoption experience and adult adopted people's contact with their adoptive and birth mothers: an attachment perspective.' *Attachment and Human Development*, 3 (2): 222–37.

Howe, D., Brandon, M., Hinings, D. and Schofield, G. (1999) *Attachment theory, child maltreatment and family support*. Mendham, Suffolk, Palgrave.

Howe, D., Dooley, T. and Hinings, D. (2000) 'Assessment and decision-making in a case of child neglect and abuse using an attchment perspective.' *Child and Family Social Work*, 5 (2): 143–55.

Hughes, D. (2009) *Attachment-Focused Parenting*, . New York: Norton.

Insel, T. R. (1997) 'A Neurobiological Basis of Social Attachment.' *American Journal of Psychiatry*, 154 (6): 726–35.

Jacobvitz, D. (2008) 'Afterword'. In H. Steele and M. Steele (eds). *Clinical Applications of Adult Attachment Interview*. New York, Guilford Press: 471–86.

Johnson, J. G., Cohen, P., Kasen, S., Smailes, E. and Brook, J. S. (2001) 'Association of maladaptive parental behavior with psychiatric disorder among parents and their offspring.' *Archive of General Psychiatry*, 58: 453–60.

Johnson, S. (2003) Introduction to attachment. A therapists' guide to primary relationshpis and their renewal. In S. M. Johnson and V. E. Whiffen (eds). *Attachment processes in couple and family therapy*. New York, Guilford Press, pp. 3–17.

Johnson, S. M. and Lee, A. (2000) Emotionally-focused family therapy: Status and challenges. In C. E. Bailey (ed.). *Children in therapy: Using the family as a resource*. New York: Norton, pp. 112–36.

Johnson, S. M., Maddeaux, C. and Blouin, J. (1998) 'Emotionally focused family therapy for bulimia: Changing attachment patterns.' *Psychotherapy*, 35: 238–47.

Johnson, S. M. and Whiffen, V. E. (2003) *Attachment processes in couple and family therapy*. New York: Guilford Press.

Juffer, F., Hoksbergen, R. A., Riksen-Walraven, J. M. A. and Kohnstamm, G. A. (1997) 'Early intervention in adoptive families: Supporting maternal sensitive responsiveness, infant-mother attachment and infant competence.' *Journal of Child Psychology and Psychiatry*, 38: 1039–50.

Kaczynski, K. J., Lindahl, K. M., Malik, N. M. and Laurenceau, J-P. (2006) 'Marital Conflict, Maternal and Paternal Parenting, and Child Adjustment: A Test of Mediation and Moderation.' *Journal of Family Psychology*, 20 (2): 199–208.

Kaess, M., Parzer, P., Mattern, M., Resch, F., Bifulco, A. and Brunner, R. (2011) 'Childhood Experience of Care and Abuse (CECA) - Validierung der deutschen Version des Fragebogens sowie des korrespondierenden Interviews zur Erhebung belastender Kindheitserlebnisse in familiaren Rahmen.' *Zeitschrift fur Kinder - und Jugendpsychiatrie und Psychotherapie*, 39 (4): 243–52.

Kale, A. L. and Landreth, G. (1999) 'Filial Therapy with parents of children experiencing learning difficulties.' *International Journal of Play Therapy*, 8: 35–56.

Keelan, J. P. R., Dion, K. K. and Dion, K. L. (1998) 'Attachment style and relationship satisfaction: Test of a self-disclosure explanation.' *Canadian Journal of Behavioural Science*, 30 (2): 24–35.

Kirkpatrick, L. A. and Davis, K. E. (1994) 'Attachment style, gender, and relationship stability: A longitudinal analysis.' *Journal of Personality and Social Psychology*, 66 (3): 502–12.

Kirkpatrick, L. A. and Hazan, C. (1994) 'Attachment styles and close relationships: A four-year prospective study.' *Personal Relationships*, 1 (2): 123–42.

Kissgen, R., Krischer, M., Kummetat, V., Spiess, R., Schleiffer, R. and Sevecke, K. (2009) 'Attachment Representation in Mothers of Children with Attention Deficit Hyperactivity Disorder.' *Psychopathology*, 42: 201–8.

Klohnen, E. C. and Bera, S. (1998) 'Behavioral and experiential patterns of avoidantly and securely attached women across adulthood: A 31-year longitudinal perspective.' *Journal of Personality and Social Psychology*, 74 (1): 211–23.

Kobak, R. and Mandelbaum, T. (2003) Caring for the caregiver: An attachment approach to assessment and treatment of child problems. In S. M. Johnson and V. E. Whiffen (eds). *Attachment processes in couple and family therapy*. New York, Guilford Press, pp. 144–190.

Kobak, R. R. and Hazan, C. (1991) 'Attachment in marriage: Effects of security and accuracy of working models.' *Journal of Personality and Social Psychology*, 60 (6): 861–9.

Lapsley, D. K. (2000) 'Pathological attachment and attachment style in late adolescence.' *Journal of Adolescence*, 23 (2): 137–55.

Leiberman, A. F. (2003) 'Treatment of attachment disorder in infancy and early childhood: Reflections from clinical intervention with later-adopted foster care children.' *Attachment & Human Development*, 5: 279–82.

Levy, K. N., Meehan, K. B., Kelly, K. M., Reynoso, J. S., Weber, M., Clarkin, J. F. and Kerneberg, O. F. (2006) 'Changes in attachment patterns and reflective function in a randomized controlled trial of transference-focused psychotherapy for borderline personality disorder.' *Journal of Consulting and Clinical Psychology*, 74: 1027–40.

Lieberman, A. F., Weston, D. and Pawl, J. (1991) 'Preventive intervention and outcome with Anxiously attached dyads.' *Child Development*, 62: 199–209.

Lopez, F. G. and Gormley, B. (2002) 'Stability and change in adult attachment style over the first-year college transition: Relations to self-confidence, coping, and distress patterns.' *Journal of Counseling Psychology*, 49 (3): 355–64.

Luthar, S. S. (1991) 'Vulnerability and resilience: A study of high-risk adolescents.' *Child Development*, 62 (3): 600–16.

Lyons-Ruth, K. and Jacobvitz, D. (1999) 'Attachment disorganisation: Unresolved loss, relational violence and lapses in behavioural and attentional strategies.' In J. Cassidy and P. R. Shaver (eds). *Handbook of Attachment: Theory, Research and Clinical Applications*. New York/London: The Guilford Press, pp. 520–54.

Lyons-Ruth, K. and Jacobvitz, D. (2008) 'Attachment disorganisation: Genetic factors, parenting contexts and developmental transformation from infancy to adulthood.' In J. Cassidy and P. Shaver (eds). *Handbook of Attachment: Theory, Research and Clinical Application*. New York: Guilford Press, pp. 666–97.

Main, M. and Cassidy, J. (1988) 'Categories of response to reunion with the parent at age 6: Predictable from infant attachment classifications and stable over a one-monh period.' *Developmental Psychology*, 24 (3): 415–26.

Main, M. and Hesse, E. (1990) 'Parents' unresolved traumatic experiences are related to infant disorganized attachment status: Is frightened and/or frightening parental behavior the linking mechanism?' In M. Greenberg, D. Cicchetti, and M. Cummings (eds). *Attachment In The Preschool Years: Theory, Research, and Intervention*. Chicago, IL: University of Chicago Press, pp. 161–82.

Main, M., Kaplan, A. G. and Cassidy, J. (1985) 'Security in infancy, childhood and adulthood: A move to level of representation.' In I. Bretherton and E. Waters (eds). *Growing points of attachment theory and research*. Monographs of the Society for Research in Child Development, 50: 66–104.

Main, M. and Solomon, J. (1986) 'Discovery of an insecure-disorganized/disoriented attachment pattern.' In T. B. Brazelton and M. W. Yogman (eds). *Affective Development in Infancy*. Norwood, NJ: Ablex, pp. 95–124.

Marvin, R., Cooper, G., Hoffman, K. and Powell, B. (2002) 'The Circle of Security Project: Attachment-based intervention with caregiver-pre-school child dyads.' *Attachment & Human Development*, 4 (1): 107–24.

Masten, A. S., Garmezy, N., Tellegen, A., Pellegrini, D. S., Larkin, K. and Larsen, A. (1988) 'Competence and stress in school children: The moderating effects of individual and family qualities.' *Journal of Child Psychology and Psychiatry and Allied Disciplines*, 29 (6): 745–64.

May-Chahal, C. (2003) 'Social Exclusion, Family Support and Evaluation.' In I. Katz and J. Pinkerton (eds). *Evaluating Family Support Thinking Internationally, Thinking Critically*. Chichester: John Wiley & Sons Ltd, pp. 45–71.

McBride, C., Atkinson, L., Quilty, L. E. and Bagby, M. R. (2006) 'Attachment as a moderator of treatment outcomes in major depression: A randomized control trial of interpersonal psychotherapy vs. cognitive behavior therapy.' *Journal of Consulting and Clinical Psychology*, 74: 1041–54.

McCarthy, G. (1999) 'Attachment style and adult love relationships and friendships: A study of a group of women at risk of experiencing relationship difficulties.' *British Journal of Medical Psychology*, 72 (3): 305–21.

McCrory, E., de Brito, S. and Viding, E. (2010) 'Research Review: The neurobiology and genetics of maltreatment and adversity.' *Journal of Child Psychology and Psychiatry*, 5 (10): 1079–95.

McMahon, C. A., Barnett, B., Kowalenko, N. M. and Tennant, C. C. (2006) 'Maternal attachment state of mind moderates the impact of postnatal depression on infant attachment.' *Journal of Child Psychology and Psychiatry*, 47 (7): 660–9.

Meaney, M. (2001) 'Maternal care, gene expression and the transmission of individual differences in stress reactivity across generations.' *Annual Review of Neuroscience*, 24: 1161–92.

Meltzer, H., Gatward, R., Goodman, R. and Ford, T. (2000) *Mental health of children and adolescents in Great Britain.* Office for National Statistics.

Mickelson, K. D., Kessler, R. C. and Shaver, P. R. (1997) 'Adult attachment in a nationally representative sample.' *Journal of Personality and Social Psychology*, 73 (5): 1092–06.

Mikulincer, M. and Florian, V. (1999) 'The association between parental reports of attachment style and family dynamics, and offspring reports of adult attachment style.' *Family Proceedings*, 38: 243–257.

Mikulincer, M., Horesh, N., Eilati, I. and Kotler, M. (1999) 'The association between adult attachment style and mental health in extreme life-endangering condition.' *Personality and Individual Differences*, 27: 831–42.

Mikulincer, M. and Nachshon, O. (1991) 'Attachment styles and patterns of self-disclosure.' *Journal of Personality and Social Psychology*, 61(2): 321–31.

Mikulincer, M. and Shaver, P. R. (2008) Adult attachment and afffect regulation. In J. Cassidy and P. R. Shaver (eds). *Handbook of Attachment. Theory, Research and Clinical Applications.* New York/London: Guilford, pp. 503–31.

Mikulincer, M., Shaver, P. R. and Pereg, D. (2003) 'Attachment Theory and Affect Regulation: The Dynamics, Development, and Cognitive Consequences of Attachment-Related Strategies.' *Motivation and Emotion*, 27 (2): 77–101.

Moffitt T. E., Caspi, A. and Rutter, M. (2005) 'Strategy for investigating interactions between measured genes and measured environments.' *Archives of General Psychiatry*, 62: 473–81.

Montague, D. P. F., Magai, C., Consedine, N. S. and Gillespie, M. (2003) 'Attachment in African American and European American older adults: The roles of early life socialization and religiosity.' *Attachment & Human Development*, 5 (2): 188–214.

Moore, K., Moretti, M. M. and Holland, R. (1997) 'A new perspective on youth care programs: using attachment theory to guide interventions for troubled youth.' *Residential treatment for children & youth*, 15 (3): 1–24.

Moran, P., M, Bifulco, A., Ball, C. and Campbell, C. (2001) 'Predicting onset of depression: The Vulnerability to Depression Questionnaire.' *British Journal of Clinical Psychology*, 40: 411–27.

Morgan, H. and Shaver, P. R. (1999) 'Attachment Processes and Commitment to Romantic Relationships.' In J. Adams and W. Jones (eds). *Handbook of Interpersonal Commitment and Relationship Stability.* New York, NY: Kluwer Academic/Plenum Publishers.

Muller, R. T. (2000) 'Social support and the relationship between family and community violence exposure and psychopathology among high risk adolescents.' *Child Abuse & Neglect*, 24 (4): 449–64.

Munro, E. (2010) 'The Munro Review of Child Protection.' *Department of Education*, June 2010.

Murphy, B. and Bates, G. W. (2000) 'Adult attachment style and vulnerability to depression.' *Personality and Individual Differences*, 22 (6): 835–44.

Murray, L., Fiori-Cowley, A., Hopper, A. and Copper, P. (1996) 'The Impact of postnatal depression and associated adversity on early mother-infant interactions and later infant outcome.' *Child Development*, 67: 2512–26.

Murray, L., Stanley, C., Hooper, R., King, F. and Fiori-Cowley, A. (1996) 'The role of infant factors in postnatal depression and mother-infant interactions.' *Developmental Medicine and Child Neurology*, 38 (2): 109–19.

NCAS (2008) *Introduction to Leaving Care.* London, National Care Advisory Service.

Norris, C. J., Coan, J. A. and Johnstone, I. T. (2007) 'Functional magnetic resonance imaging of the study of emotion.' In J. A. Coan and J. J. Allen (eds). *The Handbook of Emotion Elicitation and Assessment.* Oxford/New York, Oxford University Press, pp. 440–59.

NSPCC (2011) *Child Abuse and Neglect in the UK today.* London, NSPCC.

O'Connor, T. G. and Byrne, J. G. (2007) 'Attachment measures for research and practice.' *Child and Adolescent Mental Health*, 12 (4): 187–92.

O'Connor, T. G. and Zeanah, C. H. (2003a) 'Attachment disorders: Assessment strategies and treatment approaches.' *Attachment and Human Development*, 5 (3): 223–44.

O'Connor, T. G. and Zeanah, C. H. (2003b) 'Introduction to the special issue: Current perspectives on assessment and treatment of attachment disorders.' *Attachment and Human Development*, 5 (3): 211–22.

Offord, D., Boyle, M., Racine, Y., Fleming, J., Cadman, D., Blum, H. M., Byrne, C., Links, P. S., Lipman, E. L. and MacMillan, H. L. (1992) 'Outcome, Prognosis, and Risk in a Longitudinal Follow-up Study.' *Journal of the American Academy of Child & Adolescent Psychiatry*, 31 (5): 916–23.

Olson, J. M., Roese, N. J. and Zanna, M. P. (1996) Expectancies. In H. E. T. and A. W. Kruglanski (eds). *Social Psychology: Handbook of basic principles.* New York, Guilford Press, pp. 211–38.

Oskis, A., Loveday, C., Hucklebridge, F., Thorn, L. and Clow, A. (2011) 'Anxious attachment style and salivary cortisol dysregulation in healthy female children and adolescents.' *The Journal of Child Psychology and Psychiatry*, 52 (2): 111–18.

Padesky, C. (1994) 'Schema change processes in cognitive therapy.' *Clinical Psychology and Psychotherapy*, 1 (5): 267–78.

Paley, B., Cox, M. J., Burchinal, M. R. and Payne, C. C. (1999) 'Attachment and marital functioning: Comparison of spouses with continuous-secure, earned-secure, dismissing and preoccupied attachment stances.' *Journal of Family Psychology*, 13: 580–97.

Pearson, J. L., Cohn, D. A., Cowan, P. A. and Cowan, C. P. (1994) 'Earned- and continous-security in adult attachment: Relation to depressive symptomatology and parenting style.' *Development and Psychopathology*, 6: 359–73.

Perry, B. D. (2008) 'Child maltreatment: A neurodevelopmental perspective on the role of trauma and neglect in psychpathology.' In T. P. Beauchaine and S. P. Hinshaw (eds). *Textbook of child and adolescent psychopathology.* New York: Wiley, pp. 93–128.

Perry, B. D., Pollard, L., Blakely, T., Baker, W. and Vigilante, D. (1995) 'Childhood Trauma, the neurobiology of adaptation and 'use-dependent' development of the braIn How 'states' become 'traits'.' *Infant Mental Health Journal*, 16: 271–91.

Phelps, J. L., Belsky, J. and Crnic, K. (1998) 'Earned security, daily stress and parenting: A comparison of five alternative models.' *Development and Psychopathology*, 10: 21–38.

Prior, V. and Glaser, D. (2006) *Understanding Attachment and Attachment Disorders.* London, Philadelphia, Jessica Kingsley Publishers.

Quinton, D., Rushton, A., Dance, C. and Mayes, D. (1998) *Joining New Families – A*

Study of Adoption and Fostering in Middle Childhood. Chichester, New York, Weinheim, Brisbane, Singapore, Toronto: John Wiley & Sons.

Quinton, D., Pickles, A., Maughan, B. and Rutter, M. (1993) 'Partners, peers, and pathways: Assortative pairing and continuities in conduct disorder.' *Development and Psychopathology,* 5 (4): 763–83.

Quinton, D., Rutter, M. and Liddle, C. (1985) 'Institutional rearing, parenting difficulties, and marital support.' *Annual Progress in Child Psychiatry and Child Development,* 173–206.

Quirin, M., Preuessner, J. C. and Khul, J. (2008) 'HPA system regulation and adult attachment anxiety: Individual differenes in reactive and awakening cortisol.' *Psychoneuroendocrinology,* 33: 581–90.

Rapee, R. and Heimberg, R. (1997) 'A cognitive-behavioural model of anxiety in social phobia.' *Behaviour Research and Therapy,* 35: 741–56.

Rholes, W. S., Simpson, J. A. and Stevens, J. G. (1998) 'Attachment orientations, social support and conflict resolution in close relationships.' In J. A. Simpson and W. S. Rholes (eds). *Attachment Theory and Close Relationships.* New York, London: Guilford Press.

Roberts, N. and Noller, P. (1998) 'The associations between adult attachment and couple violence. The role of communication patterns and relationship satisfaction.' In J. A. Simpson and W. S. Rholes (eds). *Attachment theory and close relationships.* New York: The Guilford Press, pp. 317–50.

Robertson, J. and Robertson, J. (1971) 'Young children in brief separation: a fresh look.' *Psychoanalytic Study of the Child,* 26: 264–315.

Rodriguez, C. M. and Green, A. J. (1997) 'Parenting stress and anger expression as predictors of child abuse potential.' *Child Abuse and Neglect.* 21 (4): 367–77.

Roisman, G. I., Padron, E., Sroufe, L. A. and Egeland, B. (2002) 'Earned-secure attachment status in retrospect and prospect.' *Child Development,* 73: 1204–19.

Rothbard, J. C. and Shaver, P. R. (1994) 'Continuity of attachment across the lifespan.' In M. B. Sperling and W. H. Berman (eds). *Attachment in adults: Theory, assessment and treatment.* New York: Guilford Press, pp. 31–71.

Rubin, K. H. and Mills, R. S. (1988) 'The many faces of social isolation in childhood.' *Journal of Consulting and Clinical Psychology,* 56 (6): 916–24.

Runtz, M. G. (2007) 'Social support and coping strategies as mediators of adult adjustment following childhood maltreatment.' *Child abuse & neglect,* 21 (2): 211–26.

Rusby, J. S. M. (2005) *Childhood Temporary Separation: Long term effects of Wartime Evacuation in World War 2.* Florida, Dissertation.com, Boca Raton.

Rushton, A. (2003) 'Support for adoptive families, a review of current evidence on problems, needs and effectiveness.' *Adoption & Fostering,* 27 (3): 41–9.

Rushton, A. (2004) 'The outcomes of late permanent placements, the adolescent years.' *Adoption & Fostering,* 28 (1): 49–57.

Rutter, M. (1990) 'Psychosocial resilience and protective mechanisms.' In J. E. Rolf and A. S. Masten (eds). *Risk and protective factors in the development of psychopathology.* New York, NY: Cambridge University Press, pp. 181–214.

Rutter, M., Beckett, C., Castle, J., Colvert, E., Kreppner, J., Mehta, M., Sonuga-Barke, E. (2007) 'Effects of profound early institutional deprivation: An overview of findings from a UK longitudinal study of Romanian Adoptees.' *Euopean Journal of Developmental Psychology,* 4: 332–50.

Rutter, M. and O'Connor, T. G. (1999) 'Implications of Attachment Theory for child care policies.' In J. Cassidy and P. R. Shaver (eds). *Handbook of Attachment. Theory, Research and Clinical Applications.* New York/London: The Guilford Press: 823–44.

Rutter, M. and ERA team (1998) 'Developmental catch-up and deficit following adoption after severe global early privation.' *Journal of Child Psychology and Psychiatry,* 39: 465–76.

Ruvolo, A. P., Fabin, L. A. and Ruvolo, C. (2001) 'Relationship experiences and change attachment characteristics of young adults: The role of relationship breakups and conflict avoidance.' *Personal Relationships,* 8: 265–81.

Scharfe, E. and Bartholomew, K. (1994) 'Reliability and stability of adult attachment patterns.' *Personal Relationships,* 1: 23–43.

Schechter, D. and Willheim, E. (2009) 'Disturbances of attachment and parental psychopathology in early childhood.' *Child and Adolescent Psychiatry Clinics of North America,* 18 (3): 665–87.

Schimmenti, A. and Bifulco, A. (2008) Quando i gentori maltrattano I figli: le radici psicopathologiche dello sviluppo affetivo (When the parents maltreat their young: The developmental roots of psychopathology). In V. Caretti and G. Craparo (eds). *Trauma e Psicopatologia. Un approccio evolutivo-relazione.* Roma: Astrolabio, pp. 94–131.

Schimmenti, A. and Caretti, V. (2010) 'Psychic retreats or psychic pits? Unbearable states of mind and tecnological addiction.' *Psychoanalytic Psychology,* 27: 115–32.

Schleiffer, R. and Muller, S. (2004) 'Attachment representation of adolescents in institutional care.' *International Journal of Child & Family Welfare,* 7 (1): 70.

Scott, S. (2004) 'Reviewing the research on the mental health of looked after children: Some issues for the development of more evidence informed practice.' *International Journal of Child & Family welfare,* 7 (2–3): 86–97.

Scott, S., Spender, Q., Doolan, M., Jacobs, B. and Aspland, H. (2001) 'Multicentre controlled trail of parenting groups for antisocial behaviour in clinical practice.' *British Medical Journal,* 323: 194–8.

Senchak, M. and Leonard, K. E. (1992) 'Attachment styles and marital adjustment among newlywed couples.' *Journal of Social and Personal Relationships,* 9: 51–64.

Shaver, P. and Clarke, C. (1994) 'The psychodynamics of adult romantic attachment.' In J. Masling and R. Bornstein (eds). *Empirical Perspectives on Object Relations Theories.* Washington, DC, American Psychological Association, pp. 105–56.

Shaver, P. and Hazan, C. (1993) 'Adult romantic attachment: Theory and evidence.' *Advances in Personal Relationships.* London: Jessica Kinsgley, 4: 29–70.

Shaver, P. and Rubenstein, C. (1980) Childhood attachment experience and adult loneliness. In L. Wheeler (ed.). *Personality and Social Psychology,* Vol. 1. Beverley Hills, CA, Sage.

Shaver, P. R. and Brennan, K. A. (1992) 'Attachment styles and the 'Big 5' personality traits: Their connections with each other and with romantic relationship outcomes.' *Psychology and Social Psychology Bulletin,* 18: 536–45.

Shaver, P. R. and Mikulincer, M. (2002) 'Attachment-related psychodynamics.' *Attachment and Human Development,* 4 (2): 133–61.

Shore, A. N. (1994) *Affect regulation and the origin of the self.* Mahwah, NJ: Erlbaum.

Shore, A. N. (2003) *Affect dysregulation and disorders of the self.* New York: Norton and Sons.

Simpson, J. A. (1990) 'Influence of attachment styles on romantic relationships.' *Journal of Personality and Social Psychology,* 59: 971–80.

Simpson, J. A., Rholes, W. S., Campbell, L., Tran, S. and Wilson, C. L. (2003) 'Adult Attachment, the Transition to Parenthood, and Depressive Symptoms.' *Journal of Personality and Social Psychology*, 84 (6): 1172–87.

Simpson, J. A., Rholes, W. S. and Nelligan, J. S. (1992) 'Support seeking and support giving within couples in an anxiety-provoking situation: The role of attachment styles.' *Journal of Personality and Social Psychology*, 62 (3): 434–46.

Slade, A. (2008) 'The implications of attachment theory and research for adult psychotherapy.' In J. Cassidy and P. Shaver (eds). *Handbook of Attachment: Theory, Research and Clinical Applications*. New York/London: The Guilford Press, pp. 762–82.

Spencer, T., Biederman, J., Coffey, B., Geller, D., Crawford, M., Bearman, S. K., Tarazi, R. and Faraone, S. V. (2002) 'A double-blind comparison of Desipramine and placebo in children and adolescents with chronic tic disorder and comorbid attention-deficit/hyperactivity disorder.' *Archives of General Psychiatry*, 59: 649–56.

Sroufe, L. A. (2005) 'Attachment and development: a prospective, longitudal study from birth to adulthood.' *Attachment & Human Development*, 7 (4): 349–67.

Steele, H., Steele, M. and Fonagy, P. (1996) 'Associations among attachment classifications of mothers, fathers and their infants.' *Child Development*, 67 (2): 541–55.

Steele, M., Hodges, J., Kaniuk, J., Hillman, S. and Henderson, K. (2003) 'Attachment representations and adoption: associations between maternal states of mind and emotion narratives in previously maltreated children.' *Journal of Child Psychotherapy*, 29: 187–205.

Stein, H., Jacobs, N. J., Ferguson, K. S., Allen, J. G. and Fonagy, P. (1998) 'What do adult attachment scales measure?' *Bulletin of the Menninger Clinic*, 62 (1): 33–82.

Stein, H., Koontz, A. D., Fonagy, P., Allen, J. G., Fultz, J., Brethour Jr. J. R., Allen, D. and Evans, R. B. (2002) 'Adult attachment: What are the underlying dimensions?' *Psychology and Psychotherapy: Theory, Research and Practice*, 75 (1): 77–91.

Stevens, I. (2004) 'Cognitive-behavioural interventions for adolescents in residential child care in Scotland: An examination of practice and lessons from research.' *Child and Family Social Work*, 9: 237–46.

Stevens, I. and Furnivall, J. (2008) Therapeutic approaches in residential child care. In A. Kendrick (ed). *Residential child care. Prospects and challenges.* London/Philadelphia, Jessica Kingsley Publications, pp. 196–209.

Strathearn, L. (2011) 'Maternal Neglect: Oxytocin, Dopamine and the Neurobiology of Attachment.' *Journal of Neuroendocrinology*, 23 (11): 1054–65.

Suomi, S. J. (2005) 'Mother-Infant Attachment, Peer Relationships, and the Development of Social Networks in Rhesus Monkeys.' *Human Development*, 48: 67–79.

Suomi, S. J. (2008) 'Attachment in rhesus monkeys.' In J. Cassidy and P. Shaver (eds). *Handbook of attachment: Theory, Research and Clinical Applications*. New York, London: Guilford Press, 2: 173–91.

Target, M., Fonagy, P. and Shmueli-Goetz, Y. (2003) 'Attachment representations in school-age children: The early development of the child attachment interview (CAI).' *Journal of Child Psychotherapy*, 29 (2): 171–86.

Taylor, G. J., Bagby, R. M. and Parker, J. D. (1997) *Disorders of Affect Regulation: Alexithymia in Medical and Psychiatric Illness*. Cambridge: Cambridge University Press.

Thoburn, J., Norford, L. and Parvez Rashid, S. (2000) *Permanent placement for children of ethnic minorities*. London: Jessica Kingsley Publications.

Travis, L. A., Bliwise, N. G., Binder, J. L. and Horne Meyer, H. L. (2001) 'Changes in clients' attachment styles over the course time-limited dynamic psychotherapy.' *Psychotherapy: Theory, Research, Practice and Training*, 38: 149–59.

Triseliotis, J. (2002) 'Long-term foster care or adoption? The evidence examined.' *Child and Family Social Work*, 7: 23–33.

Tunstill, J. and Aldgate, J. (2000) *Services for children in need. From policy to practice.* London, The Stationery Office.

Uher, R. and McGuffin, P. (2008) 'The moderation by the serotonin transporter gene of environmental adversity in the aetiology of mental illness: review and methodological analysis.' *Molecular Psychiatry*, 13 (2): 131–46.

UNICEF (2007) *An overview of child well-being in rich countries.A comprehensive assessment of the lives and well-being of children and adolescents in the economically advanced nations.* Italy, UNICEF Innocenti Research Centre, Report Card 7.

van den Boom, D. (1995) 'Do first year intervention effects endure? Follow-up during toddlerhood of a sample of Dutch irritable infants.' *Child Development*, 66: 1798–816.

van der Kolk, B. (2003) 'The neurobiology of childhood trauma and abuse.' *Child and adolescent clinics of North America*, 12: 293–317.

van der Kolk, B. (2005) 'Developmental trauma disorder.' *Psychiatric Annals*, 35 (5): 401–8.

van der Kolk, B. A. and Fisler, R. E. (1994) 'Childhood abuse and neglect and loss of self-regulation.' *Bulletin of the Menninger Clinic*, 58 (2): 145–68.

van der Kolk, B. A., Pelcovitz, D., Roth, S., Mandeh, F. S., McFarlane, A. and Herman, J. L. (1996) 'Dissociation, somatization, and affect dysregulation: The complexity of adaption to trauma.' *American Journal of Psychiatry*, 153 (Suppl): 83–93.

van Fleet, R. (2005) *Filial Therapy: Strengthening parent-child relationships through play*, (2nd edn). Sarasota, Fl Professional Resource Press.

van Ijzendoorn, M. and Bakersmans-Kranenburg, M. (1996) 'Attachment representations in mothers, fathers, adolescents and and clinical groups: A meta-analytic search for normative data.' *Journal of Clinical and Consulting Psychology*, 64: 8–21.

Volling, B. L., Notaro, P. C. and Larsen, J. J. (1998) 'Adult attachment styles: Relations with emotional well-being, marriage and parenting.' *Family Relations*, 47: 355–67.

Wallis, P. and Steele, H. (2001) 'Attachment representations in adolescence: Further evidence from psychiatric residential settings.' *Attachment & Human Development*, 3: 259–68.

Ward, A., Ramsay, R., Turnbull, S., Steele, M., Steele, H. and Treasure, J. (2001) 'Attachment in anorexia nervosa: A transgenerational perspective.' *British Journal of Medical Psychology*, 74: 497–505.

Waters, E., Corcoran, D. and Anafarta, M. (2005) 'Attachment, Other Relationships, and the Theory that All Good Things Go Together.' *Human Development*, 48: 80–4.

Waters, E., Crowell, J. A., Elliott, M., Corcoran, D. and Treboux, D. (2002) 'Bowlby's secure base theory and the social/personality psychology of attachment styles: work(s) in progress.' *Attachment and Human Development*, 4 (2): 230–42.

Whiffen, V. E., Judd, M. E. and Anbe, J. A. (1999) 'Intimate relationships moderate the association between childhood sexual abuse and depression.' *Journal of Interpersonal Violence*, 14 (9): 940–54.

Winnicott, D. (1965) *The maturational processes and the facilitating environment: studies in the theory of emotional development*. London, International Universities Press.

Zegers, M. A. M., Schuengel, C., van IJzendoorn, M. H. and Janssens, J. M. (2006) 'Attachment representations of institutionalized adolescents and their professional caregivers: predicting the development of therapeutic relationships.' *American Journal of Orthopsychiatry*, 76 (3): 325–34.

Zegers, M. A. M., Schuengel, C., van IJzendoorn, M. H. and Janssens, J. M. (2008) 'Attachment and problem behaviour of adolescents during residential treatment.' *Attachment & Human Development*, 10 (1): 91–103.

Zeifman, D. and Hazan, C. (2008) Pair bonds as attachments: Re-evaluating the evidence. In J. Cassidy and P. R. Shaver (eds). *Handbook of attachment (2nd edition): Theory, Research and Clinical Applications*. New York/London: Guilford Press.

Index